Women and the Practice of Medical Care in Early Modern Europe, 1400–1800

Women and the Practice of Medical Care in Early Modern Europe, 1400–1800

Leigh Whaley
Professor of History, Acadia University, Canada

palgrave
macmillan

Softcover reprint of the hardcover 1st edition 2011 978-0-230-28291-9

First published 2011 by
PALGRAVE MACMILLAN

Palgrave Macmillan in the UK is an imprint of Macmillan Publishers Limited, registered in England, company number 785998, of Houndmills, Basingstoke, Hampshire RG21 6XS.

Palgrave Macmillan in the US is a division of St Martin's Press LLC, 175 Fifth Avenue, New York, NY 10010.

Palgrave Macmillan is the global academic imprint of the above companies and has companies and representatives throughout the world.

Palgrave® and Macmillan® are registered trademarks in the United States, the United Kingdom, Europe and other countries.

ISBN 978-1-349-32870-3 ISBN 978-0-230-29517-9 (eBook)
DOI 10.1057/9780230295179

This book is printed on paper suitable for recycling and made from fully managed and sustained forest sources. Logging, pulping and manufacturing processes are expected to conform to the environmental regulations of the country of origin.

A catalogue record for this book is available from the British Library.

Library of Congress Cataloging-in-Publication Data

Whaley, Leigh Ann.
Women and the practice of medical care in early modern Europe, 1400–1800/ Leigh Whaley.
p. ; cm.
Includes bibliographical references and index.

1. Women in medicine—Europe—History. 2. Medicine, Medieval—Europe. I. Title.
[DNLM: 1. Health Personnel—history—Europe. 2. Women—history—Europe. 3. History, 17th Century—Europe. 4. History, 18th Century—Europe. 5. History, Early Modern 1451–1600—Europe. WZ 80.5.W5]
R692.W485 2010
610.82—dc22 2010034822

10 9 8 7 6 5 4 3 2 1
20 19 18 17 16 15 14 13 12 11

Transferred to Digital Printing in 2012

Contents

Acknowledgements

The idea of writing about Early Modern European women medical practitioners arose when I was completing a chapter on a select group of women and their struggle to become physicians in my last book, *Women's History as Scientists: A Guide to the Debates* (2003). The battle fought by these women in the late nineteenth century to become medical students and practitioners led me to delve deeper into the past of women healers. Discussions with colleagues convinced me to examine the world of women healers in a comparative fashion.

This book would not have been written without the financial support and sabbatical leaves from Acadia University. At Acadia, I would thank Dr Beert Verstraete, former head of the Department of History and Classics, who has been very helpful and supportive with this endeavour. At Queen's University, Belfast, Northern Ireland, Professor Mary O'Dowd, and at the University of Saskatchewan, Professor Michael Hayden, read the entire manuscript and provided many useful comments.

The staff at the numerous libraries where the research for this book took me should also be given recognition. This includes the librarians at the New York Academy of Medicine's Rare Book Library, as well as the librarians and archivists at the Poynter Room at the Wellcome Library for the History and Understanding of Medicine in London, England. The inter-library loan staff at the Vaughan Library at Acadia University was able to obtain many resources otherwise not available locally.

The editors at Palgrave Macmillan have been very supportive and most helpful. In particular, I would like to thank Michael Strang, senior commissioning editor, who met with me at the AHA meeting in San Diego in January 2010, and Barbara Slater for her outstanding editing of this book.

I would also like to thank my indexer, Clive Pyne, whose professional work went above and beyond the call of duty. Finally, I would like to thank my parents for their support over the years.

Introduction

This book studies the role of women healers, their contributions and the challenges they faced in France, Spain, Italy and England from the later Middle Ages to approximately 1800. Attitudes towards the woman healer are also under consideration. This book provides an introduction to the work performed by female medical practitioners, healers and writers, and it stresses the importance of gender in the healing arts. Particularly important is to underscore the wide variety of medical practitioners employing their skills during the Middle Ages and Early Modern era. The book does not claim to be definitive, rather it is a synthesis of women's contributions to and activities in health-care and medicine.

As a starting point, we must consider the meanings of medicine and medical practitioner and the role of medicine throughout history. The standard textbook definition of medicine as found in dictionaries indicates that firstly, medicine is the science and art of preventing, treating or alleviating diseases of the human body and mind. Secondly, medicine is directly connected with drugs or pharmaceuticals in the treatment of disease. Furthermore, medicine can be understood to be a profession with various levels of specialization.[1] This work adopts a very broad and inclusive definition of medicine to mean any sort of healing and treatment by healers and non-professional health-care practitioners. Medicine must be understood within the broader social and cultural perspective, rather than constrained within a narrowly scientific view.

Intimately related to medicine is the doctor or physician. Before the Middle Ages, no clear identity to physicians, and no single name for healers existed. The university-conferred title of doctor was the first distinction.[2] With the founding of medieval universities, medicine became a profession and women were shut out. The new doctors were a university trained coterie of elite professionals. Women and other non-university trained practitioners were formally excluded from medicine, but they did not stop healing. They were forced to become more creative in order to continue their important work. With the exception of women practising midwifery, which involved much more than delivering babies, they were obliged to heal on the margins. Even midwifery would become masculinized during the later years of the Early Modern era with the rise of the man-midwife, often an obstetrician or gynaecologist.

Women have engaged in healing from the beginning of history. Well-being, care-giving and healing have always been the concern of women, often within the context of the home. The Early Modern period was no exception in spite of the institution of new regulations for healers by medical guilds and secular and ecclesiastical authorities. This era witnessed a plethora of different types of healers, both men and women. Many – among them charitable ladies and mothers taking care of the ill in the home – provided their services free from charge. Regular practitioners – healers who received payment for their work – included university trained physicians, nurses and those with an apprenticeship and licences such as surgeons, barber-surgeons and midwives. There were also those who worked outside the law. These were various types of 'quacks': itinerants, mountebanks and wise-women (often considered to be witches).[3] It is the work of these many healers – with the exception of university trained physicians – that is examined in this book.

Until very recently, the role of women healers has been largely neglected by historians of medicine, who have primarily focused on the great male university trained physicians. This attitude has changed in the past few years. Current works in the history of medicine have focused more on popular and 'marginal' healers who worked outside the university setting.[4] Most of these practitioners were on the periphery of the profession and often found themselves in conflict with and perceived as a threat to the university trained or academic physician. In addition, the newer history of medicine has explored the medical world by examining local history, illness and the experiences of patients as well as institutional healing in hospitals. Women, although often on the margins, were integral and important contributors to health-care.

This book aims to make a contribution to the history of popular medicine by examining the roles performed by and the achievements of women medical practitioners in France, Spain, England and Italy, over a period of several hundred years. Previous studies of women and medicine have tended to focus narrowly in terms of geographical concentration – for example, they deal with one country – and in terms of a limited time span. Although the problem is being addressed – one example is a recent issue of the *Bulletin of the History of Medicine* (Spring 2008), which has 'Women, Health and Healing in Early Modern Europe' as its focus – many of the current works about women and medicine concentrate on either the medieval or the modern period.[5] There is a gap between these two time periods. By dealing with the Early Modern years, this book intends to begin to fill the lacuna. This study aims to be wider in scope than most of the existing literature, which narrowly focuses on one aspect of women's contribution to medicine: midwifery, nursing, unofficial village healers or domestic medicine. This study includes all of the above and more. Finally, many of the existing studies are biographical rather than thematic in nature. This book utilizes both approaches.

In addition, this book seeks to explain why women were, for the most part, excluded from the practice of formal medicine. Why were women healers marginalized from the late medieval period? Why were women not permitted to enter the profession of medicine until the final decades of the nineteenth century? In order to discern this, I have turned to the writings of contemporary authors, both medical and non-medical men, who have written on the subject of women's proper role in society, their intelligence and their ability to understand science.

There are further important questions that this book intends to address and which have not been fully considered in the existing literature. At what point in history were women considered unsuitable to practise the healing arts? What social factors determined that women would not practise medicine? Were these factors based on ideologies, political systems, physiology (the perceived unfitness of women)? What strategies did women adopt to counteract the prevailing dominant culture when they were no longer permitted to practise official medicine?

The text is organized both chronologically and thematically. It begins with an introductory chapter, 'The Medieval Contribution', which takes a chronological and comparative view and explores the world of women practitioners in the medieval period in various European countries. A great diversity of women practised some form of medicine during the Middle Ages. Medical historians have identified a wide variety of female practitioners, from those engaged in general healing to more specialized branches of medicine including midwifery, surgery, barber-surgery and apothecary.[6] Moreover, these women practitioners had considerable freedom within the law before the advent of strict licensing regulations and the growth of medieval medical schools within traditional universities.

Chapter 2, 'New Medical Regulations and their Impact on Female Healers', analyses the significant impact that the professionalization of medicine would have on female practitioners. The development of medical licensing and a more 'scientific' approach to healing would greatly affect women healers. The chapter explores the changes in medicine beginning in the thirteenth century and continuing into the sixteenth with the growth of licensing by church and secular authorities.

Chapter 3, 'Early Modern Notions of Women: Contradictory Views on Women as Healers', discusses a wide range of societal views and expectations of women and their roles. Men contributed to the debate concerning women from many different perspectives, medical, theological, legal and philosophical. Some doctors still held the Aristotelian view of women as incomplete men and, as such, incapable of abstract thought. Ideas varied between countries and cultures, with the Spanish recommending a very cloistered life for women, either in the home or in a convent, while French writers such as the Cartesian philosopher Poulain de la Barre, who wrote a curriculum for women which included science, medicine and mathematics, recommended an academic education for women. The Spanish humanist Juan Vives also recommended an education for women, but only one that prepared them for a private rather than a public role.

In Chapter 4, 'Medical Treatises and Texts Written by Women and for Women', the noteworthy and often neglected contributions made by women to treatises on various medicines and healing substances are chronicled. Many women prescribed new therapies for ailments that were adopted by university trained physicians. This chapter investigates a variety of published medical writings by and for women from Spain, Italy, France and England.[7] As Hannah Wolley or Woolley (b. 1623), allegedly the first successful author of cookery and household management books,[8] aptly recounted in the introduction to her *Gentlewoman's Companion, or, A Guide to the Female Sex* (1673), it was no small feat for a woman to be published at this time: 'It is no ambitious design of gaining a name in print (a thing as rare for a Woman to endeavour as obtain); that put me on this bold undertaking…'[9] A Spanish woman, Doña Oliva Sabuco de Nantes y Barrera, wrote an important treatise on healing, *New Philosophy of Human Nature not Known and not Reached by the Ancient Philosophers that Improves Human Life and Health* (1587). This amazingly modern text had, until recently, been attributed to her father, Miguel Sabuco. It made pioneering contributions to the mind-body relationship in illness and the field of homeopathic medicine.[10] A shadowy Italian noblewoman, Isabella Cortese (d. 1561), published *Secreti medicinali artificiosi ed alchemici* (1561–65), a recipe book about medicine and cosmetics. In France, the vicomtesse de Vaux, Marie de Maupeou Fouquet (1590–1681), authored a book of medical recipes, *Recueil de receptes, où est expliquée la manière de guerir à peu de frais toute sorte de maux tant internes, qu'externes inueterez, & qui ont passé jusqu'à present pour incurables*, which was translated into several languages and reprinted in a number of European countries from 1675 into the mid-eighteenth century. Marie-Geneviève-Charlotte Darlus d'Arconville (1720–1805) wrote an *Essai pour servir à l'histoire de la putrefaction* (1766) in addition to translating and providing a commentary on important medical publications by other writers. In common with Sabuco de Nantes, d'Arconville's translation of Alexander Monro's *The Anatomy of Human Bones and Nerves* (1726) had also been attributed to a male author. In d'Arconville's case, the wrongful attribution was to French novelist Eugène Sue.

Chapter 5, 'Female Midwives and the Medical Profession', presents a comparative overview of the most important developments in European midwifery during the Early Modern period, including subjects such as the training of midwives, attitudes held by male practitioners of medicine, and the changes that occurred throughout the Early Modern period. Leading midwives, their contributions and treatises are also under discussion.[11] The chapter's focus is on midwives and midwifery in France and England, given the rich sources available and the important contributions made by French midwives such as Louise Bourgeois Boursier to the profession.

Chapter 6, 'The Healing Care of Nurses', explores the essential role of nurses or nursing sisters in the care of the poor and the sick from the Middle Ages to the late Renaissance. In addition to chronicling the important but neglected role of nurses in the history of medicine, this chapter aims to redress the often negative image of the nurse in the Early Modern period as incompetent and uneducated.[12] As recent experts have confirmed, despite being denied a university education, nurses performed many functions which could barely be differentiated from those carried out by university trained doctors, and often 'nursing healing activities were superior to those of physicians', presumably because the university trained practitioner received more of a theoretical than a practical education.[13]

Chapter 7, 'The "Irregular" Female Healer in Early Modern Europe: A Variety of Practitioners', studies the role and activities of the irregular or unlicensed female practitioner outside the realm of nursing and midwifery in the Early Modern period. It looks at the function of female healers after the rise of universities and the professionalization of medicine. What role could women play if they were not university trained and were unable to obtain local licences to practise medicine other than midwifery? And what part did they play in Italy where they could hold chairs of anatomy? This chapter is concerned primarily with the unlicensed female healer, and is based upon sources such as diaries and correspondence, private papers, trial records, advertisements, newspapers and published pamphlets. There are many limitations to official sources, such as records of licences or lists of physicians, barber-surgeons and surgeons and apothecaries compiled by their guilds or corporations. These lists are often inaccurate and incomplete.

Chapter 8, 'Motherly Medicine: Domestic Healers and Apothecaries', focuses on domestic or household medicine as practised by women. It provides a window onto minor illness and domestic cures. The chapter is based primarily upon a sampling of manuscript receipt books penned by mainly upper-class English women between the early seventeenth and the mid-eighteenth century. The Wellcome Library for the History and Understanding of Medicine possesses a significant archive collection of these medical receipts compiled by women. Some thirty-three manuscript collections dating from 1621 to the mid-eighteenth century provide the basis for this chapter.

Chapter 9, 'The Wise-Woman as Healer: Popular Medicine, Witchcraft and Magic' concentrates on wise-women as healers, and, to a lesser extent, as midwives,[14] in both of which roles they were often designated as 'witches'. In the Early Modern era, in many, but not all cases, they were accused of practising witchcraft even though healing was clearly their chief objective.

The witch-hunt,[15] as applied to wise-women, can be interpreted as another step in the removal of women from healing. Wise-women were important healers in Early Modern Europe and women played a pivotal role in village medicine in pre-industrial Europe.[16] In rural areas of Europe, amateur healers, many of whom were women, were ubiquitous. They cured all manner of illnesses with herbs, poultices, prayers and ointments. This healing role was threatened during the Renaissance. To cite one expert: 'During the Renaissance, however, the first concerted efforts were made to remove medicine from the realm of popular culture and establish it as the preserve of a restricted profession.'[17] Furthermore, at the time of the Renaissance when 'medicine and science lost their spiritual dimensions; as healers, magicians, and witches lost their claim to manipulate the spiritual forces of the world, the ground was prepared for a mechanization of the world picture'.[18]

1
The Medieval Contribution

This chapter explores the world of women medical practitioners in the late medieval period in various European countries. During the Middle Ages, as throughout history, women's role was to take care of the sick. Poet, treatise writer and proto-feminist Christine de Pizan (1365–c.1430), writing at the end of the fourteenth century, attested that 'if women possess such piety, they also possess charity, for who is it who visits and comforts the sick, helps the poor, takes care of hospitals and buries the dead? It seems to me that these are all women's works...'[1]

A great diversity of women practised some form of medicine during the Middle Ages. Medical historians have identified a wide variety of female practitioners from those engaged in general healing to more specialized branches of medicine including surgery, barber-surgery and apothecary.[2] Moreover, these women practitioners had considerable freedom legally to engage in healing practices before the advent of strict licensing regulations and the growth of medieval medical schools within traditional universities curtailed their work.

Prior to the establishment of universities as the centres of medical learning and the exclusion of women from the medical world through allocation of licences and degrees, women, particularly in Italy, were welcome to extend this healing and care-giving role outside the domestic sphere. Universities granted licences to physicians. Since women could not attend universities with the exception of the medical school of Salerno, they were often barred from practising medicine. However, there were exceptions in certain Italian cities where women would be granted licences to cure specific ailments and to perform minor surgery. Medieval European women contributed substantially to health-care in areas beyond the traditional female speciality of midwifery.[3] They were trained, and practised, as surgeons, empirics, anatomists and barber-surgeons.

The relatively low numbers of recorded female practitioners of medicine during the medieval period does not necessarily reflect reality or provide historians with an accurate portrayal. A 2001 study states that 'fewer than five per cent of official or licensed physicians were women'.[4] However, Monica H. Green, an expert in the history of women's health-care during the Middle Ages has noted a number of problems that face the historian of women medical practitioners, not the least of which are sources. Women do not always figure in official documents such as wills, court records and guild records, and women from this period, as contrasted with those from the Early Modern era, did not commonly leave memoirs, diaries or other personal records.[5] Other scholars have made similar comments in their works on medieval women and healing.[6] One source which has proven fruitful is that of medical treatises, which were often concerned with female disorders. These treatises were translated from the Latin to the vernacular for use by women. One such example is a fourteenth-century English version of the *Trotula* (see below). The preface clearly indicates that it was women who were practising medicine: The woman would '...help them [other women] and counsel them in their maladies without showing their disease to man...'[7] Other sources utilized by scholars include tax records and judiciary records, such as those of the Paris Parlement (highest court of appeal) and medical courts including that of the Faculty of the University of Medicine of Paris.

A starting point for discussion of the contribution made by women healers in the Middle Ages is the story of Anna Comnena, an early female medical practitioner. Anna Comnena (1081–1153), daughter of King Alexius I of Constantinople, the emperor of Byzantium, is principally remembered as the world's first female historian. Comnena was highly educated for a woman of the twelfth century, having studied Greek and read the works of Aristotle and Plato.[8] Her fifteen-volume work, *The Alexiad* (c. 1148), told the history of her father's reign. It is a rich source of ideas of contemporary medicine and astronomy and is descriptive of the role of Comnena herself as a female healer in a time of war and crusade.

Anna Comnena provides a model of the more traditional female caregiver, who, although educated – she had studied the quadrivium – and very well-versed in the medicine of her time, was not a physician, but like many women, practised medicine in the home.[9]

One of Comnena's biographers has argued that 'Anna had an unusual aptitude for medicine.'[10] She diagnosed illnesses, recommended treatments and used medical terminology to identify afflictions such as gangrene, and gout, which she described as pains in her father's feet caused by 'soft living' and 'anxiety'. She also diagnosed pleurisy.[11] Comnena understood that there were many causes to illness, from climate to diet. In keeping with the contemporary understanding of medicine derived from the Greeks, she referred to 'the humours of our animal juices, as the cause of our fevers'.[12] Hippocrates and Galen stressed the importance of the equilibrium of the humours or fluids of the body. The four humours are blood, phlegm, and black and yellow bile. They originate from the four elements of air, water, earth and fire. An imbalance of the humours was believed to result in illness.[13] In her discussion of her father's illnesses, Comnena once again mentioned 'humours' in describing his pain, 'drawing the humours to themselves...' And she wrote that he went riding 'in order that part of the flowing down matter might be carried off'.[14]

Anna Comnena described her father's illnesses in considerable detail and her narrative provides interesting insights into her medical knowledge and skills. She diagnosed his illness as 'rheumatics' which had moved to one of his shoulders. Reporting that the physicians did not take his illness seriously enough, with the exception of Nicholas Callicles, she commented that he was 'the only one who urged the cleansing of his system with purgatives'.[15] Comnena discussed in some detail the pros and cons of the use of purgatives. Pepper, one of these purgatives, she asserted, would do more harm than good.[16]

During Alexius's final illness, Anna consulted with the king's physicians, the most eminent doctors of Constantinople, who discussed various methods of treatment with her. When her father was near his death, it was Anna and her mother who carried out round the clock nursing care. In addition to nursing her father, it was Anna rather than the physicians who conducted the medical side of his care. She recalled: 'At one moment I watched the movements of his pulse and studied his respiration, then at another I would turn to my mother and cheer her up as much as possible. But ... the regions were quite incurable ... the Emperor could not recover from his last faint...' Significantly, it was Anna, rather than the doctors, who recognized that 'the pulse in the arteries had finally stopped'.[17]

In addition to treating her father, Anna performed several other medical duties. She looked after her husband who suffered from a tumour. She chronicled what she thought to be the various causes of his tumour, from the rough conditions endured by those in the military to the climate and to anxiety about his family.[18] She diagnosed duke Robert Guiscard, head of the Norman forces in Byzantium, with fever and pleurisy.[19] It is clear from her accounts in *The Alexiad* that Anna provided crucial medical care in her family and beyond.

Health-care was of great importance to the people of Byzantium. Byzantine doctors, including women, made contributions in virtually every field of medicine, including anatomy, hygiene, obstetrics, surgery, paediatrics, urology and neurology.[20] Byzantine commitment to medicine may also be demonstrated in the nature of the hospitals that they established. Scholars credit the Byzantine people with the 'first fully equipped European hospitals'.[21] Alexius I himself founded a hospital for the treatment of many illnesses, such as blindness, leprosy and orthopaedic ailments. According to Anna, 'residences for mutilated men, blind, lame, or some other defect' were constructed. Anna herself established a medical school in the Byzantine capital in 1083. The hospital had two storeys and both male and female patients and practitioners of medicine.[22]

Even more impressive was the hospital constructed by John II Comnenus and his wife Irene. John was Alexius's successor and became emperor in 1118. Founded in 1136, the Pantocrator, was a hospital, a hospice and a monastery all in one. Its mission was to treat the poor, the elderly and women. The hospital was very modern in its operation and structure. Its constitution, the *Typikon*, written in October 1136, provides details about the structure of the hospital. There were five clinics or wards, each allocated to the treatment of particular medical problems – illnesses requiring surgery, eye problems, intestinal ailments, general illnesses and a woman's clinic. There was also an emergency room and an outpatient clinic staffed by four physicians. The woman's clinic may have been a maternity ward. The constitution is not clear on its exact function.[23]

Anna Comnena was not the only woman to practise medicine in Byzantium. In the Pantocrator, health-care providers were both male and female, including the physicians. The hospital had sixty-one beds and thirty-five doctors. Clearly, the high proportion of doctors to patients indicates the importance of medical care to the people. Each evening five doctors, four male and one female, would stay in the hospital. The hospital had its own medical school where doctors were trained. Here, women were engaged in the study and practice of medicine.[24] Medical schools within the hospital existed into the fifteenth century.[25] The fact that women in Byzantium could become physicians reflects the positive societal view of women and their role. Women exercised important functions in the religious and social work of the Byzantine church. They worked as deaconesses, they baptized women, and they ministered to the sick, orphans and the poor.[26]

The *Typikon* provides evidence that the hospital possessed a support staff that was also composed of both women and men: nurses or attendants, a pharmacist and three assistants, and a midwife in the women's unit of the hospital. Nursing care was an important role for women, dating back to the fourth century AD. In hospitals, it was performed by women who were employed as 'servants'.[27] In addition to their work in the regular hospital, the constitution provided for six nurses to care for twenty-four men housed in the 'old-age home'.[28]

To John II Comnenus, the spiritual side of healing was as important as the medical or clinical element. As stated above, he not only founded a hospital, he also established a monastery. The hospital included a chapel which held regular services and the two priests heard confessions of the sick and dealt with burials. The chapel was segregated by gender with separate male and female sections. Each hospital worker was charged with carrying out his or her duties in the spirit of Christian charity. Serving the patients was akin to serving God. Nursing care was considered to be a sacred duty. The canons of the church provided for punishments for nurses who failed to carry out their duties of feeding and caring for patients in this spirit.[29]

Throughout Europe, women were, for the most part, excluded from medical schools located within universities. European universities were founded during the High Middle Ages, beginning in the later thirteenth century.[30] However, there was one medical school that accepted women. This was the School of Salerno, the *Schola Medica Salernitana*, the first western institution to introduce degrees. The *Schola* dates from the ninth century.[31] Salerno is located thirty-five miles south-east of Naples and became a health resort because of its location. It was a secular rather than an ecclesiastical establishment having received its laws from Robert I. The school itself, which has been called 'the unquestioned fountain and archetype of orthodox medicine', had a difficult course of study. Students were required to complete three years of philosophy and literature before pursuing a five-year course of medical studies. During the twelfth century, translations of Arab texts were becoming an important part of the course of study. By the twelfth century, Salerno was the leading medical school in Europe, known for the production of medical literature by scholars such as Matthaeus Platearius and Archimatthaeu. Students came from all over the European continent and England to attend the school.[32] According to the Anglo-Norman historian, Orderic Vitalis of St Évroul (1075–c. 1142), hundreds of women and men studied medicine at Salerno, 'the ancient seat of the best medical school', in the eleventh century. They were taught by monks as well as by lay practitioners, several of whom were women, and one of whom was Trotula.[33] They were known as the *Mulieres Salernitanae* (the 'Ladies of Salerno'), physicians and professors of medicine.[34]

The most prominent female medical practitioner at the School of Salerno was a woman named Trota, often cited as Trotula. What do we know about Trota and her contribution to medicine? According to existing records, Trotula was born circa 1050 and died around 1097 at Salerno. She was the wife of Johannes Platearius, a doctor and medical writer. There are extant manuscripts by her in the libraries of France, Germany, Belgium, Austria and England. France, particularly in the Bibliothèque Nationale, has a large collection.[35] She wrote a number of works concerning the female ailments, including *De Passionibus Mulierum*, also known as *Trotula Major*. It has sixty-three chapters and was copied and recopied many times. Topics under consideration include menstruation, conception, pregnancy, childbirth and general diseases. H.P. Bayon argues that in spite of the controversy over authorship, this work was the first major treatise on gynaecology in history.[36] Trotula or Trota's text, *The Diseases of Women*, remained the standard medical handbook until Louise Bourgeois began writing in the seventeenth century.

P.O. Kristeller claims that Italy continued the Greco-Roman tradition which accepted female doctors.[37] But the authors of a recent biographical dictionary of women in science assert that a good part of the reason for the controversy over Trotula as a medical doctor stems from prejudice against women in medicine. Women were simply not considered capable of practising medicine. Shearer and Shearer maintain that Trotula was indeed a historical person who taught medicine at the School of Salerno and authored a number of treatises. These included *Practica Brevis* (Brief Handbook) and *De Compositione Medicamentorum* (On the Preparation of Medicines) in addition to the two works cited above.[38] Instances of this prejudicial attitude can be traced back to the sixteenth century and Kaspar Wolff of Basel who disputed the fact that a woman like Trotula was capable of producing a medical treatise. He attributed her writing to a man by the name of Eros Juliae (a physician to Julia, Emperor Augustus' daughter). Wolff published an edition of the *De Passionibus Mulierum* in 1566.[39] The twentieth-century German medical historian Karl Sudoff maintained that Trotula and the Ladies of Salerno were not physicians but midwives and nurses. Since they were not doctors, they could not possibly have possessed the medical knowledge to produce a textbook on gynaecology. The controversy continued until the late twentieth century. Scholar Josette Dall'ava-Santucci, stated that 'currently the medical world accepts the conclusions of John F. Benton that a medical woman named Trotula existed but she was not the author of the famous treatise on female illnesses'.[40] Benton concluded that 'the professionalization of medicine in the twelfth and thirteenth centuries, combined with the virtual exclusion of women from university education, prevented them from entering the best paid and most respected positions ... Though the treatises of "Trotula" bear a woman's name, they were the central texts of the gynecological medicine practiced and taught by men.'[41] However, the authors of the 1986 *Oxford Companion to Medicine* wrote that the earliest medical school was at Salerno and that Trotula was its 'most famous teacher and practitioner'. They give her credit for classifying diseases as 'inherited, contagious and other'.[42]

The latest scholar to study the Trotula problem is Monica H. Green, who has provided a modern translation of the compendium of Trotula's works with a substantial introduction and a lucid commentary. The historical person and the texts, she maintains, are linked. *The Trotula* was originally a title; it was the 'most popular assembly of materials on women's medicine from the late twelfth to the fifteenth centuries'. These are written in Latin and their intended audience was the elite. The author, Trota, cited the medical masters, Galen and Hippocrates in her work. However, unlike many later medieval medical treatises, the book was much more pragmatically than philosophically oriented.[43]

Green posits that *The Trotula* forms three separate texts, each authored by a different person. These texts are as follows: *Conditions of Women, On Women's Cosmetics* and *On Treatments for Women*. According to Green, the first two texts were written by men and the last one by a woman from Salerno named Trota.[44] *On Treatments for Women* is a gynaecological treatise that provides guidelines for treating female diseases and gynaecological complications complete with recommended medicines. It lacks a theoretical framework in the sense that the recipes are listed in what appears to be an arbitrary fashion. A recipe to cure 'the itching and excoriation of the Pudenda' is followed by an 'ointment for sunburn'.[45] Yet, as Green argues, 'there are several consistent principles of female physiology and disease that underlie this seemingly random string of remedies'.[46] Much of the book is concerned with female problems for which Trota often recommended the use of herbs. Chapter Two, entitled, 'Concerning the Scantiness of Menses', provides a prescription to cure light periods: 'Take the red roots of willow, the kind of which baskets are woven and crush them after cleaning them well of their outer bark. When crushed, blend them by cooking with wine or water and the next day give a warm draught of the decoction for drinking.'[47] For problems in conceiving, she advised taking the livers and testicles of a pig '... and let them be dried; make a powder of this and give it in a drink to the man and woman who cannot conceive and they will procreate'.[48] In Chapter Sixteen, labour problems are discussed and the expertise of the midwife is stressed: 'It is to be noted that there are certain physical remedies whose virtues are obscure to us, but which are advanced as done by midwives. They let the patient hold a magnet in her right hand and find it helpful.'[49]

In addition to folk remedies as prescribed by midwives and in common with other medieval physicians dealing with female problems, Trota also recommended cures for ailments suffered by both men and women. Among these afflictions were the 'Protrusion of the Anus', intestinal pain, the stone, lice and scabies. She also considers problems specific to men, such as the 'swelling of the penis'.[50]

Trota is the most famous of the women of Salerno, perhaps because scholars have access to her writings today. Other women physicians authored medical treatises at this time, but unfortunately, only the titles of their works are known today. These women wrote on numerous and varied ailments, not solely female problems. Matthaeus Platearius (d. 1161), author of the *Circa Instans*, a popular medieval medical text, cites at least fourteen recipes from the women of Salerno.[51] Although some of these were for the preparation of cosmetics, others concerned medical problems such as pleurisy, haemorrhoids, female complaints and abdominal pains. Information about these women is difficult to obtain and all we know of them is when they lived and the titles of what they wrote. Judging from the titles of their texts, it is evident that they had knowledge of many branches of medicine. Abella lived during the eleventh century and wrote on black bile or madness, *De Atra Bili* (On Black Bile) and seminal fluid, *De Natura Seminis Hominis* (The Nature of Seminal Fluid). She also taught both of these subjects.

Rebecca Guarna lived circa 1200. She was a doctor who wrote on uroscopy, *De urinis* (On Urine), pre-natal development, *De febribus* (On Fever) and *De embrione* (On the Embryo). Her treatise, *De urinis*, introduced the method of using urine samples in diagnosing illnesses.[52] Mercuriade wrote treatises on pestilential fevers, *De febre pestilenti* (On Crises in Pestilent Fever), the treatment of wounds, *De Curatione* (The Cure of Wounds) and *De Unguentis* (On Unguents).[53] The titles of these works are cited in the *Collectio Salernitana*.[54] Marguerite of Naples, active in the late fourteenth century, was apparently a graduate of the school of Salerno. She became a licensed oculist in Frankfurt-am-Main.[55]

Very exceptional women received a university medical education. One of these was Costanza Calenda, who lived in the fourteenth century. She was the daughter of the Dean of the Faculty of Medicine at Salerno, Salvatori Calenda. He was a doctor of medicine who lectured at the University of Naples. Costanza studied medicine and passed an examination. Some scholars claim that she was a doctor of medicine from the University of Naples and was the first western woman to earn this degree.[56] Both Guarna, who flourished during the thirteenth century, and Calenda came from distinguished medical families.[57]

The Italians were among the most favourable of the Europeans toward medical women at this time. Italian women could receive a medical education through apprenticeship. Naples was particularly encouraging to female medical practitioners. Here, women could take a medical examination set by the royal physicians and surgeons. Women were permitted to care for other women in cases of childbirth and gynaecological matters, but they were also instructed in surgery. The illustrious Italian professor of medicine at the universities of Siena, Bologna and Parma, Ugo Benzi (1376–1439), urged midwives to expand their medical knowledge beyond the mechanics of childbirth to the treatment of illness and the understanding of human anatomy.[58] Midwives in the Middle Ages often performed medical tasks other than delivering babies and many knew a great deal more about medicine than the birthing process.[59]

Most commonly, women practising medicine were the daughters of doctors or surgeons and they were instructed by their fathers or a male relative. They would obtain a letter attesting to their medical knowledge, take it to the authorities and be examined by crown physicians and surgeons. However, this was not invariably the case, for Charles, Duke of Calabria (1296–1309), King of Naples and (nominal) Jerusalem and Sicily (1309), granted a licence that permitted Francesca, wife of Matteo de Romana of Salerno, to practise medicine and surgery: 'Francesca ... has explained to the Royal Court that she is reputed to be proficient in the art of surgery ... She has been examined and found competent by our own royal physicians and surgeons ... We grant her the license to heal and to practice ... Naples, 10 September 1321.'[60] Jacobina (medica), the daughter of the surgeon, Dr Bartholomew, who trained her, practised in Bologna.[61]

Women licensed as surgeons carried out complex surgical procedures on female patients. Francesca, for reasons of 'morals and decency', was only permitted to treat female patients. The female Neapolitan surgeon Maria Gallicia was licensed in September 1309. Her speciality was gynaecological surgery and her licence specified that she was limited to curing wounds, abscesses and hernias of the womb.[62] While treatment of women by women was very common at this time, surgical licences which were not limited to practising on female patients were also issued to female practitioners. These include Isabella da Ocre,[63] whose specialities included abscesses and wounds, and Raymunda da Taberna who treated 'cancers, simple wounds and ulcers'.[64] Margarita da Venosa and Polisena da Troya were granted surgical licences in 1333 and 1335.[65] Evidently, these women were not performing major surgical operations but were undertaking minor procedures to heal wounds, ulcers and abscesses.[66]

In most cases, women received licences to treat specific ailments rather than to practise general medicine. Clarice di Durisio da Foggia was a specialist in diseases of the eyes and treated only women. Sibyl of Benevento received a licence to treat buboes (abscesses from the plague), while Margharita from Naples was a specialist in female problems such as breast abscesses (perhaps cancer) and womb ailments.[67] Marguerite Saluzzi, licensed in 1460, was a popular doctor known for her medicinal knowledge of herbs.[68] Although there are several examples of women like Francesca de Romana practising medicine at this time in southern Italy, their numbers were still low in comparison to men: approximately three thousand to eighteen over a period of thirty-five years in Naples.[69]

Other licences received by women during this period were granted by King Robert the Wise to Trotta da Toya (1307) and Francisca di Vestis (1308). These women went through a similar procedure as male medical practitioners when applying for a licence: they were examined by the experts in the field, Trotta by a surgeon, Master Raynaldo, and Francisca by Master Giovanni, a surgeon. Francis of Piedmont, a leading physician and professor at the University of Naples, examined a female doctor by the name of Lauretta Ponte da Saracena Calabria.[70]

Women were also to be found practising medicine in other regions of the Italian peninsula during the later Middle Ages. Maestra Antonia of Florence (1386–1408) had a medical degree. Caterina of Florence (fl. 1400s) was a 'medica' at the hospital of Sancta Maria Nuova. Her signature is found on extant prescriptions.[71] Women were sometimes licensed to practise medicine on the poor who could not afford a university trained physician: Virdimura of Catania, Sicily, a Jewish woman married to a Doctor Pasquale, was licensed in 1276 for this purpose. She had passed medical tests.[72]

An Italian woman who was not associated with Naples and the School of Salerno was the anatomist, Alessandra Giliani. Although there is no evidence that Giliani treated patients, she made a significant contribution to medicine. Giliani flourished circa 1313 to 1326.[73] Educated at the University of Bologna, she was an assistant to Mondino de' Luzzi (Mundinus) (1270?–1326) who made important contributions to the practice of dissection for teaching purposes. Dissection was not a common practice in the fourteenth century.

Luzzi was a medical professor at the University of Bologna. His anatomy textbook, *Anathomia Mundini* (Mondino's Anatomy), written in 1316 and published in 1478, was based on his observations of dissections. It was the first text of this nature and remained a key instructional book for centuries.[74] Giliani studied philosophy and anatomy with Luzzi. She prepared bodies for dissection. All contemporary accounts state that she was very skilled at her craft and that she introduced the practice of filling the veins and arteries with fluids of different colours.[75] In other words, she pioneered the anatomical injection. A dedication written after her untimely death at the age of nineteen, attests to her skill in anatomy: 'In this urn enclosed, the ashes of the body of Alessandra Giliani ... skilful with the brush in anatomical demonstrations and a disciple, equaled by few of the most noted physician, Mundinus of Luzzi ... She lived only nineteen years; she died consumed by her labors.'[76]

Finally, at the University of Bologna was Dorotea Bucca (fl. 1390, d. 1436), sometimes spelled Bocchi, the daughter of a professor of medicine. She not only taught medical and moral philosophy, but was her father's successor in holding a chair in medicine at this institution. She held this chair for forty years.[77]

Italian women, unlike their counterparts in other European countries, were able to reach a similar level in medical practice to men and were thus considered equal in rights and responsibilities.

Female medical practitioners were also found in the Iberian Peninsula. Doctors (*metgesses*) and medicine women (*comadromas*) worked for the Crown of Aragón.[78] The surgeon Çahud was employed by the Crown of Valencia in the fourteenth century.[79] Records exist for five women licensed to practise medicine in Catalonia. These women received their licences from Pedro III of Catalonia and IV of Aragón, known as the Ceremonial. Four of the five women were Jewish and one was Christian. The first of these licences was expatiated in Barcelona on 20 January 1374 to Floreta of Santa Coloma de Queralt, widow of Jucef Ça-Noga, 'in arte Medicine'. According to the licence, she possessed 'sufficient aptitude' to practise. She was doctor to Leonor de Sicilia, the third wife of Pedro del Punyalet.[80] Two of the Jewish women were licensed in Zaragosa: these were Bellayne, widow of Samuel Gallipapa and mother of Jehuda Gallipapa, Jews of Lérida, her licence granted 10 September 1380, and Na Pla, wife of Jehuda Gallipapa, licence granted 5 March 1387.[81] Juana, wife of Arnaldo Sarrovira, citizen of Barcelona, native of Calda de Montbuy, was a Christian woman doctor. She received her licence on 25 May 1384. Dolcich, wife of Maymo Gallipapa, Jew, from the city of Leyda, received her licence on 28 August 1384.[82]

In common with women in other European countries, Spanish women often practised medicine with their husbands. If their husbands died, the women assumed control of their husbands' practices. This was the experience of Elicsenda who assumed her husband's herbal and apothecary business, and that of Sibilia, widow of Guillem Duran, apothecary (who died in 1313). She ran the business with her sons.[83] Unlike other European women, however, Spanish widows did not appear to have taken over their late husbands' barber practices. Instead, the widow would rent out her husband's tools to a male barber.[84]

As was the case elsewhere in Europe, women in Spain practised medicine primarily at the local and village level. Few people at this time were treated by a university trained physician, and it was the crucial role of the female practitioner to provide the meagre health-care that most people received. Historians know little in general of what these practitioners actually did; however, we have one example of a woman named Benvinguda Mallnovell. She treated heart ailments, headaches, throat problems and St Anthony's fire with magical medicine composed of chants and herbal remedies.[85] Beatriz Anaya, the wife of Dr de la Reina and 'sometime physician was paid 20,000 maravedís a year from the Zamora rents'.[86] In addition to midwifery, women also provided nursing care in the home, for instance, women cared for the sick members of the royal family of Aragón.[87]

After the passing of the *furs*, or laws regulating the practice of medicine (see Chapter 2) in Valencia in 1329, women were legally allowed only to treat other women and children, and only as long as they did not administer potions. This legislation did not altogether prevent them from treating men. Surgery, for example was not mentioned in these laws, only 'medicina'.[88]

Unlike in Italy, in France women were banned from studying at the universities and therefore had to learn medicine by practice and apprenticeship. The fact that women could not formally study medcine did not prevent them from practising it in many forms. There is evidence of many different types of practitioners in France in the Middle Ages: physicians, or *fisiciennes*, *médecines*, *miresses* (all of whom dealt with internal illnesses), leeches, barbers, *sage-femmes* (midwives) and surgeons. The first documented woman doctor was Helvidis (c. 1176), according to the record of her bequeathing a church in her name.[89]

Medical historians Wickersheimer and Jacquart have identified some 127 female practitioners in France from the twelfth to the fourteenth centuries, out of a total of 7,104, although these numbers are probably far below the actual case.[90] Our knowledge of these women and their contribution to medicine is limited and is based primarily on court cases in which they were usually prosecuted for practising some form of medicine without a licence. If the prosecution was for some other offence and they were practising legally, the court records have details of their licences. We know their names, although often just their first names, their addresses and the sort of medicine they practised in addition to the penalty they incurred, which was often just a fine. Among these practitioners were Ameline, the *miresse*, who lived in Paris and practised medicine illegally between 1324 and 1325; Antoinette de Bellegarde, living in the region of the Bouches du Rhône;

Théophanie, barber, 1291, who lived in Angers; and Jeanne d'Ausshure (d'Auxerre), surgeon, died in Chalon-sur-Sâone, 1366.[91]

Further documented evidence for the existence of female medical practitioners is in the tax rolls of Paris from the years 1292, 1297 and 1313.[92] Isabiau la Megesse, for example, was a popular healer in the Paris parish of St Opportune who paid six *sous* in taxes.[93] Denise, barber from the Paris parish of Saint-Germain-l'Auxerrois, earned more than most, paying 30 *sous* in taxes in 1292.[94] Some female barbers were paid very poorly. These included the Parisian barbers, Edeline and Jeanette du Fossé (d. 1421), who paid only 2 *sous* in taxes.[95] Ameline la Miresse (fl. 1313–25), who practised with Guillaume Porée, was charged with illegally practising surgery and was fined.[96] Outside the Paris region, we know of Marguerite la Barbière (fl. 1310) from the Pas-de-Calais who was paid 6 *sous* for healing a child's wound, Marie (fl. 1344) and Jehannette la Mareschaude (fl. 1412–16) both from Rheims,[97] Jeanne de Cusey, barber and surgeon from Dijon and wife of Girart de Cusey, also a barber. The couple were implicated in poisoning in 1438 and both practised surgery and medicine illegally.[98]

Women could combine several medical specialities. Peretta Peronne (d. circa 1411), was a 'wise-woman' and a surgeon as well as a herbalist. She was prosecuted for both witchcraft and practising without a licence.[99] Although imprisoned, she was acquitted by Charles VI.[100]

In France, as in Italy and England, women tended to learn the craft of medicine from their fathers or other family members. Stephanie of Lyon (fl. 1265), for example, was the daughter of Dr Etienne de Montaneis,[101] and Gilette of Narbonne (fl. 1300) was the daughter of a physician, Gerard of Narbonne. She assumed his practice when he died. The Italian writer Giovanni Boccaccio, called her a 'Donna Medica'. Some sources claim that she had a role in healing the king of France of fistula.[102]

We know of two women who were proficient enough in their skills and knowledge to have served royalty, as a physician and a surgeon. Hersend or Hersend la 'fisicienne' (fl. 1249–59) came from Champagne and was married to Jacques, apothecary to Louis IX. According to the records, Hersend accompanied Louis on a crusade to the Holy Land in 1249. She treated the king and was in charge of the camp followers. In return for her services, Louis granted her a life-long pension.[103]

Surgeon Guillamette de Luys (late fifteenth century) was employed by Louis XI in 1479. She is listed on the king's account book. We possess no other information about her.[104]

There are several examples of women who worked with their husbands as barbers. One of these was Catherine Ramy of Montpellier who practised from 1469 to 1480.[105] In France, widows of barbers often assumed their deceased husband's practice. Marie de Gy [de Gys] married to François, a barber, practised medicine at Dijon at the start of the fifteenth century.[106] Jeanne Pouquelin, who worked as a barber in Paris, was successfully ordered to stop working by the 'communauté des barbiers' of the city of Paris in August 1426. She was the widow of Alain Pouquelin. She had continued his work as member of a barber guild after his death. Her case was tried at the Châtelet of Paris. She appealed the case to the Parlement of Paris.[107] The Parlement ruled that she could keep her barber business open; however, she was not permitted to bleed people (conduct phlebotomies) or infringe upon the practice of surgeons unless these treatments were conducted by experts, and approved by certain commissioners as ordered by the court.[108]

Most women conducted their medical work outside the walls of the hospital, although there were exceptions to this. For example, Margot, who treated 'a sick person in their beds', at the hospital of Lectoure, and Marguerite, barber at the Hôtel Dieu of Beauvais, 1380.[109]

In general, the organization of the trades did not prohibit women from practising medicine and both sexes were admitted equally into the corporations or guilds. It was not until the late sixteenth and particularly during the seventeenth century that the trade guilds, including those of barber, barber-surgeon and apothecary began to demand some sort of instruction by its members.[110] However, the statutes of the barbers and surgeons did not anticipate what happened in the case of the death of a husband and when the widow did not remarry.

Like women in continental European countries, women in medieval England were active practitioners of medicine.[111] However, as in other European countries, with the occasional exception of Italy, they were also excluded from the upper echelons of education. They were thus confined to the lower levels of medical practice, unable to qualify for higher levels which required a university education and, usually, the study of theology. In the Middle Ages, the highest level of medical practitioner was a cleric.[112] As was the case elsewhere, there were many different types of medical practitioners, among them *medicus* or *medica*, leech, barber, barber-surgeon and midwife. The categories of these healing practitioners were far more fluid than was the case in France where demarcation was more rigid.[113] Female medical practitioners are found in medieval documents dating from 1232 to 1470. These include Agnes of Huntingdon (fl.c. 1270), Christiana (fl.c. 1313), Alice Skedyngton (fl.c. 1400), Johanna (fl.c. 1408), and Lady Beauchamp (fl.c. mid-fifteenth century). According to the records, Agnes was a very skilled *medica*.[114] Alice was a lay healer who had been a servant. Her speciality was eye care, but she also claimed to have cured smallpox by preventing pitting with the use of red cloths. Apparently this method of treatment was utilized by male physicians at the time.[115] Joan, widow of William of Lee, practised as a physic. She petitioned Henry IV for his protection after her husband had been killed in battle: 'And she has nought whereby to live save by physic which she has learned.'[116] Johanna or Joan de Sutton of Westminster practised as a leech. Lady Beauchamp is thought to be Anne Beauchamp, wife of Richard Nevil, Earl of Warwick. The name of another medical practitioner, Juliana Burdet, is found amongst recipes in the Bodleian and Wellcome Library manuscript collections. Burdet was an expert in curing icteric or jaundice.[117]

Although the English took longer than the continental Europeans to develop their medical practices, there is evidence going back to the ecclesiastical laws of Edgar, who was crowned in 973, of women possessing the authorization to heal. The law stated: 'Possent et vir et femina medici esse.'[118] Women in Anglo-Saxon England could own property, defend their rights in court, and receive enough education to run their estates. Some even had knowledge of Latin.[119]

Medicine in medieval England was often practised in families. Evidence for the existence of female doctors can be found in twelfth-century documents (writs of an endowment to Leominster Priory) of an Anglo-Norman family of physicians, John, Matilda and Solicita Ford, all siblings. All are listed as *medicus* (John) or *medica* (Matilda and Solicita). The term *medicus* means physician, someone with training, rather than a barber, bleeder or the like. Matilda and Solicita are apparently England's first female doctors.[120] *Medicus* can also be defined as 'any sort of medical practitioner'.[121]

More common than the brother and sister were the husband and wife or father and son, even father and daughter teams of family surgeons and physicians. Katherine, who operated as a 'surgeon' c. 1286,[122] was apparently followed into the family business by her female children who practised surgery without opposition from the local authorities, the monks of Westminster Abbey. There are many examples of this sort of arrangement in medieval England. One is that of Thomas and Pernell de Raysn practising medicine in Devonshire in the fourteenth century.[123] Another family team involved a mother and daughter: Agnes and Joan Collins practised as barbers in fifteenth-century Canterbury as did Agnes and Jane Goddeson in sixteenth-century Bristol. What distinguished Jane was that she had served an apprenticeship with a man. Further, we have evidence of a minimum of two London barbers, who bequeathed their tools to male apprentices with instructions that they were to be supervised by the barbers' widows.[124]

The application of potions and charms was a common healing practice among women of Europe. The famous Catalan physician Arnold of Villanova who practised medicine in Spain, France and Italy, wrote that he witnessed older local women curing 'quinsy sore throat by some secret method and a man who was threatened by death by a continual haemorrhages [sic]'.[125] Medical professor at the University of Padua, Antonio Guaineri, suggested charms and incantations as well as a plaster purgative just below the navel as cures for various ailments.[126]

Reports made by male physicians also provide insight into women healers. Gilbert of England (fl. 1230–40) wrote about Marcellus, who uses 'empirica' (treatment with herbs and plants) to help women who had been sterile to conceive a child. Her method was to take various herbs by their roots while repeating the Lord's Prayer three times and speaking to no one. She also had advice on how to conceive a male or female child: 'In silence, too, extract the juice from the herbs and write on a piece of parchment these words, "The Lord said, 'Increase' x Uthiboth x 'and multiply' x thabechay x 'and fill the earth' x amath x." Then a man should wear these words around his neck for a boy, a woman for a girl.'[127] Gilbert cited a recipe taken from an old woman that was supposed to cure jaundice using the 'cooked juice of the plantagenet [*Planta genista*: broom]'.[128] Gilbert was apparently the first physician to refer to 'red colours in the treatment of small pox'. Once again, he attributed this to the recipes of 'old-wives' with various potions and drinks.[129]

Attitudes towards non-licensed practitioners – such as the 'old wives' – hardened at the end of the medieval period. We see this in the views of the physician Conrad Heingarter, the Franciscan friar Roger Bacon and the French surgeon, Guy de Chauliac.[130] Conrad Heingarter (fl. late 1400s), who was a physician to John II, duke of Bourbon, condemned the treatments and cures offered up by uneducated practitioners – women, wandering charlatans, gypsies and other sort of quacks, ecclesiastics and monks who poisoned with snakes, old witches or vagabonds, who 'promise you with their lies health, flattering you for money...'[131] Bacon (fl.c. 1220), who was a highly influential proponent of experimental science, denounced the medicine of women who employed charms and magic in their cures.[132] Chauliac, in his magnum opus, *Chirurgia Magna*,[133] the standard surgical text for two centuries, placed 'women and many fools', in the fifth and lowest level of those engaged in surgery. According to Chauliac, this sect 'referred the suffering of all illnesses to the saints alone, basing their practice upon the belief that the Lord has given as He had pleased and the Lord would take away as he pleased'.[134] Another example of this attitude may be found in the comments uttered by John of Arderne[135] who was critical of women practitioners whose cases he assumed. One case involved a woman healer who had attempted to cure a finger wound by administering medicines through the mouth. The healer only made the finger worse.[136] The surgeon John of Mirfield (d. 1407), denounced all non-university trained practitioners, but reserved special venom for females: 'At the present time, not only ignorant men – but what is worse and must be judged yet more horrible – vile and presumptuous women usurp that office to themselves and abuse it, since they have neither learning nor skill.' He focused on the unnecessary deaths they caused 'because of their stupidity ... since they operate neither wisely nor with proper diagnosis, but casually, and are wholly ignorant of the causes and names of diseases which they declare that they know how to and can heal'.[137]

Although men in religious orders were prohibited from practising medicine from the twelfth century onwards, women in convents continued to do so throughout this period. The regulations which the church passed against monks and, later, regular clergy, who practised some form of medicine, were intended to force them to focus on their religious duties rather than on medicine.[138] While we know about famous women like Hildegard of Bingen (1098–1179), the abbess of Rupertsberg, and Harrad, or Herrad of Landsberg (1130–1195), the abbess of Hohenburg in Alsace, no definitive study has been made of medical practice within convents in the Middle Ages.[139] Women had practised informal medicine in their convents for generations. Hildegard was a special case in that she possessed a sophisticated knowledge of human biology and herbal medicine. The works of Hildegard of Bingen represent the high point of scientific and medical writings written by a European woman of the Middle Ages.[140] Harrad authored or was in charge of the writing of an illustrated encyclopaedia called the *Hortus Deliciarum* or the Garden of Delights. It was an all-encompassing work in terms of subject matter and included sections on astronomy and geography. The work was written for her convent sisters between 1160 and 1170.[141]

In France, there were a number of nuns with medical knowledge. One of these was Héloise, who was trained in blood-letting and basic medicines, and possessed the skills of a barber. Others included two barber-surgeons from the Abbaye de Longchamp: Jeanne de Crespi, a barber, who entered the abbey of Longchamp in 1334 and Macée de Chaumont who died 22 March 1485. The rules for several orders of nuns, including the Benedictines and Poor Clares, stated that convents should possess an infirmary and that nuns should be able to conduct their own medical care.[142] This was common to most convents in Europe in order to prevent a man from treating the nuns.

Although nuns were primarily nursing sisters, there is evidence for some who practised as physicians. One example is a Sister Ann who is called '*medica*' at St Leonard's Hospital, York, in 1276. The title implies that she performed more complex medical tasks than most nursing sisters.[143] In hospitals, women patients were generally treated by other women in wards separate from men. In Italy, female doctors who treated women patients were called '*magistra*' and possessed surgical skills.[144]

Religious houses with more than twenty nuns would often have an infirmary for lay people. There might be a separate building where lepers and those with mental illnesses would be treated, in addition to a room or parlour for people suffering from physical ailments. This was the case in the Syon Monastery, an English religious house in Middlesex, where the nuns looked after the sick. Founded in 1415 by Henry V, with a complement of sixty nuns and twenty-five monks, the rule of Syon indicated that the 'infirmarian' would provide both nursing and medical care. She would 'often change their beds and clothes, give them medicines, lay their plasters, and minister to them meat and drink, fire and water, and all other necessities night and day as need required'.[145]

Jewish physicians, both male and female, made substantial contributions to medicine in the medieval period. They became particularly skilled in treating diseases of the eyes and ophthalmology was often their speciality. Indeed, there were many female Jewish doctors who treated diseases of the eyes. In Seville, one Dona Leal was licensed to practise ophthalmology.[146]

The Jews were also often proficient in many languages – Greek, Latin, Arabic and Hebrew – and thus were able to read and translate a wide range of medical texts. This meant that they tended to be a more educated group of physicians than their Christian counterparts. In spite of their skill and expertise, Jews suffered from persecution and prejudice and Paracelsus (1493–1541) was not unique in his view: 'As regards medicine, the Jews of old boasted greatly, and they still do, and they are not ashamed of the falsehood; they claim that they are the oldest and foremost among all the other nations, the foremost rascals that is.'[147]

They also had to deal with restriction through papal bulls and royal ordinances which forbad them to treat Gentiles. Nevertheless, their services were used by high ecclesiastical figures such as bishops, popes and kings.[148] Although Jewish women doctors did not reach the same prominence as their male counterparts and, like their non-Jewish contemporaries, they represented a minority of medical practitioners overall, there were still a good number of Jewish women doctors in the Europe of the Middle Ages.

There is substantial evidence that Jewish women practised a wide variety of medicine as physicians, surgeons, ophthalmologists and midwives, especially between the twelfth and the fifteenth centuries in parts of Italy, Spain and France, and in Western European cities such as Paris, Florence, Valencia, Naples, Sicily and Frankfurt. Jews, like women, were prohibited from studying at universities, but as scholars have demonstrated, they still became prominent and skilled doctors. Virdimura, as mentioned above, practised medicine throughout Sicily. She successfully passed a medical examination. She specialized in treating the poor and charged them less for her services than the male doctors. Castilian royalty, most famously Ferdinand and Isabella, always used Jewish physicians. In addition, Jews worked as physicians for many cities of Spain.[149] The fact that a few Jewish women of Spain were able to become licensed physicians and not merely wise women or practitioners of domestic medicine is surprising given the attitude towards women in Spain at this time and their almost non-existent education. Perhaps the fact that they were Jews was the reason why these women could become doctors.

Jews, both male and female, received their medical education at home. They were usually taught by their fathers or other male relatives.[150] Licensed Jewish women physicians also worked for the royal family in the kingdom of Aragón-Catalonia in the fourteenth century.[151] Alfonso IV hired a medical practitioner called Francisca to care for the queen. And at the court of Aragón, there are references to three Jewish women who practised obstetrics between 1368 and 1381 during the reign of Pedro IV. Still with Aragón, two Jewish women were authorized to practise medicine for Juan I.[152]

In Barcelona in 1342, we find the case of the Jewish surgeon, Astruga, wife of Astruch, who was charged by the royal justiciar for not having tried the required examination. The king intervened in the case, arguing that she could continue her work as she was not practising medicine, but surgery and 'only on Jews'.[153]

After the persecution of the Jews in Spain in the late fourteenth century, many moved to Italy. In 1492, the Jews were expelled from Spain and Sicily, and after 1503, many settled in Sardinia and Naples. Antonia Daniello practised medicine in Florence in the late fourteenth and early fifteenth century.[154] Brunetta, a Jewish Italian woman who lived during the fifteenth century, was denounced by Bernardinus of Siena who was engaged in a campaign against the Jews. At the trial of the Jews, he accused her of having provided the needles for the bloodletting of Simon of Trent.[155]

On rare occasions, Jewish women were teachers of medicine. One such woman was Sarah of St Giles, widow of Abraham, who apparently taught Salvetus de Burgonovo. A Marseilles manuscript dating from 1326, records the agreement made between them in which Sarah would teach Salvetus, 'the art of medicine and physic', and clothe, lodge and feed him for seven months. He would pay Sarah fees for her services. He would give her the income which he made for his treatment of the sick. This seems to indicate that he already had some sort of medical training and was receiving advanced tuition from her.[156] Sarah La Migresse practised in Paris around 1292.[157] Mayrona was one of the three Jewish women practising medicine for whom we have records. Another was Fava, a surgeon, and daughter of the surgeon Astrugus (d. 1306), who worked with her surgeon son, Bonafas.[158] Fava is mentioned only once in the documents, for a particular case which took place between 19 November 1321 and 22 January 1322. She treated a man by the name of Ponçon, the hospital crier, who had suffered a blow to his testicles in an altercation. The documents indicate that she 'administered plasters and other necessary remedies'. Apparently, she was accused of touching the patient. She denied this and was supported in this assertion by her son. He told the court that he took the patient's pulse, not his mother.[159]

The Paris tax register of 1292 reveals the names of other Jewish women who were practising medicine at this time: Isabiau (la mergesse) was a popular lay healer in the parish of Ste Opportune and paid six sous in tax.[160] Adelie, a herbalist, also appears in the tax survey, listed as an 'erberière', a seller of culinary and medicinal herbs.[161]

Although much of the evidence again points to women primarily treating women, this was not always the case. Jacoba Félicie (b. 1280), who was charged with the illegal practice of medicine in the first half of the fourteenth century by the bishop of Paris and the proctor and dean of the Medical Faculty at the University of Paris, had both male and female patients.[162]

A considerable contribution was made by Arab female healers in the Middle Ages. These included primarily midwives, practitioners of folk medicine and hospital workers. Women were experts in folk medicine. They collected and cooked herbs and prepared them according to the Zodiac. There is evidence for itinerant and old women known as 'quasi practitioners' of medicine.[163]

The daughter and granddaughter of Avenaoar, or Ibn Zuhr, practised as doctors and as midwives. They were members of a great Spanish Muslim medical family.[164] Ibn Zuhr was born around 1091 in Seville. He was a Galenist and a physician to the Sultan as well as the author of several books on medicine, including on gynaecology.[165] One of the greatest medieval surgeons, the Muslim Albucasis or Abu Al-Qasim Al-Zahravi (936–1013) referred to Arab women surgeons in his *De Chirurgia* when he wrote that if a woman suffered from calculus (stone), she must see a woman surgeon.[166]

During the fourteenth century, after the plague, there was a shortage of physicians in Spain as elsewhere in Europe. The authorities relaxed some of the licensing laws which enabled Muslim as well as Jewish physicians to practise medicine legally. Among these physicians one can find a number of Muslim women, described as *metgesses*, who served the Muslim and Christian populations as midwives, physicians and surgeons. One such *metgesse* was a woman named Çahud who lived with the royal family of Valencia.[167] Muslim women also worked in Spanish hospitals during the Middle Ages. Their role as *metgesses* involved the care of infants and children. Their work went beyond nursing as one record indicates bone-setting a fracture. They were paid for their work.[168]

As the evidence offered above shows, women were actively engaged in the practice of the healing arts during the Middle Ages even though they were denied a university education – except in rare cases. They practised a variety of types of medicine, as surgeons and doctors both inside and outside the home. However, with the rise of the European university and the introduction of stricter licensing regulations for non-university trained medical personnel, women would no longer have the same freedom to practise medicine.

2
New Medical Regulations and their Impact on Female Healers

Several important changes occurred in the development of medicine from the later Middle Ages into the Early Modern era. One important transformation was the increasing trend towards the professionalization of medicine. This meant a clear demarcation between the various branches of medical practice from physician, surgeon, barber to apothecary, with the university educated physician at the apex of the medical hierarchy. The formal training of medical practitioners became part and parcel of the professionalization process. A university education became mandatory for those wanting to practise legally as physicians, and physicians in European countries would be strictly differentiated from surgeons. Only physicians received university training, while surgeons, barber-surgeons and apothecaries qualified through an apprenticeship. An example of a surgeon's apprenticeship could be four years of hospital work. Since women were banned from attending universities in European countries with the exception of Italy, they were therefore legally prohibited from becoming licensed physicians until the nineteenth century.

Specific authorities, namely Church and state, began to issue licences for the practice of specific types of medicine. Guilds or corporations, churches, the universities and, in particular, the Faculty of Medicine of the University of Paris, were crucial to the licensing process. University trained physicians actively prevented unlicensed healers, including women and minorities such as Jews and Muslims in addition to any other untrained empirics, from practising medicine. The salient feature here was the beginning of control over practice, which had not existed in such a formal way in the past. The newly founded universities, often within a church-based setting, made the most vigorous efforts to professionalize medicine and make the theoretical aspect of medicine superior to the practical side. One of the most famous cases in history of a woman medic banned from practising by the Faculty of Medicine of the University of Paris was that of Jacoba Félicie. Her case is covered in detail below.

This chapter first offers a comparative exploration of the issue of the professionalization of medicine, including licensing. Although all of the countries under consideration here introduced regulations, there were significant differences between them. Licensing practices and enforcement of licences and regulations varied from country to country. Of crucial interest is the impact that the regulation of medicine had on women healers. In other words, to what extent did licensing and a more 'scientific' approach to healing affect women practising various forms of medicine?

Licences were established as a form of official recognition and approval of a practitioner's competence in medicine.[1] As such, a licence was supposed to guarantee some level of skill, but this was not always the case. One expert has argued that rather than encouraging improvement in medicine, regulation actually held back progress and any form of innovation. Physicians used regulations to criticize colleagues and incompetence was often hidden behind them.[2] As noted above, licences to practise medicine were granted to individuals by a recognized authority – secular or ecclesiastical. As a rule, in order to obtain a licence, the practitioner was required to prove that he had passed an examination or offer some sort of testimony affirming his qualifications as a medical practitioner.

Qualifications involved some sort of training, although many who practised medicine at this time received no formal training. While in many places barber-surgeons, surgeons and apothecaries passed through an apprenticeship, in Italy they could attend universities. There was no set curriculum or stipulated plan of study for these practitioners. Surgeons were literate, and in Paris at least, they had knowledge of Latin, as much of the legislation was written in this language.[3] Barber-surgeons and surgeons were in may ways indistinguishable except for their dress – surgeons wore long robes – and prestige.[4] However, surgeons would not perform certain minor operations, considering them to be beneath their dignity. In France, these operations included the treatment of boils, tumours, bruises and minor cuts.[5] It is not known whether this is also true for other countries. We do, however, know that in France, barbers studied anatomy and herbal medicine and that they learned about ointments, salves and the treatment of wounds and sores.[6]

There are several reasons why medical practitioners sought a licence. Licences limited competition and created a hierarchy of practitioners on the basis of gender, religion and education.[7] In terms of gender and licensing, scholars have argued that in seventeenth-century England, 'gender differences in both the guild and ecclesiastical routes to becoming a surgeon ensured that relatively few women obtained "official" standing as surgeons...'[8] Male practitioners received strong support from colleagues whether or not they had served an apprenticeship and patients' opinions and testimonials seemed to hold little weight in obtaining a licence.[9] The situation was quite different for women as is explained in detail below.

Two more important reasons motivating practitioners to seek licences were economics and the law. Legally, doctors and others were not supposed to charge for their services without a licence to practise. In addition, licences provided some form of legal protection if a practitioner was sued for malpractice. In economic terms, a licence meant that practitioners could charge more for their services and possibly also attract wealthier clients.[10] Licences were supposed to ensure a certain standard of treatment and competency.[11]

Of crucial importance is the clergy's involvement in the practice and regulation of medicine in the Middle Ages into the Early Modern period. Healing was an integral part of the Christian faith. The clergy had practised medicine for years, but in the Middle Ages, they were accused of neglecting their pastoral duties in favour of medicine. As a result, the Church hierarchy initiated a series of rules in an attempt to put an end to clergy practising medicine. These included the rulings from Rheims in 1131 and the Lateran Council of 1139. Pope Alexander III prohibited regular clerics from leaving their monasteries to study medicine.[12] However, the various council rulings, which concerned the regular clergy (monks) and were aimed at prohibiting the practice of medicine that was often local in nature had only limited success.[13] Thus, in spite of various rulings from the 1100s onward, clergy continued to be involved in the practice of medicine, which could offer one reason why women were officially banned from it.[14] At the Fourth Lateran Council of 1215, clerics were prohibited from practising as surgeons. In the sixteenth century popes Paul IV and Pius V prohibited Jews from practising medicine on Christians, but this regulation does not seemed to have been enforced and, indeed, many popes had Jewish physicians.[15]

The Church's role in licensing was particularly crucial in England. In 1511, during the reign of Henry VIII, an Act of Parliament, known as 3 Henry viii c. II, granted the Bishop of London and the Dean of St Paul's the right to license surgeons and physicians.[16] York and Canterbury, however, remained under canon law.[17] Because of the technical nature of medicine and surgery, bishops had to ensure that those seeking licences had first been examined by licensed physicians and surgeons.[18] The Church remained the principal granter of licences for those without a university degree for about 250 years.[19] Surgeons were dissatisfied with this system as the Church did not always keep to its word in granting licences only to those surgeons who had been approved by the fellowship of surgeons. The connection between the Church and surgeons can be traced back to the early Middle Ages when medicine and surgery were carried out by priests.[20] On the whole, the guilds, which regulated non-university trained practitioners, resented outside involvement by either the Church or the state.

The practice of secular medical licensing arose in the context of medieval European society, which was strictly organized by occupation. Crafts, trades and professions had their own regulations, with standards of entry, codes and qualifications. Workmen and women alike were required to belong to a guild in order to practise their trade. As a rule, there was a period of apprenticeship followed by an examination. Medicine was no different from the other trades in this respect. From the eleventh to the thirteenth centuries, depending on the country, surgeons were organized into craft guilds. In addition to performing the functions stated above, medical guilds provided recourse for the patient if something went wrong. Local authorities and governments became actively involved in the control of the medical profession in Italy, Spain and France, although Spain was relatively late in guild creation.[21] The common denominator was some sort of test or examination for the practitioner by a licensed physician.

The practice of medical licensing or the requirement of a licence to practise medicine began in the twelfth century and licences were issued by both secular and ecclesiastical powers. Licensing gave greater control over the healing arts and meant that a certain group decided who could and could not practise medicine, or at least formal medicine. In addition to control over the profession, another reason stated by authorities in deciding who could and could not practise medicine was that of propriety. It was more desirable that women treat other women than that women be treated by men.[22]

Laws concerning the control of medicine pre-date the period covered in this book. There were edicts issued as far back in history as ancient Rome, as well as during the barbarian invasions by the Visigoths, but the decrees issued in the later Middle Ages may be distinguished by their 'systematic intensification'.[23] In Italy, modern medical licensing began with an edict from King Roger II of Sicily (ruled 1130–54) in 1140. This edict was severe in terms of punishment and it demonstrates that he was serious about stamping out unlicensed practitioners: 'Who, from now on, wishes to practice medicine, has to present himself before our officials and examiners, in order to pass their judgment. Should he be bold enough to disregard this, he will be punished by imprisonment and confiscation of his entire property. In this way we are taking care that our subjects are not endangered by the inexperience of the physicians.'[24] The Holy Roman Emperor, Frederick II (1194–1250) issued his own set of laws with respect to the education and practice of physicians, demanding that they should study logic for three years.[25] Physicians were to be 'certified by the judgment of the masters in the public convention at Salernum, and licensed by testimonials to his trustworthiness'. The medical school of Salerno was under his control.[26] If someone was found to be practising medicine without this certificate, he would be sent to prison for a year and his goods would be confiscated.[27] Historians have pointed out that the fact that no clerics were involved here meant that women had an equal chance to practise medicine. Nothing in these regulations mentions women or the prohibition of women practising medicine.[28]

In Italy, regional variation was the norm in terms of licensing. In northern Italy, women were recognized as physicians, surgeons and empirics, particularly the latter two, although there were fewer licensed female doctors in the north than in the south. They were not licensed in Venice, but they were in Florence and Naples, where they were limited to the practice of surgery. In southern Italy, there was a strong family trend in licensing. The daughters, wives and widows of doctors, practised medicine.[29]

In the Early Modern era, a College of Physicians was founded and the state regulated physicians, surgeons and apothecaries in the Italian peninsula. Offices of *Protomedicati*[30] or licensing boards were founded throughout Italy between the fourteenth and sixteenth centuries.[31] The Office of *Protomedici* originated in southern and central Italy for the licensing of surgeons and apothecaries in 1397, when King Martin II of Sicily, an Aragonese king, appointed the first *Protomedico*, or first physician, Ruggero de Camma. King Alfonso the Magnanimous appointed a first physician for Naples on his accession in 1444. Both kings were closely connected to the Spanish vice-royal administration.[32]

A medical guild in Florence pre-dates the licensing boards. It dates from 1293. From 1314, it was divided between apothecaries, empirics and barbers. In 1392, university trained doctors founded their own association.[33] In Florence, during the Renaissance era, the guilds of apothecaries and surgeons set the standards for admission. The doors were open to all who could demonstrate competency, even those without a university degree. This included Jews and women. However, information on female doctors in Renaissance Florence is limited.[34] University trained physicians formed a minority of practitioners, as elsewhere.

The primary task of the first physician was to visit the towns to inspect the medical practice of all types of practitioners, from physicians to apothecaries.[35] However, in the Italian city-states, especially Naples, Siena and Sicily, the first physician never possessed the same degree of power as his counterparts in Spain. The office in Spain became a massive bureaucracy. In Italy, the boards were not as rigid; fines were light and not always enforced.[36] The details of the powers of the Office of *Protomedici* were published in 1564 by the anatomist and epidemiologist Gian Filippo Ingrassia.[37] The office held a great deal of power over all areas of practice, from barbers to midwives. A licence was required to practise *physica*, surgery and pharmacy. Unlike many other European jurisdictions, even within Italy, licences from Naples in the fourteenth century, usually dispensed by the Royal Court or representatives of the king, clearly indicate that women had the right to 'exercise the profession of physician' and take care of female patients: 'Since, then, the law permits women to exercise the profession of physicians, and since, besides, due regard being had to purity of morals, women are better suited for the treatment of women's diseases, after having received the oath of fidelity, we permit...'[38] Many of the extant licences granted to women were in the field of surgery and usually licensed the holder to undertake minor surgical practices, such as the treatment of simple wounds, abscesses, ulcers and cancers.[39]

The Office of *Protomedici* also existed in other parts of the Italian peninsula. According to scholars, the establishment of such an office in Rome originated with the Rome College of Physicians, which dated from the twelfth century as a guild, although the first extant reference to it is the Papal Bull of 1471. The office took over the college's authority over time. Unlike Naples, the Roman office banned women from all medical practice except midwifery in the Instruction of 1620.[40]

Similar offices were formed in Bologna (1517) and in Siena (1562). Bologna's office was also an outgrowth from the 1378 Statutes of the College of Medicine and Arts which regulated the profession by issuing licences in order to keep out charlatans, settling disputes between patients and doctors, inspecting apothecaries and instituting fines.[41] Apparently the *Protomedicato* in Bologna was not harsh in its penalties to unlicensed practitioners. Punishments included fines, seizure of medications, and at the most, banishment from the city.[42] Women in Bologna who were midwives also performed tasks other than those related to pregnancy and childbirth, including diseases specific to women. They could treat childhood diseases, but they were prohibited from administering drugs.[43]

In Bologna, there was a three-tier system composed of physicians, apothecaries and barber-surgeons. The division between apothecaries and physicians was put into practice by the College of Medicine in 1606. The *Protomedicato* or licensing board drew up a distinction between physicians and surgeons. Surgeons were not permitted to administer oral drugs, although the physicians were not able to enforce the separation until the end of the century. Surgeons were still granted the degree of doctorate at the medical college at the beginning of the sixteenth century and were in no way considered inferior to physicians. This had changed by the end of the sixteenth century when the tripartite structure had been implemented.[44]

Apparently, the Siennese offices were the most lenient both in dispensing licences and in enforcing (or not enforcing) fines.[45] Evidently, an individual's material condition and talent in bargaining and even bribing the chief physician could relieve him from the enforcement of the edict and the paying of a fine. An example of the demonstration of compassion by the office was the case of a poor mattress-maker with three children, who also treated various ailments such as ring-worm. He was pardoned because of his poverty.[46] Nevertheless, as in other parts of Europe, women were officially banned from the practice of orthodox medicine.

In France, women were not banned from practising as surgeons and barbers, but there were numerous stipulations concerning women in the various guild edicts passed between 1258 and 1454. The first record of a medical guild dates from circa 1258. It was a surgeons' guild and was organized under the Provost of Paris, Etienne Boileau, under St Louis. The principal motivating factor in prompting surgeons to organize themselves into a corporation was the increasing competition from barbers, their major rivals.[47]

There were six edicts passed between 1311 and 1452 concerning the practice of surgery in France. In 1311, Philip IV issued the first royal ordinances for surgeons: all surgeons practising in Paris would henceforth be subject to an examination by master surgeons under the First Royal surgeon, at the time, Jean Pitard. This ordinance included male and female surgeons: 'Nullus chirurgicus, nulla chirurgia' (no male or female) could practise surgery in the city of Paris without the master's approval. By 1356, surgeons were required to know Latin in which a considerable amount of the legislation was written. In this year, King John acknowledged that the surgeons were a 'Faculty', which meant that they were considered 'learned'.[48] Thus, female surgeons were not prohibited under law from practising surgery, but they were nonetheless often perceived to be incompetent and ignorant by their peers.[49]

As was the case in other countries, there was also rivalry between barbers and the surgeons who tried to limit their practice. The first regulations for barbers were passed in 1371 under Charles V, whose 'premier Barbier Valet de Chambre' became 'the garde of the craft in Paris with the right to choose his lieutenants'. These would be the 'garde and master' of the barbers with four *barbiers jurés*. They would examine all those who practised the trade.[50] Further regulations date from 1372. These rules specified the operations that barbers could and could not perform. They could dress boils, tumours and bruises, take care of minor wounds and administer plasters.[51] Interestingly, the king did not make these regulations any more prohibitive because barbers were more likely than surgeons to treat the poor. If the poor were denied medical treatment, the public welfare would be compromised.[52] Women could practise as barbers if they were either the daughter of a master barber or married to a barber.[53]

Widows of barber-surgeons were given the same privileges as their deceased husbands in a ruling by the Paris Parlement in 1427.[54] A statute dating from 1452 concerning surgeons covered the role of both barbers and surgeons, including women. Article I stated that only those who had been examined by a master surgeon and were presented to the local authorities to whom they took an oath could practise. Article III made it clear that the surgeon was the superior practitioner: 'No barber (male or female) is permitted to undertake the healing of the sick where there is danger of death without having the advice or accompaniment of the surgeons...' As far as phlebotomy (blood-letting) was concerned, Article X made it clear that this practice was limited to surgeons.[55]

Henri de Mondeville (1260–1320), a military surgeon and later surgeon to two kings of France, Philip the Good (le bel) (1285–1314) and his son, Louis le Hutin (1314–16), protested against 'the practice of surgery by untrained empirics, lay people'. He referred to them as 'idiots, simpletons and ignorant'. Mondeville attempted to improve surgery so that only the literate would be allowed to study surgery, which would be closely tied to the principles of medicine. Surgery in Mondeville's day was filled with uneducated practitioners; those who, like Mondeville, were educated were the exception rather than the rule.[56]

Similarly, the leading surgeon of the fourteenth century, Guy de Chauliac (1300–68), a man who had studied at the most prestigious medical schools in Europe, and who had been physician to several popes, complained bitterly about the weakness of governments who allowed 'stupid women' to practise surgery.[57] Chauliac, who classified those practising surgery into sects based on the types of treatments administered to patients, put women in the fifth and lowest sect, even though many used the same healing methods as surgeons in the higher sects. As was noted above, Chauliac argued that the last sect contained 'women and many fools who referred the suffering of all illnesses to the saints alone, basing their practice upon the belief that the Lord has given as He had pleased and the Lord would take away as he pleased'.[58]

A ruling of the Parlement of Brittany from 8 October 1568 stated that 'no one could practice surgery without an examination before a doctor who was an expert in general anatomy'.[59] Widows could inherit their husbands' practices and continue their work as long as they had two years of experience. In the next two centuries, women's freedom to practise would be limited by various government rulings. A ruling of the Breton Parlement allowed widows to continue their husbands' surgical practice, but they were not allowed to reach the status of Master nor to treat patients and provide cures except under a Master's advice.[60] On 19 April 1755, the Parlement of Paris ruled against wives and daughters practising surgery. M de Martinère argued that for reasons of modesty, 'women should not be doing such operations, and that courses of Anatomy, of Osteology would be deprived to them'. On 19 April 1755 the Court ordered that in the future, 'women and girls could not be graduates of any sort of surgery except that which relates to childbirth'. Pharmacy was equally prohibited to them and for the same reasons, 'so that there remains to them only the exercise of Empirical Medicine, for which they are approved by the First Doctor or the Royal Commission, who also gives his Patents to the men and to the women for the remedies which they can invent'.[61]

England was rather late in getting into the licensing business, and the first regulations of the medical profession were passed in 1421 following a petition by the universities in which they complained about the 'many uncunning and unapproved of the foresaid science [of physic] practises'.[62] Henry VIII's statute of 1511 recognized the importance of Oxford and Cambridge in the training of physicians but it did not remove the Church's control over the profession.[63]

In England, as in France, the higher ranks of medicine were dominated by the clergy. However, unlike in France and Italy, England's major cities did not possess medical universities. This led to serious problems in the regulation of the profession of medicine.[64]

As in continental Europe, in England, non-university trained medical practitioners were regulated by guilds. The guilds could be called upon by city officials if illicit practice was suspected. They begrudged the interference of outsiders such as the Church or the Crown in their sphere of influence.[65] These English guilds or corporations were less hostile to female practitioners than was the case in other parts of Europe. The Barbers' Company dates from 1308 with the choice of Richard Le Barbour to supervise the trade. He swore an oath before the Court of Aldermen in London.[66] In England, the barbers and barber-surgeons were divided according to tasks, with barbers also practising dentistry and blood-letting and barber-surgeons practising as surgeons.[67] There is nothing in these documents which prohibits women from practising their craft. Women were found in the early organization of barber-surgeons. They were admitted to the Barbers' Company mostly through apprenticeship but also by patrimony. Women were not admitted to the Livery, but were in possession of all other privileges.[68] Women's services came at a lower rate of pay than those of men.

The city of London began to regulate surgery around the year 1369 when a board of master surgeons was appointed to control standards.[69] A document from 10 April 1390 recognized the position of women surgeons.[70] The guild or fellowship of surgeons was a smaller and more exclusive group than that of the barbers. Its members practised surgery exclusively. In 1493, it had only twelve members. The two groups were often in contention because the Barbers' Guild supervised those barbers who also practised surgery. They united in 1540 as the Company of Barber Surgeons and Surgeons.[71] Under the Act of 1540 the new company retained responsibility for the examination and licensing of surgeons. There would be a seven-year apprenticeship and 'women could be bound as apprentices and be admitted to the Freedom but not to the Livery'. They were also permitted to take apprentices in the same way as men.[72]

There is evidence for the practice of surgery by licensed women in York in the guild records. One such was Isabel Warwicke, who, according to the records, 'hath skill in the scyens of surgery and hath done good therein; it is therefore aggreed by the present that she upon her good behaviour shall use the same good sciens within this citie... 3 June 1572'.[73] However, licensing practices in Early Modern England made it very difficult for women legally to practise surgery. Even when women did acquire a licence, they were still marginalized by male surgeons. Women did not receive the same pay as men, if they were paid at all. At St Bartholomew's Hospital in London, there is evidence for two female surgeons on the staff in 1656. They were restricted to treating patients with scald-head (ringworm) and leprosy.[74]

Female barbers were more common than female surgeons. Barbers' trades were less prestigious and carried fewer benefits than those of surgeons. They could not practise surgery but they could extract teeth. Surgeons were not permitted to practise as barbers.[75] In the cities of Lincoln, York, Norwich and Dublin, women barbers were admitted as guild members. These guilds dated from the later Middle Ages, around 1299 for York, 1379 for Lincoln, Norwich and Dublin. Women appeared to be equally trained in their craft, judging by the guild's statutes.[76]

While guilds operated in urban areas, the practice of medicine in the English countryside was to all intents and purposes unregulated. Although women were admitted to the guilds, their numbers were far below those of men. Thus, we find the majority of female practitioners active in rural areas where they specialized in 'folk' medicine. They worked as herbalists, they treated cuts and bruises and broken bones and were involved in childbirth. Women were also leeches.[77] Those who were neither physicians nor surgeons and who thus received no 'education' in the formal sense, but still administered medicines, were known as quacks. They practised legally under the auspices of the Herbalists' or Quacks' Charter, Act of 34/35 Henry VIII c. 8, which allowed,

> every Person being the King's subject, having Knowledge and Experience of the Nature of Herbs, Roots and Waters, or of the Operation of the same, by Speculation or Practice, within any part of the Realm of England, or within any other the King's Dominions, to practice, use and minister in and to any outward Sore, Uncome Wound, Aposelmations, outward Swelling or Disease, any Herb or Herbs, Ointments, Baths, Pultess, and Emplaisters, according to their Cunning, Experience and Knowledge in any of the Diseases, Sorea and Maladies beforesaid, and all other like to the same, or Drinks for the Stone, Strangury or Agues, without suit, vexation, trouble, penalty or loss of their goods.[78]

The only restriction was that these unlicensed practitioners did not 'operate by cautery or incision, or prescribe internal medicines'.[79]

Medical regulation in Spain was complex. The earliest set of regulations, the *Fuero Juzgo* (Body of Spanish Laws), date from between 642 and 649. This Codex of Laws was passed by the Visigoth king Chindaswinth. As far as medicine was concerned, the laws stipulated a cash payment for penalties in cases of medical malpractice.[80] Further regulations were introduced in Spain in the later Middle Ages. The Spanish kings tended to follow similar regulations to those passed by Roger II of Sicily. King Alfonso II of Leon (1188–1230) passed a law which banned anyone from practising medicine unless he/she had been tested by a physician and licensed by town councils.[81] Northern Spain at this time belonged to the Crown of Aragón as did Montpellier where licensing dated from 1239.[82] The Cortes (court) of 1252, held at Seville, was 'an assembly of prelates, magnates and townsmen representing the estates of the realm'. At the Cortes, the leaders decided to prohibit Christian women from nursing Jewish or Muslim children and vice versa. A fine of ten *maravedís* per day of service was imposed.[83]

Alfonso III (1285–91) introduced similar laws in Aragón in the thirteenth century. These laws were passed by the court of Monzón in 1289. According to these laws, practitioners did not need a university degree to practise medicine in Aragón until the end of the thirteenth century.[84] Physicians and surgeons were examined by other practitioners.[85] With these laws, Spain followed the same rubric as other European countries. They were 'a public acknowledgement of the growing influence of medical learning'.[86]

The Spanish attempt to professionalize medicine grew more pronounced from the thirteenth to the sixteenth century. Historians have suggested the reasons for this were attempts by the Crown, the Church and municipal authorities to acquire authority over medicine and to make the profession of the university trained physician the only legitimate form of medicine. In this way, the authorities attempted to marginalize women and other non-university trained healers.[87] Despite their best efforts, the authorities were not entirely successful in this.

Alfonso IV of Valencia introduced stringent regulations in 1329. These rules are called the '*furs*' (law code), and they made it impossible for anyone to practise medicine in the kingdom of Valencia without a medical degree from a university or *stadium generale*. A medical degree took four years to complete. The towns and cities would grant the medical licences as in the past, but the decision as to who would practise was made by the university trained doctors. Physicians were appointed to hospitals and the armed forces and they regulated the publication of all medical texts.[88] These laws applied directly to women ruling that 'no woman may practice medicine or give potions, under penalty of being whipped through the town...' Presumably, this meant that women were practising in sufficient numbers to warrant a clause in the laws. Women were permitted 'to care for little children, and women – to whom, however, they may give no potion'.[89] Before these laws were introduced, historians have little evidence of official female medical practice; subsequently there is evidence of licences granted to women by kings.[90]

The kingdoms of Aragón and Navarre possessed regulating institutions such as the *confradías* of doctors, surgeons and apothecaries and municipally appointed examiners.[91] These were brotherhood organizations of skilled artisans. They grouped together doctors, surgeons and apothecaries and protected their professional privileges. Based on applications for medical licences, the majority of women practitioners were Muslims. This has led some commentators to believe that the laws were directed against Muslims practising on Christians.[92] Although some historians have theorized that these licensing laws were introduced to limit if not ban the practice of medicine by women, others have suggested that unlike the medical licensing laws in Paris, the *furs* do not appear to have been actively enforced.[93] García-Ballester provides examples of several women from the Muslim, Christian and Jewish communities who were legally practising medicine after the passage of the *furs*, and argues that there is more evidence of female practitioners after 1329 than before that date. This could well be true for Valencia, as there was a shortage of male doctors and the services provided by women were necessary. In addition, frequent plagues and other illnesses meant that the skills of female healers were needed. Male doctors also charged a great deal more than female practitioners and were thus out of reach for many. A final reason for the lack of effectiveness of these laws in Spain was the fact that they were not rigorously enforced due to various factors such as conflicts between the Crown and municipal authorities.[94]

The role of the Crown in controlling medicine was intrinsically related to the growth of the state in Spain in the sixteenth century, and in particular, under the Catholic monarchs from 1477 to 1588 and the reforms of Philip II. Royal power was exercised by secretaries who were responsible to the monarch and his advisory councils.[95] The strictest regulations were introduced by the Catholic monarchs, Ferdinand and Isabella, who issued what became permanent statutes in 1477, 1491 and 1498.[96] Evidently, the authorities were concerned that contemporary standards of medicine were very low. The preamble of the 1477 legislation stated that both the licensed and unlicensed practitioners were ignorant. It decreed that: 'the protomédicos and alcades examinadores should examine all who aspired to become physicians, surgeons, bonesetters, apothecaries, dealers in aromatic drugs, herbalists and any other persons who in whole or in part practice these professions'. The decree included both men and women. The term '*Protomedicato*' or board of examiners was first employed in this legislation.[97] After the passage of the 1477 laws, complaints against unlicensed practitioners continued. Thus, further legislation was passed in the 1490s. The 1491 law stated that physicians and surgeons 'could now be forced to appear before examiners or pay a fine of 600 marvedís if they refused'. In addition, the examiners 'could have justice on their persons and properties for their crimes'.[98] Despite the pivotal importance of this legislation, illicit medical practice continued as part and parcel of medical life in Spain.

By the seventeenth century in England, there were several types of female medical workers: nurses, midwives and regular practitioners, surgeons, barber-surgeons and apothecaries. Despite the complex web of licensing in England, women continued to be granted licences for medical practice (usually for medicine and surgery) from the Archbishop of Canterbury. Between 1613 and 1696, ten such licences were issued to women to practise medicine and surgery.[99] The information contained in many of the licences is very brief, providing only name, spouse (wife of), region and the purpose of the licence. Most women were granted licences for medicine or surgery and some were granted licences to practise both. Existing records for three women who practised medicine provide a window into the world of the female practitioner. These women were issued licences by the archbishop in the late seventeenth century and their records are unusually detailed. They were Elizabeth Moore, Jane Pemell or Pennell and Mary Rose. Moore and Rose were licensed to practise both medicine and surgery while Pemell was licensed only to practise surgery.[100]

Elizabeth Moore practised medicine with and without a licence. Many of the testimonials to her skill in healing pre-date her licence which was issued on 17 January 1690 and allowed Elizabeth Moore, widow, of Market Harborough, Leicestershire, to practise medicine and surgery in the dioceses of Coventry and Lichfield, Lincoln and Peterborough.[101] Testimonials to Moore's medical skill were written by two rectors, John Howard of Marston Trussell, Northants, and Richard Mousse of Little Bowden, Leics., as well as Isaac Laughton, MA, and Edward Moore. These men wrote that they knew, 'Mrs. Elizabeth Moore of Market Harbour in the county of Leicester to be a person of good skill in physick and chirurgery and very fit in our opinion to practice them and that we have known the good effects of her skill upon several persons.'[102] Two men with the surname of Moore who praised Elizabeth Moore's skill may have been relatives. One was Edward Moore, who signed the testimonial letter with the two clergymen. He lived in the neighbouring village of Slawston. The other letter was from one Thomas Moore who wrote: 'I do know that within Mrs. Moore to be a person of great skill and experience in the practice of physick, and very successful in the cures of agues, fevers, small pox, measles, toothache and more especially the king's evil, with other diseases incident to the country, and one whom I have often received much good in my several sicknesses. In testimony thereof I do freely subscribe my hand. Thomas Moore.'[103] The king's evil is scrofula. Moore's patients certified that they had 'received much benefit from what Elizabeth Moore has administered to us in several distempers'.[104] Nicholas Clark of Bowden Magna was cured of a dangerous impostume in his stomach and his son of the rickets by Mrs Moore. Mrs Mary Clark of Wolf Laughton was cured of pleurisy and violent fever by Mrs Moore. Mary, the daughter of Thomas Freeman, who had been twice touched by the king's evil and was left blind from it, was cured by Mrs Moore. John Wolf of Harborough was cured of various distempers and had not used another physician in twenty-five or twenty-six years. Richard Jordan (who put his mark) had been cured of smallpox. The mark of Anne A. Satchwell testifies that she was cured of a toothache. Another patient, whose name is illegible, was cured of the king's evil.

Other testimonials claim that Mrs Moore cured people of swooning fits, dysentery, palsy in the tongue with loss of speech, and malignant tumours. One patient had a sore leg for fourteen months and could not go out or stand and was cured in three months. In total, there are thirty-three signed testimonials from Elizabeth Moore's patients, all of whom were cured of a variety of illnesses. Her patients included men, women and children. Clearly, she had a very successful practice.[105]

Mary Rose of Portsmouth received her licence to practise medicine and surgery on 18 April 1696 from Peter Mews, Bishop of Winchester. There are three extant testimonial letters for Mary Rose. One of these is similar in content to a letter for Mrs Moore in that it states that Mary Rose is a 'woman of sober life and conversation and hath (under God) cured several people of diseases, wounds, strains and bruises...' This letter was signed by several medical men, including ship medical personnel: Richard Hill, surgeon of Chamber Friggitt, David Rose, sworn surgeon, London, Philip Rose, MD, Edward Patterson, surgeon of the Rose, and Henry Bayly, surgeon of the Merlyn.[106] Another testimonial was signed by various ship personnel including Thomas Acton, commander of the Merlyn.[107] Mary Rose signed the oath in her own hand using the Latin spelling of her name, Maria. That she was able to do this indicates a level of education higher than that of most of her contemporaries.[108]

Jane Pemell of Southwark was licensed to practise surgery in the province of Canterbury on 10 July 1685.[109] Three testimonial letters, dated 30 June 1685, exist in support of her application. Only one is concerned with her medical practice. Thomas Barker, surgeon of the same parish, stated that 'Jane Pemell, wife of John Pemell of St. Saviour's Southwark in the county of Surrey is very fitly qualified to practice the Artes of physicke and chyrurgery'.[110] The other two deal with her character, which was of good standing. One was from a neighbour who remarked on the quiet lives led by Jane and her husband and that he had known the couple for 12 or 14 years.[111] The third letter, signed by William Hoare, the minister, and the churchwardens of the parish of St Saviour's stated that she was a 'person of a sober life and conversation and in all things comfortable to the Church of England having lived fourteen years in the said parish, paying all the duties of the parish'.[112]

Pemell has left an extensive record of her surgical and medical activities in a fourteen-page manuscript booklet, held at Lambeth Palace Library, which provides evidence of her cures if less detail of how they were achieved.[113] She clearly had connections to the medical world which most women lacked. Her first husband was a doctor of 'physic and a man-midwife'.[114] Her second husband was Mr Henry Tyrell, surgeon, the son of a surgeon at Christ Church Hospital. Her third husband, John Pemell, who had served in the Dutch Wars, had been missing for seven years. She was thus on her own and was able to support herself through her surgical practice.

Jane Pemell had patients from many parts of what is now London, including the city of London, Shoreditch, Southwark, Wapping and Whitechapel. Some of her patients were hospitalized, but doctors had been unable to cure them. Jane Pemell transcribed a number of these cases. One was that of Bartholomew Harris who had been a patient at St Bartholomew's hospital in London where surgeons had cut his arm. Unfortunately, Pemell does not provide details on how she cured this patient, only that she did cure him, and that the patient had since married one of the sisters from the hospital. Abraham Simpson came from the same hospital and 'had it in his thigh and several bones come out'. She cured him too. From Christ Church hospital came Joseph Tyler with problems in his hand, foot and other places, and a Master Hall. She cured them all as well as some who came from St Thomas's Hospital, but she does not elaborate here saying she is already too tedious![115]

Pemell provided accounts of patients with numerous ailments, from the king's evil to eye problems. However, she is not always specific. For example, she cured the two children of a merchant in Pudding Lane. In one case, she drained a four-inch lesion to the neck. In another, she treated a Captain Hasting's son who had seen many surgeons. They had put a lead plug in the boy's back. Pennell pulled it out and syringed it with water 'which went through his body and by God's blessing cured it'.[116]

These were clearly exceptional medical women in many respects. They were able to procure licences, which presumably meant they could charge more for their services, and they were considered respectable and competent, as their testimonials prove. They were better educated than the average woman and had connections with the elite, including many in the world of medicine. These women worked primarily in the countryside away from the city of London where they could be considered a threat by male physicians and surgeons.[117]

Between the twelfth and fifteenth centuries, universities were founded in Europe. University trained physicians, unlike empirical healers, would go through an extensive theoretical training in the classical liberal arts of theology, philosophy and logic with an emphasis on the writings of Galen and Hippocrates. They would have little contact with the human body and did not perform dissections.[118] As stated above, with the exception of Italy, women were barred from attending these institutions.[119] In the fifteenth century the College of Medicine at Rome brought in a regulation that applied equally to men and women: it stipulated that 'no one, male or woman dare heal by science (*physica*) or surgery without special license'.[120]

In Spain, the universities as well as the government were involved in the regulation of medicine. In order to practise as a physician, candidates were required to finish courses for their bachelor's degree and then work as an apprentice for two years before receiving the proper certificate, which they would be required to present in order to practise medicine. Apparently Spain was the most rigorous country in Europe in ensuring that medical practitioners held university degrees.[121]

In many countries, universities came about as extensions of monasteries and cathedral schools, to which girls were not admitted. Thus, there is a direct correlation between the Church, the establishment of universities and the exclusion of women from the practice of medicine. The exact origins of the university are unknown, but historians do know that they began as independent corporate organizations in Paris, Oxford, Bologna and Padua. The actual term 'universitas' means a group of people with a 'common aim or function, or a self-governing association of citizens organized as a legal entity with a right to sue or be sued under precepts derived from Roman law'.[122]

From the end of the twelfth century, the institutional home of science was the university. Historians posit that the development of modern science went together with the establishment of these universities.[123] The chief subjects studied in the university were mathematics, astronomy and logic. Paris and Oxford reached their pinnacle in terms of scientific importance during the thirteenth and fourteenth centuries when Bologna and Padua surpassed them. The southern universities of Bologna and Padua allowed for a greater lay involvement in their universities. There were some married professors, for example, and in one case, a professor of canon law at Bologna by the name of Giovanni d'Andrea, apparently allowed his daughter Novella to lecture behind a curtain if he had to miss class.[124] Scholars seem to have accepted it as valid.[125]

The Faculty of Arts in the Italian universities was associated with medicine rather than theology. However, even the Italian universities were not free from the influence of the Church as they were ultimately under the control of the pope.[126] Unlike their northern counterparts, some Italian universities did admit women before the late nineteenth and twentieth centuries. However, as far as we know, they tended not to study science. We have documentary evidence that a certain Elena Cornaro received a philosophy doctorate from Padua as late as 25 June 1678.[127]

In England, in Oxford and Cambridge, the situation was very similar to that on the continent as far as women were concerned.[128] Only men were admitted to the universities until the nineteenth century. The monastic legacy was felt both in the communal life of the students and in the fact that there was a strong clerical presence. However, there were differences between the English and continental universities. Medicine was never a very popular subject in England and the best and brightest students went into law and theology and even general arts before medicine. The medical curriculum was borrowed from Paris and the profession suffered from a low image and poor regulation, especially outside the university towns.[129]

The founding of the Franciscan and Dominican orders in the twelfth and thirteenth centuries reinforced the celibate and all-male world of the university. Prominent scholars such as Albertus Magnus, Thomas Aquinas and Duns Scotus emerged from these orders. These all-male and generally misogynistic religious orders 'shaped European education for centuries to come'.[130]

The fact that universities grew out of the monastery and the cathedral school meant that women were barred from attending and thus from being exposed to the sciences. As Achille Luchaire has adeptly argued with respect to the French situation, 'the university was a brotherhood almost entirely composed of clerics; masters and students had the tonsure; collectively they constituted a church institution'. Further, he posited that while the 'university movement had as its principal object the replacing of the clerical schools of chapters and abbeys by corporations imbued with the lay spirit', to perceive them as centres of free-thinking 'is a gross error. Universities were ecclesiastical organizations and were organized accordingly.'[131] Underlying the attempt by university trained physicians to exclude women and Jewish healers from the practice of medicine were sexist and racist theologically based ideologies and a desire among Christian male physicians to stop others, and in particular, clinically experienced female healers, encroaching on their territory.[132] The cases cited below of women who were prosecuted for practising medicine without a licence provide ample evidence of this.

The Faculty of Medicine at the University of Paris was one of the most prohibitive, although not entirely effective, organizations in its attempts to prevent women and other non-licensed healers from practising medicine. Between 1271 and 1272, it passed a series of regulations for practitioners and delineated the requirements for acquiring a licence to practise medicine. This licence was granted by the Chancellor of Notre Dame.[133] Here we see the importance of the Church in keeping women from practising medicine. Students at the medical school at the University of Paris were required to take clerical vows. Since women were banned from the priesthood, the study of medicine was closed to them. Empirics were denounced by the faculty as those persons who were doing acts harmful to the health of the people of Paris and who lowered the reputation of all practitioners, themselves included. Thus, according to the official documents, to prevent further abuses from such charlatans, regulations were written by the faculty which were claimed only as confirming a statute that had existed for many years. The faculty insisted that this statute had been supported by letters from the Bishop of Paris, by the king, and by oaths taken by members of the faculty. Unlicensed healers were brought before the bishop's court.[134] Jews, women, apothecaries, herbalists and surgeons were specifically referred to in the regulations:

> No Jew or Jewess [shall…] presume to operate surgically or medicinally on any person of the catholic faith … Therefore we strictly prohibit that any male or female surgeon, apothecary, or herbalist, by their oaths presume to exceed the limits or bounds of their craft secretly or publicly or in any way whatsoever, so that the surgeon engage only in manual practice and as pertains to it, the apothecary or herbalist only in mixing drugs which are to be administered only by masters in medicine or by their license. ... Also none of the aforesaid shall visit any sick person to administer him any alternative medicine or laxative or anything that pertains to a physician.[135]

Strict enforcement of the faculty's new regulations began in the early 1300s. Again, the formally stated reason provided for these new regulations was the upgrading of medical education and standards, but as scholars have pointed out, the formal prohibition of women was certainly an important motive.[136] A royal ordinance against the illicit practice of medicine was issued in December 1352 because of the petition by the Dean and Masters of the Faculty of Medicine of the University of Paris. Included in the petition were, 'women and old wives, monks, rustics, some apothecaries and numerous herbalists' who were practising medicine 'ignorant of the science of medicine and unacquainted with human constitutions, the time and method of administering and the virtues of medicines, particularly laxatives...'[137] However, women who were not widows, but trained by their fathers could still be barber-surgeons, according to a judgement passed by the Paris Parlement in 1347.

The University of Paris was very active in prosecuting illicit medical practitioners, including women, and one of the earliest cases brought before the bishop's court was that of Clarice de Rothomago which took place from 17 January to 15 June 1312. Charges against her originated with the Dean of the Medical Faculty of Paris for the illegal practice of medicine. He ordered her arrest, and following the trial she was excommunicated. When she appealed this ruling, the court also excommunicated her husband, Peter Faverel, an empiric. Churches were ordered to denounce them and anyone who supported them was threatened with similar treatment.[138] Apparently, this ruling, however harsh, was not very successful as a deterrent and this case was only one of many prosecuted during this period.[139]

The most famous case of a female practising medicine illegally that was brought before the faculty was that of non-licensed practitioner Jacoba Félicie de Almania.[140] According to the trial records, Jacoba was a woman in her thirties who had neither studied in Paris nor at any other *Stadium*.[141] Three other women and two men were charged with her, also with practising medicine illegally. The women were Juana, a convert, a surgeon, Marguerite of Ypres, and a Jewess, Belota; the men were maestros Esteban Burgondo and Jacob Lepelé. The 'inquisition (was) made at the instance of the masters in medicine at Paris ... to the end that they be punished and that this practice forbidden them'.[142]

Félicie, who treated both male and female patients, was charged with examining sick and poor people by taking their pulse and inspecting their urine; telling patients that she could cure them by giving them various drugs; that she had been warned to stop practising by the Chancellor of Paris and the dean and magistrates, but did not. Although six out of the seven witnesses at her trial supported her and spoke to the effectiveness of her treatments, which worked when those of the graduates from the faculty did not, this did not deter her accusers. They never denied the success of her medicine, but the fact that she was not trained by books meant that she could not legally practise medicine. The Masters of Medicine argued that she was 'completely untrained in the practice of medicine', that she was 'uneducated and not approved by those who have jurisdiction over that...'[143] Further, they argued that because she had not studied medicine, she risked causing the death of a patient by prescribing her potions. They even argued that she was more of a risk to the public than an untrained lawyer:

> It is much worse to kill a man through drink and clysters than to lose civil court cases as a result of the ignorance and lack of training of lawyers and since such murders are a mortal sin, jurisdiction is an ecclesiastical matter on the grounds that it is a sin and therefore the regulations of the aforementioned legal are binding on this subject since as a matter before the law she should have been able to practice medicine, she ought to have acquired the approved training.[144]

Witnesses at the trial included the respected physician John of Padua, a military knight and surgeon to King Philip IV of France. He spoke for the prosecution, supporting the argument that Félicie was not a university trained physician and thus ignorant in the practice of medicine. He posited that she did not understand the medicaments she was using and thus could easily kill a patient. For the defence, John of St Omer and his wife in addition to other patients whose fevers had been cured by Félicie, spoke on her behalf. They claimed that various liquids and poultices she administered to them had been very effective remedies. One witness, Jehan de Saint-Audemer, a tavern owner and citizen of Paris, told the court that Jacoba had visited him several times and examined his urine with great care. She assured him that if she could not cure him, he would not need to pay her. He paid her forty Paris sous and stated that she cured him when the doctors could not. He reported that Félicie gave him a 'tisane, that is, a clear liquor, agreeable which she drank herself before administering it to me'. Another witness, Jean Faber, claimed that he had suffered from headaches and earaches and Félicie administered various drinks, one of which was green in colour. He stated that he did not know their ingredients. They agreed that he would not pay her unless she cured him. Faber alleged that he 'had been treated by Masters Johannes de Turre, Martin Hermanus and many other masters of medicine. He continued by stating that he went to Félicie only after he'd seen the trained doctors. He described her treatment of a herbal poultice which cured his ailments. He finished his testimony by praising the medicine practised by Félicie, telling the court that 'he had heard it was said she was wiser in the art of surgery than the physicians or surgeons of Paris'.[145]

At the end of her defence, Félicie explained why she believed that it was preferable for a woman to treat other women than for men to treat women: 'It is better and more seemly that a wise woman learned in the art should visit a sick woman and inquire into the secrets of her nature and her hidden parts, that a man should do so, for whom it is not lawful to see and seek out the aforesaid parts...' In addition, the defence explained that often a woman would choose to die rather than 'reveal the secrets of her infirmity to a man out of a sense of modesty and even of shame'.[146] However, Félicie had treated both male and female patients. The court's final ruling on 22 November 1322 stated that: 'Her plea that she cured many sick persons whom the aforesaid master could not cure ought not to stand, and is frivolous, since it is certain that a man approved in the aforesaid art could cure the sick better than any woman.'[147]

The records of the trial stated that Félicie was 'wiser in the art of surgery and medicine than the greatest master or doctor in Paris'.[148] Her success as a medical practitioner must have caused jealousy amongst the university trained professionals and hence been a determining factor in banning her from practising medicine. However, this was not discussed at the trial. Félicie was found guilty, along with the four other empirics, and was prohibited from practising medicine under the pain of excommunication and a fine of sixty Paris pounds.[149] Juana, Marguerite of Ypres and Belota received the same penalty as Jacoba, threat of excommunication and a fine.[150]

The Faculty of Medicine of Paris continued its battle against female physicians into the Early Modern period. The Parlement ruled on 12 April 1578 that women were prohibited from medical practice. The particular case which brought about this ruling was against a woman from Anjou.[151] However, in spite of the regulations, women continued to practise.

Correspondence between Pope John XXII and the various bishops of Paris indicates that despite the cases cited above and the prosecution of other non-university trained practitioners, the illegal practice of medicine continued to be a problem for the authorities. In a letter to Stephen, Bishop of Paris, dated 21 June 1325, the pope indicated the persistence of untrained people practising in Paris and the surrounding areas. His information was based on a petition drafted by various university masters and scholars which stated 'persons ignorant of the medical art, old women particularly, and even more to be detested, soothsayers ... were presuming to practice medicine in the city and environs of Paris, and that these charlatans were causing many deaths'.[152] Another letter, written five years later to a new bishop of Paris, Hugh, demonstrates that the problem of illegal practitioners had not been solved. The pope instructed the bishop 'to make every effort to see that henceforth no one was permitted to practice medicine in the city or suburbs of Paris unless he was a master or was licensed in the art, or was otherwise known to be qualified by having been approved by a council consisting of the dean of the medical faculty and two of the masters then lecturing on medicine in the university'. People who did not comply with this ruling would be 'subjected to ecclesiastical censure'.[153] The University of Paris was not alone in prosecuting cases against women healers. In 1558, the governors of the University of Montpellier ruled against a 'woman empiric' practising medicine and surgery. The governors decreed that 'people practicing the art of medicine and surgery, including those dispensing beverages and drugs, without the approval of the Faculty, would be punished and banished from the provinces and areas where they were found practicing'. Included in this decree were apothecaries who were not approved by the faculty.[154]

Concerning the practice of surgery, the University of Paris's rules of 1271 were directed against surgeons and other practitioners to whom the statutes referred as 'certain manual operators' (herbalists and apothecaries) who did not understand how to administer medicines with respect to particular diseases. No surgeon, male or female, no apothecary nor herbalist, was to exceed or overstep the limits or bounds of his craft, either secretly or publicly. The surgeon was to engage only in manual practice. He or she could not visit the sick and could not 'administer to him any alternative medicine or laxative or anything else' which was in the realm of the university trained physician.[155] Further regulations were inaugurated by Philip IV (1268–1314) in 1311, stating that 'neither male nor female surgeons could practice in Paris without having been examined by a board with the king's first surgeon presiding'. These statutes did not prevent people from practising 'illegally', so in 1352, John II (1319–64), reiterated these regulations and specifically mentioned that they applied to both men and women. No man or woman was 'to administer any medicine, alterative, laxative, sirup, electuary, laxative pills, or clysters of any sort'.[156] Apparently, illegal practice by surgeons and apothecaries continued as before. Charles VI, on 3 August 1390, informed the officials of the university that several persons had been visiting patients and promising to cure them. They were to be investigated and if found practising medicine, would be charged.[157] Finally, in 1484, during King Charles VII's regency, women were no longer granted licences to practise surgery. They were permitted to practise as barber-surgeons: they could blood-let and cauterize, but they could not accept fees for their services.[158]

The case of an illiterate female surgeon, Perretta Petonne (sometimes given as Peretta Peronne), of Paris and Rouen (1360–1411), demonstrates that numerous women were practising surgery without a licence. Petonne appeared before the Parlement of Paris on 9 and 16 June 1410. In her testimony, she revealed that many women of Paris were practising the art of surgery without a licence. In addition, she informed the court that she 'was working for God' and that it was unfair that she had been summoned when many others practising had not. According to the court proceedings, the major complaint against her was not that she was a woman surgeon, but that she was 'practising without a licence, without the approval of the commission of municipal surgeons'.[159] Although Petonne spent time in prison, she was subsequently acquitted by Charles VI.[160]

University trained physicians came increasingly to view surgeons as a lower form of practitioner. From 1436 onwards, surgeons were permitted to attend university lectures, but they were not awarded degrees. The university curriculum focused on the theoretical aspects of medicine and surgery was given short shrift. Women were not permitted to attend university, and medical and surgical studies were thought not to be appropriate for them. Barbers were also admitted to the lectures at the Faculty of Medicine from January 1494, but this was stopped after a year, following complaints by the surgeons.[161] It seems that the combined efforts of popes, medical faculties and kings could not prevent the illegal practice of medicine.

From the later Middle Ages into the Early Modern era, the common denominator in all of these countries was the formal regulation of medicine through laws emanating from various authorities. These laws usually stated that those who could legally practise medicine should be trained in some way (normally at a university), and examined by the proper authorities before receiving their licence to practise medicine. There is no doubt that throughout this period, greater control over healing was attempted by those in power. Depending on the region and country, however, controls were enforced differently. As we have seen, in parts of Spain the need for doctors and medical care demanded that the regulations were more loosely enforced. Whether or not these ordinances were successful in stamping out 'illegal' practitioners is questionable. The laws were a reflection of the general societal view of women which saw the female as weaker, more fragile and less intelligent than the male.[162]

3
Early Modern Notions of Women: Contradictory Views on Women as Healers

This chapter will survey the varying societal views of women and their roles with respect to how these affected the prospects of women healers. Men contributed to the debate concerning women from many different perspectives – biological, theological, legal and philosophical. It is the more scientific views that are the focus here. Questions raised concerned to what extent women were capable of practising medicine, and if they were, was it anyway an appropriate role for them. To what extent did women's biological and, by extension, societal constructions preclude them from the healing arts? In order to respond to these questions, we must turn our attention back to the Classical era when the debate on the nature of women and their appropriate roles originated.[1]

Two major ideological influences dominated ideas about women in Early Modern Western Europe. One was that of biological difference between men and women and originated with the reproductive function. This view was propounded by classical philosophers and physicians. The other perspective, also stressing the inferiority of women, was the Christian worldview. Early Christian thinkers, particularly the Patristics, were influenced by the classical biological justification of female inferiority.

The interpretation of reproductive and biological differences centred on seed theories based on the Hippocratic Corpus and the works of Aristotle and Galen. According to these texts, the biological function influenced the societal. During the Renaissance, medical writers continued to be influenced by these theories regarding respective male and female reproductive roles even though they were over 1300 years old. This is not to say that experimental anatomy had not developed since the fifth century BC, but even clinicians based their work on classical theorists. New translations and commentaries of Greek writings appeared in the late sixteenth century reviving awareness of theories that originated with the Greek writings of Hippocrates and the unknown authors who contributed to the Hippocratic Corpus and Aristotle. The Galenists were influenced by Hippocrates, Aristotle and Avicenna.[2]

The Hippocratic Corpus is what remains of a library of thirty-four medical texts dating from the sixth and fourth centuries BCE. These writings formed a collection written by various authors at different times primarily on the subject of human reproduction and female gynaecological disorders.[3] The Corpus presented an overwhelmingly negative view of the female, in keeping with the majority view of the time. Menstruation was characterized as 'mysterious, dangerous', and a 'contaminating' event.[4] Its authors described the phenomenon of the 'wandering womb' as a very powerful organ.[5] Scholars have argued that the wandering womb theory was another factor in the diminution of the female contribution to generation, while others have stated that 'by concentrating on certain functions of the female', there was an assumption that she needed special treatment.[6] The writers of the Hippocratic Corpus did subscribe to the doctrine of two seeds: the female seed was vaginal secretion.[7] Nevertheless, the female was still inferior, as a stronger seed produced a male child and a weaker one, a female.

A further interesting point about the female that made her different from the male was the idea put forth by Hippocratic writers that the female was a being set apart. She was a creature entirely different from man in terms of the substance and feel of her body: it was cold, moist and passive, corresponding to her reproduction purpose.[8] One expert on the Hippocratic Corpus has demonstrated that, according to these writers, the female was abnormal in comparison to the normal male, that she was 'structurally a sick being'.[9]

Aristotle's views on women are of primary importance for it is his views that came to dominate western civilization. He alleged that he had found a scientific basis for female inferiority. Aristotle was the first philosopher and physician in western civilization to present a 'single theory of the concept of woman'.[10] He inaugurated a 'revolution' in the sense that he provided a new definition of what it meant to be male or female. His views on women superseded those of earlier thinkers and persisted well into the Early Modern era.

According to Aristotle's definition of the female, and in accord with the Hippocratic Corpus, the female was a deviation from the norm, or the male: 'The first departure indeed is that the offspring should become female instead of male; this, however, is a natural necessity.'[11] For Aristotle, the female was a 'mutilated male', lacking in the 'principle of the soul'. In other words, the female was a defective or incomplete male. She was produced when something went wrong, when nature failed to follow its path properly.[12] The normal body was a male body. The female was an inferior form, too cold to transform blood into semen and thus unable to reach perfection.[13] Females were deficient in comparison with men. The characterization of the cold and wet female and hot and dry male in Aristotle's system originated with the Hippocratic Corpus, but Aristotle applied a value system to the distinction. Females did not mature as quickly in the womb as males because of their lack of heat. This meant that they were defective. And that they matured faster out of the womb was also a flaw. As one expert concluded: 'Women can't win with the supposed "empiricist;" all apparent differences between male and female are attributed to the "natural deficiency" of the female sex.'[14] In order to understand Aristotle's reasons for this view, it is necessary to examine his theories concerning generation.

Aristotle formulated a biological theory for the basis of female inferiority in his assertion that the woman did not contribute to conception. He refuted the idea put forth by the authors of the Hippocratic Corpus that females possessed seed and thus contributed to generation.

> ...We may safely set down as the chief principles of generation the male [factor] and the female [factor]; the male as possessing the principle of movement and of generation, the female as possessing that of matter. One is most likely to be convinced of this by considering how the semen is formed and whence it comes; for although the things that are formed in the course of Nature no doubt take their rise out of semen, we must not fail to notice how the semen itself is formed from the male and the female, since it is because this part is secreted from the male and the female, and because its secretion takes place in them and out of them, that the male and the female are the principles of generation ... Now it is impossible that any creature should produce two seminal secretions at once, and as the secretion in females which answers to semen in males is the menstrual fluid, it obviously follows that the female does not contribute any semen to generation; for if there were semen, there would be no menstrual fluid; but as menstrual fluid is in fact formed, therefore there is no semen ...[15]

This theory may be contrasted with the view of Aristotle's predecessors who believed in the double-seed theory. If the female did not provide the seed, what did she supply? She furnished the womb, or the matter, which provided nourishment for the foetus in the form of menstrual blood. Aristotle concluded, 'It is clear that the female contributes the material for generation, and that this is in the substance of the menstrual discharges and they are residue.'[16] The uterus was a passive receptacle.

Aristotle took his theory of the male (active) and female (passive) roles in the reproductive process and applied it to the psychological make-up of woman, and by extension, to her role in society. In psychological terms, because only men produced semen, they were perceived as 'effective and active', while the female was 'passive'.[17] With respect to reasoning faculties, both male and female possessed a soul with the ability to reason; however, in the female the irrational power dominated. For the male, the opposite was the case. Furthermore, although the woman, unlike the slave possessed a 'deliberative faculty', it was 'without authority'.[18] Women were not able to control themselves physically and psychologically through the exercise of reason as men could. Therefore, women must submit and obey.[19] His advice to pregnant women provides further clues into his thinking about female reason. A pregnant woman should refrain from 'rational activity...'[20]

This leads to Aristotle's ideas on the role of women in society. Because the woman was inferior by nature, and her irrational side dominated, the man ruled the woman because 'the male is by nature fitter for command than the female ... The relation of the male to the female is always of this kind.' The woman should obey the man and keep quiet: 'Silence is a woman's glory.'[21] It is important to note that Juan Vives and other Renaissance humanists would reiterate the concept that the ideal woman was silent and virtuous, if not virtually invisible. The primary purpose of woman for Aristotle was the production and nurturing of children, preferably sons. The family was the key institution in the Aristotelian system, providing man with fulfilment of his needs and wants. Aristotle did refer to the husband and wife as 'friends', each with his or her own functions, but the man still rules over the wife.[22] According to Aristotle, woman possesses limited capabilities and is the weaker sex: 'For nature had made the one sex stronger, the other weaker...' Thus her capacities for work are limited and she must be kept indoors: 'In the performance of work, she [nature] made one sex able to lead a sedentary life and not strong enough to endure exposure...'[23] The female is 'irrational', the male 'rational' by nature, so it is also logical that the male commands.[24]

The Greek philosopher and physician Galen (c. 129–200CE) built upon the wandering womb theory of the Hippocratic Corpus and on Aristotle's views on the inferiority of women. Galen's medical theories, particularly those dealing with the nature of disease, dominated European medicine for about 1500 years.[25] He hypothesized that women were inferior because 'their smaller size produced scantier, colder and wetter semen'.[26] Although Galen gave women some credit in the reproductive function, he still considered them to be less fully developed than men. Women's tissues were cooler and moister than those of men thus their sexual organs remained internal. This in turn made 'her incomplete, colder and moister in dominant humours, and unable to concoct perfect semen from blood'.[27]

Prominent Arab physicians Avicenna (980–1037) and Averroes (1126–98) kept western thought alive during the Dark Ages. Avicenna was a Persian medical writer whose work was translated into Latin in the twelfth century. He is significant because his medical writings influenced such western thinkers as the Dominican theologian Albertus Magnus, who was Thomas Aquinas's teacher. Avicenna argued that male power was stronger than that of the female, an idea that he borrowed from Galen. He wrote that the process of reproduction was akin to making cheese – the male sperm was the clotting agent of the milk while the female sperm acted as a coagulating agent. Thus, the male sperm, as the stronger part, was the more significant.[28]

Averroes echoed Avicenna in his *Commentary on Plato's Republic*. He theorized that men and women were different, but only by degree. What this meant was that 'men were more efficient than women'. He did concede that women might excel in music, but men must write the music and women perform it.[29]

Throughout the later Middle Ages and the Renaissance era, the biologically or anatomically based consensus continued to be that women were physically, morally and mentally weaker than men. The views of the Italian medical professor at the University of Pavia in the early fifteenth century, Anthonius Guainerius (fl. 1413–48), author of the *Treatise on the Womb*, were typical. He held that the male was superior and the female inferior. The female's nature was determined by her uterus: a hot uterus produced a hot character while a woman with a cold uterus was lazy and faint-hearted.[30]

Historian Ian Maclean argues that the Galenist camp superseded the Aristotelians in their views on the female contribution to reproduction: the female sperm existed and was effective. However, female sperm was colder and less active than that of the male, and male sperm determined the sex of the child.[31]

In 1593 the Parisian doctor André Du Laurens (1558–1609) published an account of the dispute between medics over the female role in reproduction entitled *Anatomica humani corporis historia*. Du Laurens rejected the Aristotelian view, arguing against the idea that one sex was incomplete. After 1600, most medical writers held that both male and female played a role in reproduction, although this did not make for a less scathing view of females and there were still some doctors who followed Aristotle's views. By 1700, however, the majority of medical men had renounced the Hippocratic and Aristotelian notions about the nature of male and female biology and had accepted Galen's theories. Although these theories understood women 'to be equally perfect in her sex', women continued to be held as inferior for 'she does not seem to achieve complete parity with man ... Her physiology and humours seem to destine her to be the inferior of man, both physically and mentally...'[32] Indeed, some historians have argued that the acceptance of Galen's views led to eighteenth-century Enlightenment notions that sex differences pervaded all aspects of life: biological, intellectual and moral.[33] Woman's role was to bear children and raise them. She did not have a purpose outside the home. Although commentators rejected Aristotle's seed theory, his notions concerning women's nature and role remained dominant until the twentieth century.

The second persistent concept of woman in Western European society derives from Christian thought.[34] Christian theologians inherited Greco-Roman views and during the Middle Ages, one finds the ubiquitous Aristotelian view newly combined with Pauline Christianity, which asserted that woman was an inferior or deformed male, irrational and incapable of reason. On the other hand, there was the contradictory assertion that women and men are equal in Christ. These two views led to some interesting conflicts from the time of the later Roman Empire to the late Middle Ages. The debate during the medieval period centred on the question of the nature of woman, and what should be done about women in terms of their public/private role.

Saint Augustine of Hippo (354–430)[35] was arguably the pre-eminent Christian scholar whose ideas became the accepted worldview and influenced later church fathers such as St Thomas Aquinas. Augustine wrote several treatises that contributed to the debate about the nature and role of women. His ideas, although based on biblical texts, primarily those by St Paul, were clearly also influenced by the medical treatises of the day. This is particularly the case when he was writing about women and reproduction. According to Saint Augustine, there was a direct correlation between the female body and female inferiority. She is the receptacle and provider of nourishment for male sperm.[36] And the fact that the female body was visibly different confirmed that there were fundamental differences between male and female and to deny this 'would be a manifest absurdity'.[37]

Augustine's *The City of God*, written between 413 and 426, together with his *De Genesi ad litteram* and *De genesi contra Manicheaos*,[38] are pertinent to the debate because they deal with his view of women as human beings and of their role in society. Augustine believed that man and woman were both created on the sixth day and were equal before the Fall and unlike Aristotle, he did not see woman as a defective male. In addition, he wrote: 'You created man male and female, but in your spiritual grace, they are one. Your grace no more discriminates between them according to sex than it draws distinction between Jew and Greek or slave and freeman.'[39] But Augustine argued that the sin of Adam was brought on by Eve's lust. Woman allowed herself to be seduced and then tempted.[40] In other words, Eve was responsible for the first sin. Augustine's emphasis on Eve's weakness against temptation was a continuation of the classical myth of Pandora who released vice and passion into the world.[41]

Parts of the *De Genesi ad litteram* are more favourable to women. Here Augustine celebrated the union of male and female as instituted by God. If woman is made from man, that is a sign of the love that should unify male and female. However, he still argued that even before the Fall, woman was made to be submissive to man, although not ruled by him.[42] He concedes that woman in as much as she was a human being, 'had a rational mind and therefore she was made to the image of God'.[43]

It is worth noting that Jewish women, who were important practitioners of medicine in late medieval and Early Modern Europe, were held in even greater contempt than Christian women. Christian thinkers such as Saint Augustine held extremely negative attitudes towards Jews in general and Jewish women in particular. If Christian women were evil, then Jewish women were barely human. Jews 'were perceived as being not only marginal ... but also outside the very notions of human and social structure'.[44] Underlying this perception are the biblical story of the Fall, blamed on Eve, and the notion that Jews killed Christ. Although Christ's death redeemed humankind, only the conversion of Jews would hasten Christ's return. Jewish women were unclean and impure. Women's menstrual blood was associated with all sorts of evil from killing animals to harming plants. Jews posed a constant threat to Christian society. They were in concert with the devil. Unlike Christian women, who, although inferior to men, had a chance of salvation, Jewish women did not. These views persisted well into the Early Modern period.[45]

Medical and scientific writers of the early Christian era and the Middle Ages reinforced and complemented Christian views on the nature and role of women. Their views, along with those of the Christians, have persisted in the history of western civilization. All Christians put forth similar views: that the female was inferior to the male due to the reproductive organs and that women needed to be kept under male authority.[46]

Thus, according to biological and theological dictums, women were perceived as imperfect males. Based upon this notion, we shall now examine the views held by physicians about women and medicine. Not surprisingly, the prevalent view among these medical men was that women should not treat the sick. However, there existed a small minority who dissented from this. Proponents of the ubiquitous negative side will be examined first. One of these was the French physician, Franciscan monk and man of letters, François Rabelais (c. 1494–1553). Rabelais was particularly critical of all non-university trained practitioners of medicine. Himself a graduate of the prestigious University of Montpellier's medical school, Rabelais was keen to keep competitors out of the profession. He argued that empirics, charlatans and 'doctors of the old school' all lacked proper medical training.[47] Medical impostors, sedentary or nomadic, were anathema to Rabelais. They haunted the countryside of Poitiers. He described a certain type: the old woman who meddles in curing with her herbal medicines.[48]

Rabelais's views on women were commonplace in his time and familiar to medical men of his generation. They were part and parcel of the biological explanation for the differences between male and female based on the ancient Greek concept of the wandering womb. Briefly summarized, Rabelais contended that woman was inferior to man and thus must obey him: this was the way of nature. The female sex was fickle and impertinent in nature. The only possible reason for woman's creation was to please man and for the perpetuation of the race. Woman's destiny was to be wife and mother. Women have meditated evil against men since the beginning of the world because they wished to control men.[49]

In common with other university trained physicians, André du Breil of the University of Paris and Thomas Sonnet de Courval, also a graduate of the University of Paris medical school, condemned all manner of folk healers.[50] Both du Breil and de Courval attacked the Swiss physician

Paracelsus (see below) and other 'magicians', empirics and 'charlatans', village wise men and women. These physicians wrote treatises from the moral, medical and political perspectives stipulating the dangers posed by empirics. Both men maligned untrained practitioners, who, although literate, relied on their 'wits' and 'imagination' more than empirical knowledge to heal people. Breil alleged that these 'healers' were in concert with the devil; that they poisoned and did more harm than good. He claimed that midwives were most likely witches.[51] De Courval, author of *Satyre contre les charlatans et les pseudo médecins empyriques* (1610), warned the public against 'pseudo-doctors-empirics', arguing that these people committed errors and abuses in the practice of medicine. They were found in great numbers in France. They ignored medical theory, and poisoned the public.[52] Women were numbered among these charlatans. De Courval specifically referred to nuns and 'witches', or older women. Nuns, whose task was to keep watch over the sick, prepared medicines without the supervision of a doctor. Old and wrinkled women meddled in medicine by conjuring out fevers and exorcizing ulcers and haemorrhoids.[53] De Courval also condemned the affectations of noblewomen who tended to the sick, asking: 'How many grand dames and young ladies ... have medicine cabinets all stuffed and full of make-up, unguents, distilled water and a great number of drugs of which they use without knowledge, experience and judgment to the ruin of the poor sick?'[54] Women were categorized as magicians and witches who had stepped beyond the boundaries of their role in practising medicine and reading French medical texts.

Gui Patin (1601–72), Dean of the Faculty of Medicine of the University of Paris from 1650 to 1652 and later professor at the Collège de Paris, wrote in a similar tone in letters to fellow physicians. He argued that women had no place meddling in their profession, that medicine belonged to only those who possessed a higher capacity for intellectual processes.[55] For domestic medicine, usually practised by women, he had nothing but contempt: 'In the majority of the grand houses there are no longer apothecaries; it is a man or chambermaid who makes and gives the enemas and the medicines also which we have reduced to the laxative juice of prunes or bouillon.'[56]

The views expressed by Dr Juan Huarte de San Juan (1529–88) on women practising medicine reflect the general Spanish trend during the Renaissance–Reformation era. His highly influential treatise on pedagogical psychology, the *Examen de Ingenios par alas Ciencias* (1575), held a negative position on women based on their physiological composition. His opinions were informed by Hippocrates, Aristotle and Galen. Women were an imperfect version of men; they were cold and moist, while men were hot and dry. Women's ability and wit followed the temperament of the brain. Cold and moist were qualities that 'impaired' the rational soul. Their opposites, 'hot and dry render it more perfect, and improve it'. For those reasons, he felt that women should not be practising medicine.[57]

Jaume Roig of Valencia (d. 1478) wrote in a similar vein. Roig, a physician from Valencia and the son of a physician, studied at the prestigious Faculty of Medicine at the University of Paris. After returning to his native Spain, he became the official examiner of physicians, a post which he held for some forty-three years. Roig's capacity as official examiner of physicians made him particularly sensitive to illicit practitioners of whom there were many. He inveighed against them, depicting them as 'evil and inept', and focused on female healers in his invective against women, the *Spill*.[58]

Roig's personal experience with incompetent unlicensed female practitioners may well have underscored his already negative perceptions. His second wife sought the assistance of female doctors (*metgesses*) when attempting to become pregnant. Unfortunately, their efforts were in vain. Roig claimed that rather than effecting a conception, these women practitioners made his wife sick 'with their baths, ointments, bandages, perfumes and suppositories'. She developed everything from physical ailments such as ulcers to psychological disorders including hysteria.[59]

Roig wrote the *Spill* in the context of one of the many plagues that ravaged populations during the Early Modern era. His work reflects the fear of competition from unlicensed practitioners, particularly women, who were threatening not only official doctors, but also, as he saw it, the whole patriarchal order of Early Modern Spain, in which women were powerless.[60] The official rationale behind his work was to educate the public in how to maintain health and avoid illness. Unfortunately, Roig's misogyny led him not only to castigate women for their ineptitude in curing illness, they were also blamed for it – they were carriers of disease, moral and physical – and men should be protected from this pestilence.[61]

There was no shortage of university trained physicians in England who crusaded against the unlicensed and formally untrained practitioner. Women were of the worst sort among this coterie of charlatans. James Hart, James Primrose and John Cotta, all seventeenth-century physicians, wrote treatises in defence of their profession against women and other popular practitioners. Hart declared that he had 'detected and laid open some errors and impostures practiced by some ignorant practitioners in physic in that of disease'.[62] His list of 'empiricks' (untrained practitioners) included Women Physicians, Surgeons, ignorant Apothecaries, fugitive Physicians, Mountebankes, Quack-Salvers, Ephemerides-masters and others.[63] He reserved special venom for the 'Woman Physician' who 'injuriously usurps upon the Physician's calling…' According to Hart, women were acting 'against modesty and decency befitting that sexe; as against good order and against the laws of God and Man…' while being 'altogether unfit for so weighty an employment'. If they were tending to the sick, they were neglecting their 'place and calling whereunto by this Maker they were ordained like busy bodies intrude upon so sublime a profession, in administering physicke to the sick and to others by way of prevention…'[64]

James Primrose, doctor of 'Physick' and author of *Popular Errours or the People in the matter of Physick*, thought that the role of women was to care and serve men, and to this end, 'they should know how to make a bed well, boyle pottage, cullices, barle broth, make Almond milke and know the remedies for sundry diseases'.[65] However, women should not meddle in the treatment of serious illnesses as 'they usually take their remedies out of English bookes, or else make use of such that are communicated to them by others, and then they think they have rare remedies for all diseases'. Citing Galen as his authority, Primrose wrote that 'remedies should be altered according to the person, place, part affected, and other circumstances...'[66]

John Cotta practised medicine in the county of Northamptonshire. He was concerned of the 'dangers if medicines fall into the wrong hands'.[67] He warned against 'vile people and unskillful persons without restraint ... who make gainful traffic by botching in physic...' The variety of this sort of practitioner was endless: 'It is a world to see that swarmers abound in this kind, not only of Taylors, Shoemakers, Weavers, Midwives, Cooks and Priests, but Witches, Conjurers, Jugglers and Fortunetellers.'[68] He referred to women as 'unfitting counselors and commenders of medicine'. He recommended that they 'be either prohibited or better governed'.[69]

Similarly, Dr Richard Whitlock, a fellow of All Souls College, Oxford, criticized those he termed the 'kitchen physick', in other words, people practising medicine from their homes.[70] He chided women who dispensed 'syrups, conserves, waters, powders, etc...' The chapter of his book entitled, 'The Quacking Hermaphrodite or Petticoat Practitioners Stript and Whipt' is a scathing indictment on female practitioners. Women's role was not to be 'preaching and prescribing or administering...'[71] He made plain his rationale for this perspective: 'Blind is their administration of remedies because to an unknown disease and especially where one Remedy shall serve not only the several Times of the same Distemper, but several diseases in causes, subjects and wherein they are sexe, age, constitution, etc. and maketh no matter with them.'[72] In common with other medical men, Whitlock mocked the amateur pharmacist and physician, usually a well-meaning woman of the aristocracy: 'There is a virtuous, knowing, well-disposed Lady, Gentlewoman, or the like, that by God's Blessing can cure all diseases from Aries, head and face, to Pisces with Feet, with water and a Powder...' And he continued that the 'Shee Dr and Apothecary' is a danger to the patient and 'an injury to other Professions...'.[73]

Thomas Gale, surgeon to Queen Elizabeth I, blamed women and witches for the 'sickness of some three hundred people suffering from sore arms and legs, feet and hands, with other parts of the body so grievously affected that one hundred and twenty of them could never be recovered without the loss of limb'.[74] British physician and preacher, Dr Thomas Fuller (1654–1734) maintained that they 'infested the sacred precincts of medicine'. Clergyman and Oxford scholar, Robert Burton (1577–1640), criticized the 'common practice of some to first go to a witch and then to a physician'.[75]

There appeared to be no hope of reconciliation between the university physicians trained in Galenic medicine and the popular healers. A diploma from the university denoted knowledge and knowledge meant the right to practise medicine. The view that a proper education was vital to becoming a physician became widespread in the eighteenth century amongst the medical profession. Jean Verdier, doctor of medicine and a magistrate at the Paris Parlement, underscored this perspective. He posited that the practice of medicine belonged exclusively to those who had studied and passed an examination proving their competence. Verdier did not believe that women were intellectually incapable of understanding science and medicine; however, he felt that the 'different inconveniences particular to their sex puts them in a position where their work would be interrupted; the difficulty of running the household and this is their most important function, distracts them from studying...'[76] On the subject of amateurs – in which group he included queens and heroines whose medicines are known to many – he listed historical figures such as Cleopatra, Artemesia and Marie of Palestine, and contemporaries including Marie de Maupeou Fouquet and the Duchesse d'Aiguillon in France, the Countess of Kent in England, and Anne Wecker of Germany. Although he admitted that 'some of these women have enriched our Pharmacopeia with many recipes and our libraries with useful Treatises, the great majority of them practice medicine by empiricism. The effects of their medicine are more pernicious than useful...'[77]

According to Verdier, the one field of medicine where women were equal to men was surgery. Surgeons did not require a university diploma to practise. The various royal ordinances concerning surgeons, which dated from 1311, avowed that surgeons of both sexes exercised the art of surgery, that they received the same education, and that this proved that women were approved for this art equally to men.[78] Midwifery was an aspect of medicine which some physicians, among them Verdier and Philippe Hecquet, thought should be left to women.[79]

There were exceptions to the dominant view of non-university trained healers. Anthonius Guianerius acknowledged in his *Treatise on the Womb*, that he employed the skills of midwives to carry out much of his practical work, particularly the examination and even administration of drugs to female patients. He consulted with other popular healers, but he set himself apart from those to whom he referred as 'vulgar practitioners'.[80] The Swiss alchemist and physician, Paracelsus,[81] who disagreed with the Galenists in believing that the body was a chemical rather than humoral system, and thus diseases were best cured by administered chemicals, also borrowed medical receipts from women healers. Female healers, he argued, had more practical experience than learned physicians. He wrote that the best of his learning came from old wives or witches, traditional remedies and procedures taken from village barbers.[82]

Ambroise Paré (1510–90), a French army surgeon who served four kings of France, tended to be supportive of midwives and other female practitioners except for physicians. His general opinion of women was positive, believing that 'sex is no other thing than the distinction of male and female, in which this is most observable, that for the parts of the body and the site of these parts, there is little difference between them, but the female is colder than the male'.[83] He instructed midwives in the difficult delivery of babies and urged them to seek the assistance of a surgeon in the case of breech births.[84] Paré revealed in his *Apology* that he had learned the technique of treating burns with raw onions beaten with salt from an old country woman. He wrote that no blisters appeared on the burned leg of his patient where he had applied the onions.[85] The great seventeenth-century physician Thomas Sydenham (1624–89), founder of clinical medicine and epidemiology, favoured 'old women's experience over learned men's theories'.[86]

Jean Liébault, a university trained physician, was amenable to women practising medicine. He wrote that the farm wife should be knowledgeable on matters of 'natural medicine for her own family and others, when misfortune strikes...' People did not need to consult a physician for all physical problems. It was costly and unnecessary.[87] Women should be experts in herbal remedies and skilled in treating basic complaints such as headaches, toothaches, minor injuries, asthma and epilepsy. A physician should be consulted for more complicated diseases.[88]

Men of science outside the medical profession also supported women practitioners of medicine. One of them, Olivier de Serres (1539–1619), a famous French agriculturalist and author of *Le Théâtre d'Agriculture* (1600), argued the opposite to Sonnet de Courval, maintaining that 'several great lords and ladies have not disdained such a divine science [medicine]...They have engraved their names in the medicaments which they have invented.' Serres posited that 'women are more equipped than men ... to care for the sick, especially in the countryside where physicians were scarce'. In addition, Serres declared that women had read medical texts which had been originally published in Latin, Greek and Chaldean.[89]

Henri Corneille Agrippa de Nettesheim, who had studied medicine, but did not hold a medical licence, held a very different view on the nature and role of women. Born in Cologne in 1486, Agrippa tried to prove female superiority over 450 years ago. He mastered eight languages and earned a doctorate in civil and canon law.[90] In 1499, he enrolled at the University of Cologne, where he studied law, medicine, 'magic sciences' and theology. He claimed to have a medical degree, but this is uncertain.[91]

Denounced as a heretic by the Franciscans before Marguerite of Austria, Agrippa wrote the treatise, *De Nobilitate et praecellentia foeminei sexus* (A Treatise of the Nobility and Excellence of Womankind) to win her favour. It was written in Latin in 1509, presented to Marguerite in 1529, and translated into French in 1537.[92] The pamphlet was published in London first in 1542 and then again in 1652, 1670 and 1684. Marguerite was a learned woman who had written several works of prose and poetry. In this pamphlet by Agrippa, we find the nature of women discussed from the theologian's perspective. Agrippa deals firstly with creation, arguing that things were created in order of rank, with human beings created last. Man was created before woman. Eve was the last creature to be formed in Paradise and directly from God. God gave man and woman the same form and the same nature. He even argued that original sin came from Adam rather than Eve. This was a radical departure from previous writers. Following the views of Galen and Avicenna, Agrippa posited that the female contributed more substance and intelligence to the offspring than the male. Women have even been able to conceive without men – witness the example of the Virgin Mary. All of these points were made in an effort to prove female superiority.[93]

***

In addition to the debate over the study and practice of medicine and science and their relationship to women's roles, Early Modern Europeans inherited a debate which had been raging since the late fourteenth century and which was literary and philosophical in nature, called the 'querelle des femmes'. At the centre of this debate was a woman, Christine de Pizan (1364–1430). She was European history's first feminist writer in that she consciously wrote against the contemporary misogynist views of women. She is the dominant feminist figure of the fourteenth and fifteenth centuries.[94]

The 'querelle des femmes' was a debate over the role and value of women in European society. It lasted for 300 years and was debated in thousands of tracts, treatises and pamphlets on the 'nature of woman', her intellectual abilities and role in society. The 'querelle des femmes' was a development stemming from an earlier debate, 'the querelle de la rose', based on the allegorical poem, *Le Roman de la Rose*. The 'rose', by convention of courtly love, was at liberty to demand feudal obedience from her lover. The *Roman de la Rose* was written by two authors almost forty years apart. The poem was started by Guillaume de Lorris (1212–37) about whom we know almost nothing other than that he wrote the first part of the poem in 1225. It was respectful of women and celebrated courtly love. Lorris died before he could complete the poem.

The second part was written by Jean de Meung, who took an entirely different view of women. Meung was part of a new generation of writers who did not celebrate courtly love. He was a product of the University of Paris, educated in the law, medicine, theology and philosophy. His attack on women was composed in the form of a fable and expressed an extremely negative attitude toward women. Women were vicious, perfidious and evil animals who must be controlled. The 'rose' should be possessed by a man and bear children.[95] The 'querelle' was connected to the whole idea of controlling women. Initially, the debate centred on the themes of love and marriage. Defenders and detractors of women tried to demonstrate the goodness or evilness of women rather than debating their intellectual capacity. Eventually, the debate broadened to include women's ability to reason.

Christine de Pizan, the only female who participated in this debate, entered into the debate with her *Epistre au Dieu d'Amours* (Epistle to the God of Love), written in 1399. In this poem, Christine described a group of outraged women who had asked the God of Love to transmit their complaints to an assembly of gods. Their main concern was the moral rehabilitation of women – they discussed the responsibility of each sex in love. They did not state that all women were virtuous, but the gist of her address was that not all women were bad, as claimed by Meung in the *Roman de la Rose*. There are good and honest women as well as the not so honest. Christine sent copies of her letter to many important figures, Jean de Montreuil, Gontier Col and even to Queen Ysabeau of Bavaria and to Guillaume de Tignonville provost of Paris and counsellor to King Charles VI.[96] Her goal was to 'sustain the honour and praise of women'.[97] Christine defended the intellectual capacity of women in an argument whose ideas would be more fully developed in her later work, *The City of Women*.[98] Pierre Col responded to Christine's *Epistre* in a letter outlining the incapacity of women. Col accused her of forgetting to guard her modesty.[99]

These exchanges prompted Christine to expound her views in a fuller form in two books, both dated 1405, *La Cité des Dames* (The City of Women) and *Le Livre des trois vertus* (The Book of Three Virtues). In these texts, she protested against the view and treatment of her sex. She created a city of women aided by three female goddesses: Reason, Uprightness and Justice. In this city, women would be educated. Although de Pizan did not specifically discuss medicine, she did argue that women were as capable as men of scientific learning. Pizan called herself a 'fille d'estude' or a servant of science.

Christine asked Reason whether God had ever wished to ennoble the mind of woman with the loftiness of the sciences. Did God provide women with a 'clever enough mind for this?' Christine went on to state how much she wanted to know the answer for men claim that 'women can learn only a little'. Lady Reason replied: 'You know quite well that the opposite of their opinion is true... If it were customary to send daughters to school like sons, and if they were taught the natural sciences, they would learn as thoroughly and understand the subtleties of all the arts and sciences as well as sons...' She concluded with the premise that women were actually more capable than men of inquiry: 'Just as women have more delicate bodies than men, weaker and less able to perform many tasks, so do they have minds that are freer and sharper whenever they apply themselves.'[100] Although women have at least equal intelligence to men their knowledge is much less. When Christine asked Lady Reason why this is the case, Reason responds that society's expectations of women are that 'it is enough for them to perform the usual duties to which they are ordained ... The public does not require them to get involved in the affairs which men are commissioned to execute...'[101]

Pierre Dubois (c. 1250–1312), a lawyer and writer, supported the views of Christine de Pizan, and himself wrote favourably about women studying and practising medicine. He was well ahead of his time in his thinking. He was the author of a treatise entitled, *De Recuperatione Terre Sancte: Traité de Politique générale* (1306), which was presented to the king of France, Philip IV. It dealt with the required conditions for a successful crusade and then how to establish peace among the Christian nations of the West. Education was an important part of his plan. Both male and female children would be educated free of charge in Latin, Greek or Arabic and theology. All girls were to be taught basic medical and surgical skills. These were 'feminine skills'. Male doctors and surgeons 'should have wives similarly instructed, in order that they can more fully look after the sick'. Although his scheme was never implemented, the Council of Vienne (1311–12) stipulated that schools of Hebrew, Greek, Arabic and Chaldaic be established at the Roman court and at the universities of Paris, Oxford and Bologna.[102]

The Cartesian philosopher and French theologian François Poulain de la Barre (1647–1723) was among the first Europeans to write treatises on the subjects of female equality and education. He wrote a curriculum for women which included science, medicine and mathematics in addition to other academic subjects. He interpreted Descartes's philosophy to prove the equality of the sexes, applying the Cartesian method by examining everything, judging everything and putting reason above all else.[103] The ideas contained in *The Discourse on Method* forced him to renounce his previous ideas about women. The methodology of doubt and scepticism made him re-examine his previously held prejudices about female inferiority. In the Preface to *De L'Egalité des deux sexes* (1673), Poulain wrote that his purpose was 'not to prove that women are better than men, but to provide a way of comparing the arguments for and against and then making the best decision based on the reasons on which they are founded'.[104]

Part I of *De L'Egalité* was concerned with contemporary and past prejudices against women. Part II challenged the prevailing view of women by employing Cartesian methodology. In the Preface, Poulain stated the thesis that he planned to refute: 'The happiest thought comes to those who work to acquire a solid science after having been instructed in the popular method; this is to doubt that which has been taught and to desire the discovery of truth for oneself. In the progress of their research, they discover that we are filled with prejudices and that we must completely renounce them to arrive at clear and distinct knowledge.'[105]

Poulain provided explanations for the exclusion of women from science and medicine. 'Everyone, those who are learned and those who are not learned at all, and even women themselves agree and say that they take no part in the sciences and public life, because they are not capable of these duties; that they have less intelligence than men, and that they should therefore be inferior to them in everything as they are...'[106] He summarized statements made by Clement of Alexandria and Saint Basil which indicate that male and female are of the same nature.[107]

Nature did not intend women to be in a subservient position in society. Custom, instead of natural law, made women inferior to men. On the basis of his experience, and discussions with women from all social classes, he refuted the supposed inferiority of women. In a sense he carried out his own empirical research. He also provided examples of female competence in the past, such as that of nuns running monasteries.[108]

In his marginal notes, he wrote that, 'the mind has no sex ... not acting differently in one sex than in the other; it is in each equally capable of the same things'.[109] Physical differences between males and females mean nothing when dealing with the mind: 'it is easy to notice that the differences between the sexes concern only the body; that being the only part necessary to the production of men to which the mind does nothing but lend its consent'.[110] Again on physical differences, he wrote that men are not necessarily stronger than women, 'that there are some organs in one which are not in the other. In all that, it is not necessary ... that women have less strength and vigor than men.'[111] This was a bold statement for its day since most writers exploited physiological differences and supposed female weakness to justify female intellectual inferiority.

Based upon his belief and demonstration that women were equal to men in all ways, he then proposed that all fields of endeavour should be open to women. These ranged from the law, both civil and canon, to medicine and education. He was the first modern writer to advocate the right to work for all.[112]

Although the 'querelle des femmes' was dominated by French writers, it was not limited to them. In Spain, there are texts on the subject of woman going back to the middle of the thirteenth century with Catalan texts translated from the Arabic.[113] Like the earlier French texts, these are primarily concerned with morality rather than with intellectual abilities. The major theme of these texts is the subordination of women to men, their duties as wives and mothers.[114] However, it is interesting to note that Spanish women had enjoyed a significant amount of freedom with respect to the public sphere during the Middle Ages. They owned businesses, they could inherit and dispose of property, which was often in the woman's name, and a wife continued to have complete ownership of her dowry after marriage. This rule of equality was established in the *Liber Judicorum*.[115] Why and how this changed has been explained primarily in economic, religious and medical terms. Mercantilism, which began to be practised in the sixteenth century, left women with fewer avenues of employment and less pay than men for their work.

The Renaissance and the Catholic Counter-Reformation took place almost simultaneously in Spain, and the former was greatly influenced by the latter. By 1575, 'entrenched forces of conservatism were in control', and progressive scholars ran into problems with the Inquisition.[116] While Renaissance man was encouraged to develop to his potential, Renaissance woman was taught to be a good wife and mother. Indeed, in Spain, the most pervasive attitude towards women was that they were inferior creatures in every sense of the word. This attitude of female inadequacy may be summarized in the words of Fernando de Valdés, author of *Excelencias de la fe* (1537), who was a professor of canon law at the University of Salamanca and a member of the supreme council of the Spanish Inquisition: 'No matter how learned a woman may be, put a padlock of silence on her mouth of the mysteries of the fathers of the church. For it is certain what the ancients said, that the jewel which makes a woman prettiest is the padlock of silence on the doors of her lips for all conversation...'[117]

The Counter-Reformation curtailed female equality as women came to be blamed for many of the evils that afflicted society, and the combined influence of the Counter-Reformation and the Renaissance resulted in the publication of a series of manuals or handbooks on the subject of the proper behaviour of a Christian woman. The most influential of these was that of humanist writer Juan Luis Vives, whose ideas towards women are discussed below. Silence and obedience to men were held to be key objectives.[118] Scholars maintain that the influence of Vives's handbook on female education and appropriate roles for women spread beyond the borders of Spain to become the 'most important voice' in sixteenth-century Europe.[119]

Many scholars hold Juan Luis Vives to be the most noteworthy of the Renaissance humanists who contributed to the debate on the nature, role and education of women because of his *Institutione Foeminae Christianae*, or *The Instruction of a Christen Woman* (1524).[120] Vives based his notions about women primarily on Aristotelian thought as delineated above. In addition, he turned to the Bible and the Church fathers, particularly Saint Ambrose and Tertullian for inspiration.[121] Vives depicted women as 'weak in reason, passion and body ... Woman's thought is swift and for the most part unstable...'[122]

Vives was the leading exponent of Erasmian views in Spain, although Erasmus was more progressive in terms of female education, stating that 'education and learning are as desirable in a woman as a man'.[123] Nevertheless, Vives was the Spanish humanist who paid the closest attention to education. He was employed by the court of Katherine of Aragon and drafted an educational proposal for Katherine's daughter Mary. Vives advocated education for women, but his education was more in the line of training. It was designed to prepare girls for a private role and included learning to read and write and the acquisition of the domestic skills of sewing, cooking and spinning.[124] For Vives, whose ideas were typical of the age, female education meant preparation for marriage. He was adamant that women should remain in the private rather than the public sphere.

Intellectual education played a part, but the emphasis was on the domestic arts such as sewing and cooking. He wrote: 'I am of the opinion that we should take care of the education of young girls more than is generally thought ... They should be taught to be modest and sober.'[125] His principal objective was to teach women to be chaste and virtuous. Women must be taught to be silent if not virtually invisible, and they should not occupy any position of authority. Here his ideas are very similar to other Spanish writers of the sixteenth century. Women were not to be teachers, 'nor to have the authority of the man but to be in silence'.[126] His justification is based on the nature of woman, derived from Eve, who was tempted by the serpent even though his argument was weak.[127]

Spanish theologian and poet Fray Luis de Léon (1528–91) wrote in the same genre as Vives, but was more positive towards women in the sense that he viewed women as soldiers protecting the home and castle for their men.[128] He was well-acquainted with Vives's works. De Léon, author of *La Perfecta Casada* (1583), was a humanist scholar remembered more today for his poetry than his scholarship. He held chairs in theology, the Bible and moral philosophy. Experts have asserted that he 'does not write for or against women, but writes about the married woman from the perspective of Christian and moral philosophy'.[129] This view, however, could be contested, for he sees women as morally, intellectually and physically inferior to men, basing this perspective on the Old Testament book of Proverbs, Chapter 31: 10–31. His focus was on the married woman cloistered in the home – hence the title of his book, *La Perfecta Casada*, the ideal wife. According to de Léon, 'a good wife' would be 'industrious and housewifely'.[130] Her duty was to maintain harmony in the home and serve her husband.[131] As with Vives, silence was to be cultivated in women.[132]

For many writers, the debate about women in Spain revolved around the 'excesses of courtly love' which some 'feared as a new aristocratic religion'.[133] The courtly gentleman ruined himself in pursuit of the love of his lady, who was secretive and inconstant. These notions of the female character are derived from Aristotle. Men who wrote in this misogynistic vein included Alfonso Martínez de Toledo, author of *El Archipeste de Talvera que fabla los vicios de las malas mugeres e complexiones de los hombres* (1498) and Pere Tororella, a fifteenth-century Catalan poet and author of *Coplas de Las Calidades de Las Donas*.[134]

Although Mosén Diego de Valera (1412–88) wrote a defence of women, he still saw women's role as limited. His *Tratado en defensa de las virtuosas mugeres* (before 1448), was written in reply to the 'nueva secta' (new sect) of slanderers, 'and which draws on a corpus of conventional arguments and historical examples of virtuous women'.[135] Valera was a member of the minor nobility, a diplomat and courtier. He attacked the 'malice and ignorance'[136] of those he opposed. Like Vives, he wrote a didactic treatise instructing an imaginary male friend. He inquired as to what the appropriate role was for women and what were male expectations of women? What, indeed, did men expect from women?[137] Although the treatise was dedicated to Queen Maria, she was an observer who had no voice of her own and the dedication serves only to legitimize the male voice. Enrique de Villena also challenged the traditional ideology of woman as evil, devoting a chapter in his *Doce trabajos de Hércules* (1417) to the merits of woman insofar as she could bring the best out in man.[138]

Although there had been defences of women written before the eighteenth century, such as that of de Valera and Enrique Villena, Fray Benito Jerónimo Feijoo y Montenegro (b. 1676) was the first Spanish author to write a text in favour of women and their abilities. He held the Chair of Theology at Santo Tomás Oveido University. His attitudes were very similar to those of Poulain de la Barre and he must have been aware of Poulain's works, although there is no direct reference to them in his treatises. In France, Feijoo's works were cited in such prestigious journals as the *Mercure de France* and his eight volume *Teatro crítico universel* (1726–40), was partially translated into English and Portuguese. His *Defensa de las mujeres* (1726), which is contained in Volume I of the *Teatro*, and is his most significant work, was based on both his observation of women during his own times and historical figures, such as women rulers.[139] He set out to prove that woman is the intellectual equal of man and therefore should be entitled to the same education.[140] He refuted three major arguments made against women: asserting that they were not morally corrupt, nor physically and intellectually weaker than men. He rebutted Aristotle's imperfect male theory. Male and female both possessed good and bad qualities and complemented each other.[141]

Feijoo devoted the greater part of his essay to female intelligence. Women, he argued, do not lack ability, but they do lack information and confidence – they believed themselves to be less intelligent than men. He even promoted the idea of women making good doctors, citing the Spanish doctor Oliva Sabuco de Nantes as a fine example.[142] He attempted to answer the question: 'If women are equal to men in their aptitude for the Arts and the Sciences, for governing, running a country politically and economically, why did God establish the dominance and superiority of men, with respect to Chapter Three of Genesis?' by stating that governance belongs to each sex whoever recognizes the major capacity for this.[143] Feijoo questioned the literal meaning of the Old Testament in addition to accepted versions. Women were originally equal to men, but Eve's sin led to her political subjection. She was the first to sin – this rather than her natural inferiority in intelligence – led to man's predominance. To infer male superiority was simply untrue.[144] Feijoo did not go as far in his 'feminism' as did Poulain de la Barre, for he recommended the political subjection of woman to man, although he never fully explained his reasons for advocating this. To sum up, Feijoo accepted male and female equality in terms of intelligence, morality and spirituality, but women remained politically subject to men.[145] The family, for reasons of defence and welfare, required a strong decision-maker – this was the man's role. Unlike Poulain de la Barre who proposed a public role for women, Feijoo, more conservatively, clung to female suitability for the domestic role. Women should be good wives and mothers, albeit he did not think this function to be inferior to man's more public role.

Early Modern Europeans held varying societal views of women and their roles and these affected the prospects of women healers. Thinkers from many different perspectives, including the medical, theological, legal and philosophical, contributed to the debate concerning women. Views also varied between countries and cultures with the Spanish recommending a very cloistered life for women, either in the home or in a convent, and the French often advocating much greater openness, even in the later Middle Ages. Although the majority of commentators thought that woman's place was not in the world of medicine, there were still some significant dissenting views.

4

Medical Treatises and Texts Written by Women and for Women

Women contributed significantly to the literature on medicine during the Early Modern period. They wrote treatises on medicines, treatments and therapies, chemicals and the impact of chemistry on medicine, and healing substances. Some women even prescribed new therapies. Although women were denied a proper medical education during the Early Modern period, this did not prevent a number of determined women from learning from their relatives or male friends and acquiring enough knowledge to write on scientific matters.

Women's reasons for writing medical treatises were diverse. Some wanted to disseminate their medical knowledge to wider society, while others were motivated by more personal reasons, such as Mary Trye, who wished to vindicate her doctor father in a quarrel with another physician. Her treatise in defence of her father reveals her own knowledge of medicine.

This chapter investigates a variety of published medical writings by and for women from a variety of European countries, most significantly Spain, Italy, France and England.[1] As English writer, Hannah Wolley or Woolley (b.1623), allegedly the first successful author of cookery and household management books,[2] aptly observed in the introduction to her *Gentlewoman's Companion, or, A Guide to the Female Sex* (1673), it was no small feat for a woman to be published at this time: 'It is no ambitious design of gaining a name in print (a thing as rare for a Woman to endeavour as obtain); that put me on this bold undertaking...'[3]

In Spain, we find the noteworthy contributions to medical knowledge by Doña Oliva Sabuco de Nantes Barrera (1562–?), an expert in psychosomatic and homeopathic medicine, and in Italy, Isabella Cortese (d. 1561), author of *Secreti medicinali artificiosi ed alchemici* (1561–65), a recipe book concerned with medicine and cosmetics. In France, the vicomtesse de Vaux, Marie de Maupeou Fouquet (1590–1681), authored a receipt book, *Recueil de receptes, où est expliquée la manière de guerir à peu de frais toute sorte de maux tant internes, qu'externes inueterez, & qui ont passé jusqu'à present pour incurables*, that was reprinted several times and in several languages from

1675 into the eighteenth century and Marie-Geneviève-Charlotte Darlus Thiroux d'Arconville (1720–1805) wrote an *Essai pour servir a l'histoire de la putréfaction* in addition to sixteen other medical publications.[4]

During the Renaissance, women were more likely to devote themselves to literature, poetry and philosophy than to medicine. If women received an education at all – and those who were educated tended to be daughters of the nobility – it was a humanist education. However, there were clearly exceptional women who dedicated themselves to medical subjects. Oliva Sabuco de Nantes Barrera, born in 1562 in Alcarez, near Toledo, was one such. Sabuco de Nante's field of expertise was mental hygiene and psychotherapy.[5] Her fundamental premise was that illnesses were caused by 'passions'. Her medical theories were published in *New Philosophy of Human Nature*,[6] which was reprinted a number of times during Sabuco's brief lifetime; she died in her late twenties. The first edition was published in Madrid in 1587. The second edition, dating from 1588, fell into the hands of the Inquisition and several sections of the text in this edition were deleted by the inquisitors. The book was published in Portugal in 1622.[7] An edition of 1707 was censored by the Roman Catholic Church, and the Inquisition endeavoured – unsuccessfully, in that there are two copies extant – to destroy all the copies of the book. The *New Philosophy* was published three times in the nineteenth century and once in the twentieth, in 1981. The first English language edition was published in 2007.[8]

Oliva Sabuco de Nantes was the daughter of a pharmacist, Miguel Sabuco y Alvarez, who was an expert in herbal medicine and had a great knowledge of botany which he passed on to his daughter. Scholars believe that she was educated in the sciences by him and by her brother who was a pharmacist. There is no doubt that the greatest influence on her choosing the natural sciences as her vocation was her father,[9] although her godfather, a medical doctor, might also have played a role in her education. Pedro Simón Abril, a local philosopher of renown, a grammarian and teacher, was also instrumental in her academic training. An expert on Aristotle, Abril introduced Sabuco de Nantes to many of the philosophical ideas contained in her *New Philosophy*.[10] Scholars do not know if she received any formal education. She may have received some schooling at a Dominican convent near her home, but there are no records to support this speculation. The convent did, however, possess a rich library to which Sabuco de Nantes had access.[11]

Her medical ideas, well ahead of her time, are contained in her *Nueva Filosofía*, translated as *New Philosophy of Human Nature neither Known to nor Attained by the Great Ancient Philosophers Which Improves Human Life and Health*, which was published in 1587 when she was twenty-five years old.[12] Sabuco de Nantes preceded university trained British physicians, Thomas Willis (1621–75) and Francis Glisson (1597–1677) in their work on the nervous system by about thirty years. The editors and translators of the *Nueva Filosofia* note that neither of these scientists credited Sabuco de Nantes for her ideas even though parts of their works – especially those dealing with psychosomatic illnesses – are very similar in content.[13]

Until recently, Sabuco de Nante's authorship of the book was contested. Prior to 2006 and the publication of the new translation and study of the *New Philosophy* by Mary Ellen Waithe and her coterie of scholars, the text was attributed to Sabuco de Nante's father, Miguel.[14] Given the contemporary attitude towards female scholars and scientists, and the fact the Sabuco de Nantes lacked a formal education, suspicion of her authorship is neither surprising nor unusual. Marie Charlotte d'Arconville suffered from a similar prejudice as her translation of Alexander Monro's *The Anatomy of Human Bones and Nerves* was for many years erroneously attributed to Eugène Sue.[15]

The New Philosophy is organized in two volumes, with the first volume written in Spanish, the second in Latin. Volume I is concerned with subjects as wide-ranging as men's health, politics and society, while Volume II, written in the form of a dialogue between two shepherds, concerns the impact of emotions on the body in addition to a discussion of various illnesses, such as the plague. The text is further divided into chapters entitled 'Colloquy on Human Nature and Knowledge of One's Self', 'Treatise on The Composition of the World', 'Treatise about Things which will Improve the World', 'Colloquy on Remedies' and 'Colloquy on Errors of Traditional Medicine'. In addition, there are two *Opuscula* written in Latin, 'About Human Nature' and 'True Philosophy'.

A great portion of the book deals with philosophy, although the 'Colloquy on Remedies' and 'Colloquy on Errors of Traditional Medicine' are concerned with health. Medical experts such as Hippocrates and Galen are cited as well as philosophers including Plato and Pliny the Elder. Pliny's *Historia Naturalis* in thirty-three volumes is the most frequently cited source. It provided Sabuco de Nantes with details of plants and foods valuable in promoting good health.[16]

Sabuco de Nantes is significant for producing an entirely secular work (it is not surprising that it was condemned by the Spanish Inquisition) based upon empirical and rational philosophy, which questioned contemporary medical ideas concerning the connection between mind and body. She challenged prevailing medical views concerning pain, anger and disease.

The salient theme running through Sabuco de Nantes's work is the connection between the mind and the body and its consequences for health. Sabuco de Nantes explored the relationship between human emotions and disease. She insisted that there is a powerful relationship between the body and soul, and that if humans understand this relationship, their health can be considerably improved. She was interested in how mental health impacted physical health, for example, the physiological impact of fear on the body. She deduced that:

> Because humans have a rational soul (that animals do not have), and from it they possess the powers, reminiscence, reason and will, located in the head, divine part of the body that Plato called the seat and home of the rational soul. They love and desire, fear and hate ... only humans have

spiritually understood pain of the present, sorrow about the past, fear, dread and worry about the future ... for this reason ... they have so many kinds of illnesses, and so many sudden deaths when anger and sorrow are so grave that are enough to kill in one moment. And when is minor, kills them in a few days ... and if it is so minor ... it leaves behind ... ill-humors in the body that are the causes of diseases.[17]

Sabuco de Nantes provided an original anatomical description of the human body in terms of an 'upside down tree', where the brain, 'the vegetation of trunk and branches' (body and limbs), has a superior part in controlling behaviour. She called the various bodily fluids – white blood cells, lymph, spinal fluid, digestive juices – 'vitality-milk'.[18]

According to Sabuco de Nantes, a major problem with physicians was their failure to provide a cure for the plague which repeatedly devastated European populations. Sabuco de Nantes diagnosed the cause of the plague as a poison carried in the air. Infections of the eye, blood and skin were carried through the air. Inhaling 'bad air' was the route by which infections entered our bodies.[19] Sabuco de Nantes's theorizing of airborne infection was clearly centuries ahead of her time.

Other aspects of medicine that she examined were the impact of pain on the body, the effect of the brain on sleep, and reasons for miscarriage, which could include emotional upset such as news of the death of a loved one. She prescribed a healthy diet for pregnant women and children.[20] Physical threats to good health included the emotional upset from relocation, moving from one country to another, changes in the weather (excessive cold and heat were serious threats) and the moon, excessive fatigue and poison from animal bites.[21]

Sabuco de Nantes's book influenced the thinking of contemporary French physicians and chemists including Charles le Pois (Carolis Pisonis) (1563–1633) and Etienne de Clave (fl. 1624). Charles le Pois was first Professor and Dean of the Faculty of Medicine at the University of Pont à Mousson, a Jesuit University, in 1598. In his treatise entitled *Choix d'observations*, le Pois based his remarks on the relationship between hysteria and the uterus on Sabuco de Nantes's book. He posited that there was no relationship between the two.[22] The chemist, Etienne de Clave, who challenged the Aristotelian view that all materials are composed of the four elements of heat, cold, moisture and dryness, praised Sabuco de Nantes in the preface to Book II of his *Paradoxes ou Traités Philosophiques des Pierres et Pierreries* (1635). He called her 'a learned Spaniard ... who refutes Aristotle aplenty, and goes as far as branding certain Aristotelian opinions as gags'.[23] In 1604, a Spanish physician and poet, Francisco Lopez de Uveda, also praised Sabuca de Nantes, predicting that she would soon be more famous than writers like Cervantes.[24]

In Spain, the medical doctor and university professor of surgery in Alcala, Miguel Marcelino Boix y Moliner (1633–c.1720), was also influenced by

Sabuco de Nantes's philosophy of medicine. In his *Hippocrates aclarado, y sistema de Galeno impugnado* (1716), he claimed that he had discovered the works of a controversial scholar of seventeenth-century Spanish medicine, and he lauded the author as a 'philosophical genius'.[25] The Enlightenment era medical doctor, professor of anatomy and philosopher, Martín Martínez (1684–1734), wrote a eulogy for Sabuco de Nantes, *Elogia a Doña Oliva Sabuco*, in celebration of the fourth edition of the *New Philosophy*, published in 1622 in Portugal.[26] Martínez held important positions in the Spanish medical world. He was examiner for a *Protomedicato* board whose job was to examine all physicians before they received their licences. He was Felipe V's personal physician, and president of the Royal Society of Medicine. He authored several books on anatomy and surgery. In his *Eulogy*, he applauded Sabuco de Nantes's invention of new terminology, such as 'suco nérveo', to describe certain bodily fluids. This new term, meaning, 'the nervous sap, or original neurotransmitting substance',[27] could be found in the *Diccionario de Autoridades* (1713) published by the Royal Spanish Academy.

Finally, Sabuco de Nantes anticipated later philosophers including René Descartes and his philosophy of mind–body dualism. She did not locate the interaction between the soul and the body in the pineal gland, but she did locate it within the brain.[28]

In Italy, Isabella Cortese (d. 1561), an Italian noblewoman who lived during the Renaissance, wrote the first cosmetic handbook, published under variations of the title *I Secreti Cosmetici* (Cosmetic Secrets). This work also contained some medicinal remedies. The complete title of the first edition was *I secreti della signora Isabella Cortese ne' quali si contengono cose minerali, medicinali, arteficiose, alchimiche et molte de l'arte profumatoria*, translated as 'The secrets of Signora Isabella Cortese. In which are included mineral, man-made and alchemical things and many [things] concerning the art of perfumery, suitable for any lady'. Cortese's book is known as a 'Book of Secrets'. 'Books of Secrets', or 'how to' books were both common and popular during the Renaissance.[29] Typically, they were composed of recipes and formulae for preserving, for making dyes and for medicines. 'Books of Secrets' claimed to 'reveal, to anyone who could read them, the secrets of nature and the arts'. In reality, they were compendia of medicinal, cosmetic and general household recipes and instructions, including those for making jewellery and cleansing substances.[30] What is interesting for our purposes is that Cortese was the only woman to compile such a text at this time.[31]

Biographical details about Cortese are scarce. According to her book, she had studied alchemy for over thirty years and this left her with little money. Historians maintain that Cortese lived in the Venice area as the first edition of her book, dated 1561, was produced in this region. Like Madame de Fouquet in France, Cortese had great success with her book which was a best-seller in its time. It was printed fifteen times in Italian between 1561 and 1677 and a German edition was published in 1592.[32]

Cortese was an enthusiastic advocate of alchemy, although she claimed to have discovered that the theories of 'the famous philosophers', who she believed to be alchemists, were ineffective. At the start of Book II, she cited various philosophers, including Arnold of Villanova (c. 1235–1311), Geber, an Arab chemist from the eighth century, and Raimondo Lullo (1235–1315) dismissing their theories in favour of practice and stressing the close connections between the ingredients of her medicines and the philosophical concepts of matter (body) and spirit. In a letter to her brother-in-law, Mario Chaboga, she critiqued the works of the experts and revealed that she had studied their ideas for thirty years. She believed that there was 'nothing good in them', that she had 'wasted time and almost lost my life and possessions' by devoting her life to studying their books. Rather than focusing on the theories of Villanova, Lullo and Geber, she urged Chaboga to 'follow the rules I write down for you'.[33]

I Secreti is a curious combination of science and medicine, popular beliefs, astrology and magic. It reflects the Italian Renaissance cult of physical beauty and aesthetic perfection. The text is approximately two hundred pages in length and organized in three books: Book I contains medical remedies covering everything from various plagues to calluses to warts on the penis. There are twenty-eight medicinal remedies. Book II deals with alchemy and provides instructions for the preparation of dyes in seventy-five different ways, while Book III is composed of cosmetic recipes for creams, scents and dental pastes. Later editions contain four books. The fourth book is composed of recipes for perfumes, face powders, soaps, deodorants and bleaches for whitening the skin. Among the ingredients she used were eggs for the removal of freckles, honey and lemon to clear up acne, face masks composed of vegetal and tuber flours rich in saponin combined with clay, egg whites, Arabic gum and honey or almond. There are four recipes against the plague, various unguents and plasters made of oils and waxes.[34]

Cortese invented remedies of her own which 'restored her health, honor and wealth'.[35] She prepared treatments for various ailments in addition to soaps, face creams and poultices. One medicinal receipt that she prepared was an ointment made from a combination of almond oil and milk to treat a wound. Another was for medicinal lozenges that soothed the stomach and the mind as well as providing freshening for the breath. The receipt was composed of 'fine Muscat wine, lavender spikes, cedar bark and aloe wood. Added to this was an eighth of an ounce of fine musk.' This mixture was to be made into coin shapes and stored in a scented glass container in a cool place. One would take one lozenge before bed, 'placing it under the tongue until dissolved, and another in the morning, to be repeated as you pleased'.[36]

While the book is primarily remembered as a compilation of cosmetics and medicinal cures, *I Secreti* is also a philosophical treatise. Cortese demonstrated that she had received some education in the contemporary debate about philosophy and alchemy, particularly the relationship between the body and the spirit and the importance of the investigation of the 'secrets of nature'.

In some instances, women combined medicine with charity. This was the case with Marie de Maupeou Fouquet and the *Remèdes Charitables*. Madame Fouquet lived during a tumultuous period of the seventeenth century in which the War of the Fronde[37] disrupted the lives of many ordinary French people, increasing the misery of the poor. This was also a time of religious upheaval with the Counter-Reformation taking hold in France, and of renewed spirituality and the founding of new religious orders such as the Carmelites and the order of Vincent de Paul. Religious works were one arena of public activity open to women and Madame Fouquet took advantage of this. She was motivated by Christian piety and was called the 'mère des pauvres' by the courtier and historian Louis de Rouvroy, Duc de Saint-Simon, who praised her in his memoirs. He wrote that, 'The virtue, courage and singular piety of this Lady, mother of the poor, whose name still lives was unshakeable…'[38]

Marie de Maupeou Fouquet, vicomtesse de Vaux, was born in 1590 into a prominent aristocratic family belonging to the Nobility of the Robe. Her father, Gilles de Maupeou, seigneur of Albeiges, was a counsellor in the Paris Parlement, the highest court of appeal in France before its abolition in the French Revolution of 1789. Gilles de Maupeou held various positions in the service of the French monarchy: in 1579, he was appointed auditor and the next year, *maitre de requêtes* (Master of the Requests in the Council of State, an adviser to the king). He was the Intendant of Brittany from 1598 to 1599, secretary in the king's chamber, counsellor of state and Intendant of finances. On 22 February 1622, Marie de Maupeou married François Fouquet, also a member of the Paris Parlement. She was the mother of sixteen children, eleven of whom survived. Her five daughters became nuns (this tended to be a family affair in the seventeenth century) and two of her sons became bishops.[39]

Marie de Maupeou Fouquet's charitable career began in the 1630s with her participation in *Les Dames de la Charité*. The group, *Les Dames de la Charité*, was created in 1634 by a set of aristocratic women similar to Madame de Fouquet in background and social status.[40] Initially composed of fourteen women, married or widowed, the Ladies of Charity would later grow to between 100 and 120 women.[41] The principal motivator in establishing the group was Madame Goussault who asked Vincent de Paul to organize a company of ladies 'to instruct and exhort the patients of the Hôtel Dieu'. Initially, Vincent de Paul refused to be involved – he claimed that the spiritual welfare of the sick was the business of the chapter, but Madame Goussault persisted, speaking with Vincent's superior, the Archbishop of Paris, Jean François de Gondi, who ordered Vincent to comply with her request. The Ladies of Charity met for the first time at the home of Madame Goussault in the rue Roi-de-Siècle. Present were women from some of the most prominent and oldest aristocratic families in France, including the duchesse of Aiguillon who was Richelieu's niece, and lady-in-waiting to the queen; Anne of Austria, Madame de Lamoignan; Elisabeth Chappelier; dame d'Aligre; the Princess of Condé; the Duchess of Nemours; and Louise Marie de Gonzague, the future queen of Poland. At the second meeting of the ladies, Madame Séguier and Madame Fouquet attended[42] and formal officers were elected: Vincent de Paul was elected perpetual director, Madame de Goussault president. The ladies would put into practice Vincent de Paul's first rule of the co-fraternity: 'to aid the body and the soul by nourishing and medicating the body and the soul...'[43] The purpose of this group was to work with the Sisters of Charity at the hospitals, such as the Hôtel Dieu. They would distribute food, including meat, and, dressed simply, they would visit the sick in hospital. Their daily visits would begin at 2.00 p.m. and last until 4.00 or 5.00 p.m. depending on the season. The women worked in pairs with an Augustinian sister who would indicate the sickest patients who were in need of the most care.[44] They only took care of female patients. The women were also exhorted to have patients make a confession and if they so desired, a priest was called. If one of the ladies died, they made sure she would be replaced.

As an extension of her charitable work, Marie de Fouquet put together a compendium of medical receipts. The preface stresses the pre-eminence of charity, because of 'the continual action of doing good, and that it is the connection which unites all virtues to achieve perfection'.[45]

Madame Fouquet's intended audience was the public, the ordinary person by way of priests and nursing sisters, rather than educated physicians and apothecaries. The Daughters of Charity, who ran pharmacies in hospitals, carried a copy of Madame Fouquet's anthology.[46] Madame de Fouquet compiled the text in conjunction with a university trained physician M Delescure, a doctor from Montpellier. The first edition of Fouquet's *Recueil de receptes choisies experimentées & approuvées. Contre quantité de maux fort comuns tant internes q'uexternes inveterés, & difficiles à guerir*, was published in Villefranche-de-Rouergue by Grandsaigne in 1675. Sixteen further French editions were published, the last in 1740, under various titles, primarily versions of the *Recueil* title. The 1695 edition was entitled 'Disinterested medicine',[47] and thus more clearly conveyed the charitable message.

The book was popularized as *Recueil de remèdes faciles et domestiques*. This work certainly promoted Madame de Fouquet's name and her mission. Historian of medicine Matthew Ramsey has argued that 'The most prominent of the charitable handbooks and perhaps the most successful of its kind in early modern Europe was the *Charitable Remedies* of Madame Fouquet...'[48] It became the principal *vade mecum* for every parish priest and nursing sister.[49]

The anthology remained in use in rural areas of France until at least the middle of the nineteenth century.[50] It was also re-edited and reprinted in several European countries and languages. There are Belgian editions dated 1684 and 1699 (both in French); and a Dutch edition, published in Amsterdam in French in 1704, 1720 and 1738. The recipe collection was published in Italian, Portuguese, Spanish and German. In Italy, the book was published in several different cities (Milan, Bologna and Venice) in various editions between 1683 and 1750. The 1697 Italian edition contains a translation of the *Méthode que l'on pratique à l'Hôtel des invalides pour guérir les soldats de la verole* which was added to part two of the *Recueil* in the Lyons edition of 1685. As far as the Iberian Peninsula is concerned, the book was translated into Castilian Spanish in 1739 and 1750 and there was a further Spanish edition as late as 1872, published in Valencia. The book appeared in Portuguese in 1712, 1714 and 1749. The German edition was published in Dresden, by Bey Johann Jacob Wincklern in 1708.

Madame Fouquet was not the only individual to publish a book of traditional remedies in Early Modern France, but she was the only woman to do so. Moreover, many of these remedy books had little to do with charity, despite the word's appearance in their titles. One example of this is a very popular home remedy book published between 1623 and 1639, authored by Dr Philbert Guybert (1579?–1633), doctor regent of the University of Paris. His text possesses a very similar title to Madame Fouquet's book, *Le médecin charitable, enseignant la manière de faire & préparer en la maison avec facilité & peu de frais les remèdes propres à toutes maladies, selon l'advis du medecin ordinaire. Augm. de rechef de plusieurs remèdes tant pour les riches que pour les pauvres ...* (Paris: Denys Langlois, 1626), but it is actually exclusively concerned with medicine, surgery and pharmacy. It says nothing about charitable medicine. Guybert's interest was in promoting the authority of the physician through the preparation of home remedies with the aid of a physician. This method of treatment would also lower the costs borne by the physician.[51] Guybert's collection, like Madame Fouquet's, was published many times, but unlike her collection of remedies, his was also translated into English as *The charitable physician, shewing the manner to make and prepare in the house with ease and little paines all those remedies which are proper to all sorts of diseases*, published in one volume with the *The charitable apothecarie and The charitable physitian, sheuuing the manner to embalme a dead corps* (London, 1639). His book was published with the approval of the Faculty of Medicine at the University of Paris. Even if his intentions were less charitable than those of Madame Fouquet, Guybert also attempted to provide the ordinary person with a simple way of treating common ailments.[52]

Dr Delescure, who assisted Madame Fouquet in the preparation of her book, recognized the value of addressing this collection of medical recipes to the public. Delescure, who wrote the Preface to the *Recueil*, put the stress on simple remedies which were 'easy to prepare and comfortable in their application'. He commended the book as a 'rare and rich present from one of the most holy and Charitable Ladies of the kingdom'.[53] The triple collaboration of Madame Fouquet, her son Louis Fouquet, bishop of Agde, and the doctor, Delescure, lent weight to the publication of the *Recueil de receptes*. Today, the medical value of this collection may seem doubtful and the science primitive: nothing surprising and modest cures. Nevertheless, the book had a remarkable success; its innumerable editions are witness to this fact.

Many of the recipes in the book, such as those for salves and unguents, were devised by Fouquet herself from her experience as the mother of eleven children. The book is organized into two volumes: one for remedies for internal ailments and one for external disorders. The 1696 edition (expanded) is in two volumes and contains almost 600 receipts. She provided cures for ailments including headaches, apoplexy, epilepsy, paralysis, nerves, melancholy (depression), sore eyes, ears, nose, bad breath, sore teeth, rheumatism, canker sores, pimples, calluses in the hands, stomach problems, jaundice, colic, all sorts of fluxes, dysentery, female problems – breast-feeding, childbirth, the prevention of miscarriages, plasters for pregnant women, inflammation of the breast – fevers, sciatica, various types of plasters and poultices for everything from stomach aches, colic, tumours, vomiting and liver problems to haemorrhoids. Receipts for various ointments for minor wounds, burns and bites are also provided.[54] Several pages are devoted specifically to stomach problems, from colic to tumours.[55] She employed traditional pharmaceutical ingredients such as excrement, olive oil and aloe, as well as more recent remedies such as mercury.

Fouquet dedicated her book to the clergy. A 'Dedicatory Epistle' precedes the book of remedies. She wrote that 'the God who created us commands us to discuss the hidden causes of all illnesses and ailments; that he gave us the intelligence to understand the symptoms and the perfect knowledge of the properties which compose the medicines'.[56] She insisted that she would never advise priests to 'usurp the rights of any person', but 'in the freedom that I have in dedicating this small book, my entire goal and design is to persuade you, having in hand the Receuil de receptes choisis, and finding urgent and pressing occasions to employ the receipts, especially in the places where the sick poor can do nothing, or find it difficult to obtain help'. Priests were to prepare the mixtures faithfully and to dispense them charitably.[57] She admitted that quite possibly the clergy would be surprised by her collection, but that her recipes were designed for everyday illnesses. Fouquet wrote of the priests' 'noble ministry', their 'Power and the Faculty to heal the most noble part of man'. She would assist them in the healing of illnesses which attack the body every day. Comparing the priests with the apostles, she beseeched them to 'walk exactly in their steps, and to take the same route'. She pressed the clergy to relieve the sick among their suffering flock and to 'lead them by a Charitable administration and the remedies well-known and assured...' In no uncertain terms, Madame Fouquet informed priests of their duty: they were commanded not only by Christ, but also by the Church, and Charity obliged them to get out and heal.[58]

Madame Fouquet believed that the sacred character that the priest dedicated to spiritual vices should be extended charitably to corporal ills (sickness). In other words, the clergy were not doing enough to help the sick, particularly those who were both poor and sick. She wrote that she would employ all of her energy to convince the clergy to carry her book with them, to visit the poor sick, and to ensure that they did not use her remedies for profit. According to Madame Fouquet, medical care for the sick poor was 'in no way incompatible with the priesthood ... It is certain that the priests, clerics and all types of ecclesiastics who already have the direction of souls ..., are obliged according to their power to assist the people, not only through spiritual aid, but also by all means of temporal assistance or help and by consequence the preservation of life for the restitution of health...'[59] She continued by conveying to the priests that they were under an obligation to teach the seminarians not only how to prepare the remedies but also to make use of them. There is no doubt that Madame de Fouquet was a courageous woman who was not afraid to assert her authority before the Church and the medical profession. The Church, through a number of rulings, since the later Middle Ages, had ruled that priests should no longer engage in the practice of medicine. Yet, Madame de Fouquet was appealing to the priesthood to visit the sick in their homes, those she described as covered in ulcers and lesions. She was untrained in the medical profession, a woman, and she was telling the clerics that they had a responsibility to use her book of remedies. In the 1676 Lyon edition, she reiterated the idea that the secular role of remedying to the sick was not incompatible with the priest's clerical duties. She even cited a Papal Bull intended for the Jesuits, which explicitly stated that priests were permitted to perform this function when there is no access to a doctor.[60]

The influence of Madame de Fouquet's book spread well beyond the world of the poor. Members of the Faculty of Medicine in Paris examined Fouquet's 1701 edition and approved it as useful for the public. Speaking on behalf of Madame Fouquet, Monseigneur de Treguier attested to the fact that in his episcopal city of Agde, twenty-eight people had received remedies from Madame Fouquet's book in a week, and twenty-four of the twenty-eight had been cured. Monseigneur de Gap wrote that the priests in his diocese attributed the healing of illness to her remedies and that they had the effect of miracles in curing the sick.[61]

Jean Pecquet, personal physician to Madame de Fouquet's son Nicolas and Madame de Sévigné, worked with various ingredients that she used in her recipes. In particular, he conducted an analysis on the positive impact of various mineral waters when studying the circulation of the lymph system.[62] Pecquet discovered the 'chyle reservoir' which helped to confirm Harvey's important breakthrough in discovering the circulation of the blood.[63]

Madame de Fouquet was also credited with having miraculous power in curing the queen's ailments, which doctors had been unable to remedy. According to Madame de Sévigné,

> Mme Fouquet ... gave the Queen a plaster which cured her of her convulsions, strictly speaking, they were vapors. What is astonishing is the fuss everyone makes about the plaster, saying that Mme Fouquet is a saint and can work miracles ... In less than an hour her head was relieved, and there was such an extraordinary discharge of matter, so putrefied and so likely to have caused her death in the crisis of the following night, that she herself said, for all to hear, that it was Mme Fouquet who had cured her and that it was the matter since discharged that had caused the convulsions which had almost killed her the night before. The Queen Mother was convinced of it and had told the king so. ...[64]

Details of the life of Marie-Geneviève-Charlotte Darlus Thiroux d'Arconville (1720–1805), anatomist and author of *Essai pour servir à l'histoire de la putrefaction* (1766), are not as well known as those of Madame de Fouquet, although both women were from the French nobility and both were involved in charitable works.

The daughter of a government financier, d'Arconville was married at the age of fifteen to Louis Lazare Thiroux, a lawyer and member of the Paris Parlement. Their marriage produced three sons. After a bout of smallpox at the age of twenty-two, which left her disfigured, she devoted herself to her education.[65] At the Jardin du Roi,[66] d'Arconville took courses in medicine, physics, botany, chemistry, natural history and anatomy. These courses were open to the public and there were no examinations, although attendants did receive a diploma. Among those who attended these courses were the distinguished Enlightenment thinkers Diderot and Rousseau. Voltaire, Diderot, Turgot, Condorcet and Lavoisier were among d'Arconville's friends,[67] as were some important eighteenth-century scientists, including the naturalist Bernard-Germain Lacépède and the chemist Antoine Fourcroy.[68] D'Arconville produced three important scientific works: an *Essai pour servir à l'histoire de la putréfaction*; a French translation of Peter Shaw's[69] *Chemical Lectures* with extensive notes and corrections to his work; and a French translation with commentaries of Alexander Monro's *The Anatomy of Human Bones and Nerves* (Edinburgh, 1726).[70] D'Arconville translated Shaw's *Chemical Lectures* as *Leçons de chymie, propres à perfectionner la physique, le commerce et les arts*. These public lectures were delivered by Shaw from 1731 to 1733 in London and Scarborough,[71] although they were not published in Paris until 1759. The lectures focused on a wide variety of subjects including heat, air, earth, waters, solvents, fermentation and putrefaction (which would be the topic of d'Arconville's own work), analytical chemistry (animal, vegetable and minerals), wines and spirits, oils and salts, with each lecture supplemented by experiments. Presumably d'Arconville was qualified to comment on these subjects with her background education from the Jardin du Roi and her close connection with some of France's leading scientists. With respect to Shaw's 'mistakes', she commented: 'I believe that it is my duty to correct some mistakes by notes which I have added to sections which are not entirely clear or where I believed to perceive some errors.'[72] Her corrections were primarily concerned with the preparation of medicines and the making of syrups, where she would alter ingredients for potions designed for ailments such as constipation.

In addition to making revisions to Shaw's work, d'Arconville provided a lengthy preface in which she wrote that the work included a history of chemistry, types of chemistry, the goals of chemistry and comments on chemistry's relationship to medicine and pharmacy, stressing the importance for a physician to understand the intricacies of pharmacy in order successfully to practise medicine.[73] Her attention to detail reveals her knowledge of the science of chemistry. One specific example she provides relates to a recipe for purges where Shaw recommends a pint of Dulwich water. The water was named after Dulwich, at that time a village near London, where minerals were found. Shaw argued that purgative mineral waters were effective only in concentrated form by ebullition. D'Arconville countered that 'the ebullition that the author proposes here to concentrate the mineral waters and to increase their strength, appear to be ineffective, as to the contrary, there are very few mineral waters which can support the ebullition and even a degree of heat without decomposing'.[74]

D'Arconville's major work, *Essai pour servir à l'histoire de la putréfaction* (1766), is a description of approximately 300 experiments concerning meat conservation and decomposition with small sections discussing eggs, fish and human bile. She was very thorough in her research, repeating her experiments many times, not merely to be certain of her results, but to compare the results with analogous substances in terms of reaction to heat, cold, humidity and dryness.[75] She provided detailed tables listing the solutions employed in her experiments, from various wines and liquors to vinegars and waters. Her principal objective was to analyse the impact of various liquid substances on meats and vegetables.

D'Arconville's work opened with a Preface explaining her reasons for the work, its methodology and its application to medicine. In tune with the spirit of the Age of Enlightenment, d'Arconville began by stating that the primary goal of her study was usefulness, its practical use for physicians and surgeons in the cure of diseases such as smallpox, of which she had been a victim. 'Chemistry', she posited, 'has greatly contributed to the discovery and essence of many substances...'[76] She praised the scientific theories of Newton, Boerhaave, Winslow, Haller and others. She stressed how their love of science had brought great benefits to mankind.[77] She referred to the work of botanist Bernard de Jussieu (1699–1777), who had shared his knowledge of plants with her.[78] Jussieu, who invented a method of plant classification, had been one of her teachers at the Jardin du Roi where he was a demonstrator.[79]

In terms of her subject matter, the putrefaction of materials, d'Arconville argued that the knowledge of the 'substances themselves in slowing down or accelerating the process of putrefaction is important in itself'.[80] Very little research had previously been conducted and thus the field was open for observation. According to d'Arconville, the only person to research putrefaction was Dr John Pringle (1707–82),[81] general physician to the armies in England, whose results had been published by the Royal Society of London.[82] Although she intended that her work serve as a corrective to his conclusions, she denied being his rival. D'Arconville's comments concerning Pringle's experiments are lengthy and substantive, indicating her sophisticated knowledge of chemicals. With respect to Pringle's observations on septic and antiseptic substances, she noted the power of quinquina in the preservation of animal matter. However, her results were not always the same as Pringle's, especially those experiments using chamomile.

D'Arconville alleged that her work would also serve as a corrective to botanist Joseph Pitton de Tournefort's findings.[83] De Tournefort (1656–1708) was a French botanist who studied medécine at the University of Montpellier and was appointed a Professor of Botany at the Jardin des Plantes in 1683. He was the author of *Histoire des plantes qui naissent aux environs de Paris avec leur usage dans la medécine* (Paris: De L'Imprimerie Royale, 1698). D'Arconville maintained that the most precise observations and the best followed instructions were mistaken from time to time even by the most enlightened and scrupulous observers. She inquired: 'Did they not believe that coral and madrepores [mother of pores, a type of coral], and many other animal substances were made from plants composed of silt from the sea?' Even the illustrious Tournefort made this error. She claimed that coral and other similar materials seemed to belong to the 'reign of minerals' because of their durability and incorruptibility, the barnacles, the polyps and other animals of this nature belonging to this genre.[84] The table of contents in her study lists thirty-two classes of substances used to perform experiments dealing with meat preservation for periods of one day to eight months.[85]

D'Arconville might have wanted her work to be a corrective to much that had gone before, but she appears rather self-effacing in her Preface and seems in many ways to have underestimated her knowledge of the sciences: 'I am far from thinking that I have acquired on this subject the right to reconnaissance men. The little experience and research I have done on this subject have not furnished me with the assistance necessary in such a vast enterprise.' She continued by explaining that she was 'aware of all that is lacking in this essay'. She attempted to convey to her readers the difficulty in 'making great experiments in which results always differ' under circumstances in which she had limited sources available to her. These sources were those she had been able to garner from the experts. She hoped that the work would be of benefit to the public.[86] A lack of self-confidence in ability and achievements was not uncommon among women scientists of this era. Emilie du Châtelet, an important physicist of the eighteenth century also expressed considerable self-doubt.[87]

D'Arconville's third scientific and medical contribution was a French translation of Dr Alexander Monro's classic textbook, *Traité d'Ostéologie* (Paris: Guillaume Cavelier, 1759), with illustrations and accompanying notes. This work was intended to serve as a commentary on dissections and demonstrations and contained original descriptions of the cranium. D'Arconville was the first woman to make illustrations of the human skeleton.[88] The translation of *The Anatomy of Human Bones* has been attributed to John Joseph Sue (1710–92), a professor of anatomy at the Royal College of Surgery; however, historian of science, Londa Schiebinger, has recently provided convincing evidence to dispute this attribution. She concludes that the introduction and illustrator were the same, quoting the author: 'The plates were drawn under my eyes, and there were many that I had redone many times in order to correct the slightest fault.'[89] In addition Schiebinger, who has conducted extensive research on this issue, states that the introduction to the translation can be found reprinted in other works by d'Arconville. What is intriguing is that d'Arconville's drawings of the female pelvis show it as much wider than the male pelvis, while the female skull is much smaller than its male counterpart, thus stressing the differences between male and female. Schiebinger calls this a 'sexist portrayal' of the female, which was not uncommon in the eighteenth century.[90] Finally, scholars point to the fact that d'Arconville preferred to publish anonymously – perhaps reflecting her lack of confidence and modesty and attitudes towards women in eighteenth-century France – thus adding to the difficulty of determining the identity of the author.[91]

D'Arconville wrote many more works than these, often published anonymously. In addition to her scientific works, she was a prolific humanist author. She produced seventy volumes of fiction, history, poetry, drama and biographies as well as several translations of English literary works. Among these works are *Pensées et réflexions morales sur divers sujets* (Avignon, 1760), *De l'amitié* (Paris, 1761), *L'Amour éprouvé par la mort ou Lettres modernes de deux amants de vieille roche* (Paris, 1763), *Des passions* (Paris, 1764), *Mémoires de Mlle de Valcourt* (Paris, 1767), *Dona Gratia d'Ataïde* (Paris, 1770), *Vie de Marie de Médicis* (Paris, 1774, 3 vols), *Mélanges de littérature, de morale et de physique* (Amsterdam, 1775, 7 vols) and *Histoire de François II* (Paris, 1783, 2 vols).

The inclusion of Hannah Wolley among this illustrious group of female medical writers may, at first glance, appear to be rather odd. She was not of noble birth, nor was she well-connected. She was not educated by some of the finest minds of her generation as was d'Arconville. Yet, her published works focus on many aspects of medicine. It is this which she has in common with the others cited here.

Hannah Wolley was born in 1622 and what she knew of medicine she learned from her mother and elder sister who were 'skilled in physic and chirurgery'.[92] She worked in the household of a noblewoman from the age of seventeen until she was twenty-four, and with the assistance of her employer, she began to develop her expertise in cookery and medicine. She was married twice and her first marriage, to Benjamin Wolley in 1646, produced four sons. He was the master of Newport Grammar School where she also worked until he died. In 1666, she re-married, this time to Francis Chaloner, but was widowed around 1669, after which she became a governess.[93] At one point in her life, she ran her own household with great success.

Wolley was the author of seven books, mainly cookery manuals containing medical recipes and household management instructions. These include *The Ladies Directory* (1661, 1662), *The Cook's Guide* (1664), *The Queen-like Closet or Rich Cabinet* (1670, 1672, 1675, 1676, 1681, 1684; German translation, 1677), *The Ladies Delight* (1672) and *A Supplement to the Queen-like Closet* (1674, 1681, 1684). Two works which contain her medical writings include *The Queen-like Closet* and *The Gentlewoman's Companion, or, A Guide to the Female Sex*, first published in 1673 and again in 1682.[94] Not only did she write about medicine, she also practised it successfully.[95]

In common with d'Arconville, Wolley's self-declared purpose in writing was utility. Pragmatic by nature, she considered 'the end of life to be usefulness nor I know wherein our sex can be more useful in their generation than in having a competent skill in Physick and Chyrurgery, a competent estate to distribute it, and a Heart willing thereunto'.[96] Like Madame Fouquet, her work describes many waters and ointments designed to remedy all sorts of afflictions.

Her intended audience for the *Gentlewoman's Companion* was all female, 'From the Lady at the Court, to the Cook-maid in the Country.' She claimed that there was no other book like hers in any language. Her sources included her 'own experiences' in addition to 'all the books I could meet with that kind (i.e. Physick and Chyrurgery)'.[97]

The medical subjects she focused upon may be divided into three categories as set out in the table of contents: diagnosis of diseases, cures for diseases and female ailments. In the introduction she maintained that her greatest skills were in 'making salves, ointments, waters, cordials, healing any wounds not desperately dangerous; Knowledge in discerning the Symptomes of common diseases and giving such remedies as are in such causes...'[98]

The Queen-like Closet or Rich Cabinet contains 'rare recipes for preserving, candying and cookery Very Pleasant and Beneficial to all Ingenious Persons of the FEMALE SEX'. The book is dedicated to 'My much Honored Friend Mrs. Grace Buzby'[99] and contains remedies for a wide variety of ailments, including rickets in children, caudle for a sick body, cough of the lungs, consumption, colds, smallpox and infections. It lists useful pills such as Dr Lionel Lockyer's Universal Pill, curing any 'Disease curable by Physick'. Wolley claimed that it 'operates gently and safely ... subduing All Diseases, whether internal or external, as hath been experimented by persons of all sorts and sexes, both young and old, with admirable success'. She also recommended 'Mr Matthew's Diaphoretick and Diuretick Pill, purging by Sweat and Urine'.[100] Also recommended are various waters including, 'A very sovereign water' which seems to cure all manner of illnesses from the palsy to failure to conceive,[101] and 'heart water, various pastes, and plague water'.

Mary Trye, a contemporary of Wolley, was a practising physician in Pall Mall, London. She was the daughter of Thomas O'Dowde, an Irishman and self-professed chemical physician. O'Dowde was the head of a group who attempted to obtain a charter for the Society of Chemical Physicians, a newly formed medical organization in the 1660s,[102] and the author of *The poor man's physician, or the true art of medicine, as it is chymically prepared and administered, for healing the several diseases incident to mankind* (London: F. Smith, 3rd edn, 1665). This was a pamphlet of approximately one hundred pages which offered recipes for cures that had been successfully employed and a condemnation of traditional Galenic medicine. O'Dowde was a physician to the poor and often did not receive fees for his services. He might have supported himself through service to Charles I as an agent for the royalist cause. After Charles's execution, O'Dowde left England but returned to serve Charles II.[103] Unlike many physicians, O'Dowde remained in London during the plague of 1665. He died treating plague victims, although he claimed to have found a cure for the disease.[104]

The pamphlets written by Thomas O'Dowde and his daughter, Mary Trye, reflect the contemporary division and conflict in the medical world of seventeenth-century England between university trained physicians still practising Galenic medicine and empirics or *medicus*, general practitioners of physick (as Trye describes herself and her father).[105] Traditional medicine was dominated by Galenic theories which held that the treatment of disease should be through purges by bleeding and laxatives. However, from the late 1640s, English medicine was highly influenced by important continental scientists. These were the Flemish chemist Jean-Baptiste van Helmont and his son Francis Mercury, and the Swiss physician and chemist Paracelsus. Van Helmont taught that physicians should employ remedies and medicines specific to the disease. He was prosecuted by the Roman Catholic Church for applying ointment to a wounded individual rather than to his weapon. As stated above, Paracelsus was a pioneer in the use of chemicals and minerals in medicine.[106]

Mary Trye's pamphlet was directed against Henry Stubbe (1632–76),[107] a Warwick physician who had written many medical treatises in which he had attacked O'Dowde along with other practitioners of non-Galenic medicine.[108] Trye and her father were chemical physicians, non-university trained, who focused on medicines and experimental philosophy rather than academic natural philosophies.[109] Stubbe was a university trained physician, having attended Christ Church College, Oxford. He served as the king's physician in Jamaica in 1661 but returned to England in 1665 because of ill-health.[110]

He was a member of the College of Physicians and was associated with the group of physicians who would found the Royal Society.[111] Stubbe was a Galenist who claimed that good health was derived from the purification of the blood and 'by evacuations through the several emunctories of the body'. These 'evacuations' occurred through sweat, urine, faeces, saliva and phlebotomy.[112] Stubbe was an advocate of the use of chocolate as a medicine maintaining that it was a mild aphrodisiac which encouraged evacuation. He published an attack on chemists' methods.

In the mid-1660s, competition for patients between the chemists and the university trained physicians was heating up. The proposed Society of Chemical Physicians resulted in a bitter pamphlet war between the chemists and the university trained physicians. Men like O'Dowde considered themselves to be superior practitioners because of their knowledge of medicines.

In addition to his opposition to chemical physicians such as O'Dowde and Trye, Stubbe was engaged in a pamphlet war with members of the newly founded Royal Society. Many members of the Royal Society promoted a new philosophy called 'virtuosi'. 'Virtuosi' physicians were those members who considered physic to be practical in nature rather than theoretical.[113] Stubbe was opposed to this idea and wrote to one of these 'virtuosi' physicians, Jonathan Goddard, who was a member of both the Royal Society and the College of Physicians, about the dangers presented by empirics and practitioners such as O'Dowde, asking: 'Did his brethren the Experimentators first disparage ye Anceint practise of Physic as inutile; ye Censure ye Company as useless, and advance ODowds Colledge.'[114] Stubbe also complained about the support that he believed chemical physicians were receiving from members of the Royal Society. He wrote: 'but then they promoted the Anti-College of Pseudo-Chemists encouraging O'Dowde and his ignorant Adherents in opposition to the Physicians...'[115]

Mary Trye and Thomas O'Dowde were practitioners of the new chemical medicine and Mary's work was a continuation of her father's practice in London. Thomas O'Dowde dedicated his pamphlet to the most 'Reverend Father in God Gilbert by Divine Providence, Lord Archbishop of Canterbury and Metropolitan of all England'. In his 'Epistle Dedicatory', he stated the purpose of his work: 'I have published the ensuing relation of cures, together with a copy of the engagement subscribed by those learned Practisers and Professors of Chymical Physick, who under the favour and protection of his most gracious Majesty, desire to join in a Society to practice and promote the Said Art, for the relief and comfort of the kingdom after a long abuse of peoples' patience and purses by the common road practice of Galenical methods of medicines.' All chemical medicines were prepared in his own laboratory.

Mary Trye was particularly critical of the university trained physicians' lack of training in 'practical and experimental knowledge'.[116] The physicians, she claimed, 'have great learning and come to be famous in repute and yet not able to cure diseases so well as physicians of less esteem'.[117]

As she explains at the start of her book: 'I received a medicinal talent from my father; which by the instruction and assistance of so excellent a tutor, as he was to me, and my constant preparation and observation of medicines, together with my daily experience by reason of his great practice ... I made myself capable of disposing such noble and successful medicines and managing so weighty and great a concern.'[118]

The title page of Trye's pamphlet describes its purpose and content *Medicatrix, or the Woman-Physician* (1675). Part I is a vindication of her father and his medical practice: 'Vindicating Thomas O'Dowde, a Chymical Physician, and Royal Licentiate; and Chymistry; against the Calumnies and abusive Reflections of Henry Stubbe a Physician at Warwick ... A Recital of some Publications Mr. Stubbe makes in his own Life. His malice against ingenious Scrutinies, and the advantage thereof. The Life of Mr. O'Dowde: His Promotion of the Chymical Society: His noble Acquirements in Medicine: His Practice in the last great Plague.' Part II deals with her own practice of medicine and also criticizes Stubbe's practice of phlebotomy as a cure for smallpox, pleurisy and scurvy. She challenged him to cure these diseases and others such as 'gout, stone-agnes, dropsy, consumption, griping of the guts', with 'chemical medicines'. She offered the case of the gout to further her attack on Stubbe in particular and learned medicine in general. She argued that there were people who died from this disease not because there was no cure but because remedies were scarce and few physicians could master them. Attacking Stubbe, she wrote: 'for we use learning, though so useful, yet it may be mis-employed; and a man may be a scholar and yet not cure the gout, nor many other great diseases'.[119]

Trye dedicated her book to 'Lady Fisher, Wife to Sir Clement Fisher Knight and Baronet of Packington-Hall in the County of Warwick'. Lady Jane Fisher, née Lane, helped the future Charles II to escape after the Civil War. In addition to vindicating her father and advertising her own remedies, Trye provided a 'Defence of the Female Sex' and its ability to refute Stubbe's arguments. She wrote: 'And since I must take liberty to tell Mr. Stubbe that I am satisfied there is ability enough in my sex, both to discourse his envy, and equal the arguments of his pen in those things that are proper for a woman to engage.'[120] She claimed to have twelve years of experience and great skill in medicine.[121] During the years of her practice, she had met with the 'Physician of Warwick' and claimed that her 'medicines are ten times better than his'.[122]

Thus her treatise contains a justification of her own medicines and cures against those of Stubbe, to whom she sarcastically refers as Mr Medicus and Phlebotomy. In treating the 'Ladies': 'what remedies I can afford them, and what good I can do them, not by him to be pretended too, much less performed, notwithstanding all his Oratory and Trincketts: And all this great benefits is done by a few Chemical Medicines, such as he calls purgatives, diaphoreticks and Cordials...' Trye condemned Stubbe's treatment of smallpox: 'I will cure the disease of the Small Pox without Phlebotomy, or taking one drop of blood from the patient ... by my method of medicines...' She did not elaborate on the contents of her medicines but she maintained that eight women who had become ill from the pox had been cured by her. She also saved them from scarring.[123]

In order to prove her case against Stubbe and that her cures were effective, Trye provided great detail in describing one of her cases dealing with a patient named Mr Abrell, who was suffering from 'Aploxey' (sic; she was referring to epileptic fits).[124] His symptoms included speechlessness, foaming at the mouth and convulsions. She administered her liquid medicine, 'carefully and particularly prepared for him' and claimed that his condition improved within a quarter of an hour. After three to four more doses of her medicine, she reported that he was cured.[125] Directly attacking Stubbe, she wrote: 'And now Mr. Stubbe may see what a direct madness is to think that an Apoplexy can be cured without Phlebotomy.'[126] Her conclusion was that she provided safe, effectual and quick remedies.

Unlike other women discussed in this chapter, Madame Fouquet, for example, Mary Trye did not provide the reader with recipes for her curative medicines, but she did list their names in a postscript. These were 'medicinal milk', 'radiant pills', various cordials, 'balsamic drops' and other 'cleansing potions'. She stressed the fact that her medicines were pleasant and that patients were safely cured from their diseases.

Two English women authors who should be mentioned in the context of medical writing are the almanac writers Sarah Jinner (fl. 1658–64) and Mary Holden (fl. 1680s). Almanacs were best-selling publications containing astrological prophecies, predictions of all kinds, tables of sunrises, sunsets, tides, and other similar information. They were also a common source for the dissemination of medical cures and both Jinner and Holden covered diverse medical subjects in their own almanacs. According to one commentator, 'their medical advice does represent a desire to develop, organize, and preserve a body of medical knowledge specifically directed toward women and their needs, since Sarah Jinner's almanacs, for example, helped to preserve classical knowledge of abortifacient drugs increasingly omitted from male-authored texts'.[127] However, the quote about abortions is speculative. The nearest recipe for an abortion was for pills to expel a dead child.

Sarah Jinner, a self-defined 'student of physick', was a 'female radical' (presumably referring to her political activity during the English Civil War) who published a number of almanacs beginning in 1658. According to contemporary sources, she was a 'well-known practicing London astrologer'.[128]

It seems likely that Jinner's *The womans almanack: or, prognostication for ever: shewing the nature of the planets, with the events that shall befall women and children born under them. With several predictions very useful for the female sex* (1659) was the first almanac published by a woman and intended for a female audience.[129] All that remains is a fragment of the original almanac. Based upon Jinner's comments in the 'To the Reader' introduction to her

1659 almanac, the woman's almanac appears to have been an early modern version of a sex manual. She provides information to couples on how to conceive: 'I recommend the most excellent piece of Levinus Lemnius, his secret Miracles of Nature modestly treating generation and the parts thereof, and how one may be fruitful that is barren.' She urged women to know their own bodies in a not so subtle advertisement for her book: 'The reason why I commend this piece, is that our sex may be furnished with knowledge: if they know better, they would do better.' Her advertisement for the woman's almanac includes an attack on a physician for not knowing what 'a pain in the bottom of their bellies' means, calling him a 'dunce'. In terms of female complaints, the doctor is of no help.[130]

The actual medicinal recipes in this almanac are now missing, but later editions, such as that of 1660, contain comments which indicate that there were medicinal receipts in the first edition: 'To the Reader, here presented the most excellent Receipts for many things physical: we are not ignorant what, abundance of good hath been done by the Rules of Physick we have formerly published.'[131] Jinner offered both cosmetic and medical recipes. Problems tackled by her cosmetic recipes ranged from 'the removal of freckles, sweat and unwanted hair to good water for sunburning'. Her medical recipes were composed of treatments for children's problems: rickets, worms, teething, bed-wetting. Her specialities were 'cures' for reproductive issues which encouraged conception. These included ointments to prevent miscarriages, falling down of a womb, 'confections to cause fruitfulness in man or woman', 'a potion to further conception in a woman', and ailments to relieve sore nipples from breastfeeding.[132]

Jinner's impressive knowledge of human anatomy is demonstrated in the discussion of her remedies for hernias. In her description of a hernia she wrote: 'Hernia or rupture is said to be when any tumor appears in the purse of the testicles proceeding either from something descending into the cods, or from some matter going there and causing them to swell.'[133] Not only did she provide a cure, but she also specified the various types of ruptures, and how they were defined. In addition, she provided remedies for minor complaints from rotting teeth, colds and indigestion to earache and eye aches.[134]

Mary Holden was a midwife, astrologer and 'physician for female diseases' from Sudbury in Suffolk. She advertised her services in her 1688 almanac in the following manner: 'I have Excellent Remedies for all Women troubled with Vapours, Rising of the Mother, Convulsion fits ... and all other Diseases incident to my own Sex.'[135]

As an astrologist, she made predictions about diseases as well as claims to cure them.[136] Holden's almanacs, entitled, *The womens almanack for the year of our Lord 1688 being the bissextile, or leap-year: calculated for the meridian of London and may indifferently serve for any part of England*, and *The womans almanack, or, An ephemeris for the year of our Lord, 1689 being the first after bissextile, or leap-year, and from the creation of the world, 5638 ... calculated for*

London ... and may serve for any other part of England were published in 1688 and 1689. Like Jenner, Holden described herself as a 'student in Physick and Astrology', claiming that she could cure fits, cankers of the mouth and other ailments.[137] She also provided cosmetic advice, for example, 'How to make Hair as red as a foot, a lovely brown', on curing 'a Lady's Red Face' and to make 'Love Powder'.

In addition to their almanacs, both women supplied herbal remedies and gave sexual advice. As astrologers, they provided a number of services from helping with people's emotional problems to supplying information about the seasons, tides, stars and planets.[138] Astrology was a respected trade at this time with a close link to medicine. Most kings and queens had an astrologer at their court. The University of Paris even decreed that every physician have in his possession a copy of the latest almanac 'as the necessary aid to medical practice'.[139]

Largely forgotten by historians of medicine,[140] Scottish herbalist and artist Elizabeth Blackwell (1707–58), made a significant contribution to medicine and pharmacy through the illustrations and accompanying commentary in her book of medicinal herbals, *A curious herbal, containing five hundred cuts of the most useful plants, which are now used in the practice of physick ... To which is added a short description of ye plants; and their common use in physick*, 2 vols (London: J. Nourse, 1739–51). Blackwell, who was the daughter of William Blachrie, a wealthy Aberdeen businessmen, received some training in art as a child. She had a great interest in botany. Her husband and second cousin, Alexander Blackwell, had studied medicine in Leiden and no doubt Elizabeth learned something of the subject from him. He contributed to her book from debtor's prison. She wrote the book to pay for his release from prison.[141]

Elizabeth Blackwell was the first woman to produce an illustrated description of medicinal plants intended for the medical community.[142] She explained the purpose of her book in the introduction, stating that she was 'desirous to make this Work more useful to such as are not furnished with other Herbals...' She would provide 'a short description of each plant, the place of growth and time of flowering with its common uses in Physick, chiefly extracted from Mr. Joseph Miller's Botanicum Officinale with his consent and the ordinary Names of the Plant in different Languages'.[143] One example is that of the Creeping Birthwort or *Aristolochia dermatitis*. The description reads: 'The stalks grow about two foot high. The leaves are a yellow gray green, and the flowers a dull Yellow. It is a native of Spain and Italy and flowers here in May. The roots accounted opening and attenuating, good to cleanse the stomach and lungs of tough phlem [sic], promote the menses, the lochia and the birth.'[144] The Bistort or Snakeweed, which she described as [having] 'stalks of one foot, leaves of dark grape green colour', were useful for all 'fluxes and haemorrhages, incontinence and making of bloody water'.[145]

Blackwell based her drawings on plants found in the Chelsea Physic Garden.[146] She was assisted by the curator, Sir Isaac Rand, who suggested that she move her lodgings closer to the gardens so that she could maintain a more constant observation of their growth.[147] Blackwell's efforts were supported by a number of prominent medical men including Sir Hans Sloane, Dr Richard Mead and Sir James Douglas.[148] Unlike women who attempted to practise medicine, ladies who studied and contributed to natural history were respected. Botany was particularly encouraged.[149] Elizabeth dedicated her herbal to Richard Mead, MD, 'in Ordinary to his Majesty and Fellow of the Royal College of Physicians of London and Fellow of the Royal Society', and to Isaac Rand, 'Apothecary and Fellow of the Royal Society'. To Rand she wrote, 'You must know that I had no skill in Botany ... that it is you I am obliged for every compleat part of this work...' Previous herbals, such as those written by Patrick Blair and Joseph Miller, upon whose book Blackwell's was partially based, were not illustrated.[150] Before publication of her book, Blackwell sent her drawings to Sloane and Mead who offered her words of encouragement.[151] Blackwell gave a copy of her book to the College of Physicians, who commended her work, as is demonstrated on the front piece of her book.

As testified by contemporaries, medical treatises authored by women made significant contributions to scientific knowledge in Early Modern Europe. Although the women who wrote these treatises were neither properly educated in medicine nor were medical practitioners, they nonetheless made an important impact on Early Modern medicine.

5

Female Midwives and the Medical Profession

No examination of female medical practitioners would be complete without a discussion of midwives, who have been crucial medical practitioners throughout history. In the past few years, scholars have taken a new look at the role of midwives, perhaps because of the growing popularity of home births and the contemporary engagement of midwives rather than physicians in the realm of pregnancy, birth and postnatal care.

This chapter will provide a comparative overview of the most important developments in European midwifery during the Early Modern period, including subjects such as the training of midwives, attitudes held by male practitioners of medicine, and the changes that occurred throughout the Early Modern period. Leading midwives, their contributions and treatises will also be considered.[1] The chapter's focus is on midwives and midwifery in France and England – on both of which there are rich sources available – and the important contributions made by French midwives to the profession.

The term 'midwife' is an old English word which means 'with woman'. Other terms associated with midwifery are obstetrician, which means 'to stand by', and the French *accoucher*, meaning to put to bed. In French, midwives are *accoucheuses*, *sages-femmes* (wise-women) and *matronnes* (matrons – older women).[2] In Spanish, midwives are called *partenas* or *comadres de parir*, and *madrinas*[3] and in Italian, they are known as *mammane*.

Throughout history, the profession of midwifery has been dominated by women. By tradition, birth was an exclusively female endeavour. During the Middle Ages, women preferred female attendants, even female surgeons or physicians. An example of such a multi-faceted practitioner was the female physician 'Hersend' who accompanied a group on the Crusades to take care of the female camp followers.[4] Throughout the Early Modern era, men were rarely present in the birthing chamber. A physician was summoned if the birth was not going well, but even in difficult births, many midwives carried on with the assistance of local women. Physicians were not always readily available, particularly in rural settings. This scenario of a female centred birthing process continued until the seventeenth century and even into the twentieth century in some parts of Europe.[5]

Before the nineteenth century, two types of midwives can be identified in Europe: 'traditional' and 'urban'. 'Traditional' midwives received no formal training. For the most part, they were older women, often widows, whose only training came from other women, from relatives and from having had children themselves. In other words, they learned their trade by trial and error. They often worked without receiving compensation. According to one expert on the subject of midwifery, these women should not be characterized as midwives even though they delivered babies. Often they did more harm than good.[6]

Midwives carried out all of the tasks associated with birth: many provided pre-natal advice and post-partum support, they prepared special herbal teas to reduce pain, and they cut the umbilical cord. They might have taken the infant to the church for baptism or baptized the child themselves if the baby's life was in danger. Midwives were experts on diseases related to pregnancy, childbirth and childhood illnesses.

Midwives often dealt with problems other than those directly related to pregnancy and birth, such as menstrual problems.[7] Their knowledge and experience were relied upon in questions of infanticide and doubtful virginity. In France, midwives were employed by the Châtelet of Paris to examine these medical-legal questions.[8] Midwives could also be employed in cases of alleged rape, such as that of eighteen-year-old Henriette Pellicière, who had accused Simon le Bragard of rape. Three midwives, sanctioned by the city of Paris, visited the girl, examined her and found evidence of rape.[9] Before the eighteenth century, midwives were frequently more knowledgeable about pregnancy and birth than most physicians and surgeons.

Some midwives also performed abortions. This was certainly the case in seventeenth-century France where records exist of midwives who were convicted of performing this procedure. If the authorities learned of the abortion, the midwife was put to death. In one recorded abortion case, three deaths resulted: that of the mother and the foetus and of the midwife, who was sentenced to death for her crime. This was the case of Marie Le Roux, wife of Jacques Constantin, 'la dame Constantin jurée matrone de Paris', who provided an abortion for a Mademoiselle de Guerchy. Madame Constantin had been a midwife to many of the nobility who called her 'the midwife to the Queen's daughters'.[10] According to Gui Patin, Professor of Medicine at the Royal College of Paris, Constantin's house was a 'public brothel, and where a quantity of ladies go to have their babies or abortions'.[11] Patin, it seemed, was privy to information about this case as he was the confidant of the prosecuting attorney, Jacques Tardieu. Patin provided not only medical information but also theological and juridical arguments. The court case revealed that Mlle de Guerchy was seeking an abortive potion.[12] According to Patin's letters, written between 22 June and 16 August 1660, Madame Constantin was imprisoned in the Châtelet. Upon questioning, the midwife admitted that Mlle de Guerchy had died at her home, but she denied having administered any beverage. According to Madame Constantin's testimony, Guerchy died in a great deal of pain, crying about a certain beverage. Guerchy had consumed the beverage, but Constantin attested that she 'did not know what it was, nor who had made it'.[13] The foetus died in the mother's womb. The potion failed to induce an abortion. Although the court did not have any tangible evidence against Madame Constantin, she was condemned to death and hanged.[14] She was found guilty of 'having destroyed by illicit and pernicious means, the young girl's fertility'.[15] Her goods were also confiscated.

The training and regulation of midwives varied from country to country, as will be shown below, but there were also some common practices. Until the eighteenth century, most midwives were trained through some form of apprenticeship. Often this was informal and empirical and involved watching an experienced midwife practising her craft. This was particularly true for rural midwives. Some in urban centres received hospital training and a minority read the midwifery manuals which began to be published in the sixteenth century. As time went on, midwives were increasingly criticized and scrutinized by male medical practitioners for their lack of proper training and professionalism.[16] Given the diversity in training and knowledge, the quality of care provided by midwives varied widely.

The Enlightenment's emphasis on educating midwives would eventually eliminate the older, traditional rural midwife in favour of the urban trained professional. In the eighteenth century, midwifery courses were provided by the travelling midwife and instructor, Marguerite Angélique le Boursier du Coudray (1712–94). Low birth rates as well as midwifery practices were of great concern to the French state in the eighteenth century. In an effort to combat high infant mortality and infertility among women, Louis XV appointed Le Boursier du Coudray in 1759. She was the best known and most successful eighteenth-century midwife to teach obstetric practice to peasant midwives in the countryside. This royal midwife spent more than thirty years training country women in the art of childbirth, beginning her royal assignment at the age of fifty. Du Coudray trained two hundred lecturers – although only five of these were women – worked in more than fifty towns and had more than 10,000 students. She founded midwifery schools, training not only midwives, but also surgeons and doctors who would be in charge of the schools.[17] She was well-paid for her work: from 1769, she received 8,000 *livres* per year while she worked, with a retirement pay of 3,000 *livres* per annum.[18] Male surgeons did not approve of her work, but the Church did, and permitted her to baptize any babies she delivered.[19]

As a teaching aid, Madame du Coudray invented an obstetric machine, a model of a woman's pelvis carrying a foetus. This was the first life-size obstetric mannequin for the simulation of live births. Du Coudray explained her methodology and rationale for the anatomical model in her popular how-to book on delivery techniques. She wrote: 'I took the task of making my lessons palpable by having them maneuver in front of me on a machine I constructed for this purpose...' The model 'represented the pelvis ... the womb, its opening, its ligaments, the conduit called the vagina, the bladder ... I added the model of a child of natural size...' With her 'machine', Madame du Coudray demonstrated how the child could be removed from any position. The model was made from various materials, including wicker, leather and sponges.[20]

Education and training for midwives became more common in Italy after 1760. The movement towards universal public training was inaugurated by the surgeon Galli of Bologna in 1753 where he started courses first for obstetricians and then for midwives.[21] Ten years later, a physician named Antonio Piccoli, proposed the establishment of a training school for midwives in Verona. These schools would teach midwives the methods of Galli and Robert Manningham (see below). Galli began public courses, with the support of Pope Benedict XIV, at the Institute of Sciences in Bologna in 1760. Although these courses were initiated by medical men, the public authorities soon assumed responsibility for them, particularly at the municipal level. The lack of a unified nation-state in Italy meant that the local and regional authorities were able to exert considerable power.[22]

After the mid-eighteenth century, midwifery courses in Italy were influenced by Madame du Coudray. Italian courses tended to be at a higher level and last longer than those in France: at least one semester longer and with superior instruction in anatomy classes, which included dissection of cadavers not only by surgeons, but also by the midwifery students. In addition, older experienced midwives were preferred to younger women.[23]

However, as one expert argues, Italy diverged from other European countries during the eighteenth century in the sense that females still tended to dominate the midwifery profession. Men remained theoreticians rather than practitioners in part as a result of the lack of maternity homes in Italy. Public opinion and the Roman Catholic Church were also opposed to the involvement of men in obstetrics, and women themselves were strongly averse to the presence of men during birth. Midwives in Italy were held in much higher regard than in other European countries, England in particular. The Church, and later the state, both aimed at controlling midwives' activities, but were at pains not to provoke conflict with other medical practitioners.[24]

In Spain, the only training that midwives received was that gained through experience until the eighteenth century, when the *Protomedicato* recommended that an examination – that had been suspended in the mid-sixteenth century – should be reintroduced.[25] In the mid-eighteenth century, the Spanish system changed again when King Fernando VI eradicated all previous laws pertaining to the medical profession. From 1750, midwives were to be examined by the *Protomedicato*. A textbook written by Dr Antonio Medina was published to assist them with the examination. Towards the end of the eighteenth century, midwifery schools were established in the larger cities, such as Madrid and Barcelona. These schools were sponsored by two scientific societies. In 1787, a 'chair of childbirths' was established at the College of Surgery in Madrid and in 1795, Barcelona College began courses for midwives. Men could not become midwives unless they had surgical training. Although the female training for midwives was shorter and less rigorous than the male training for surgery, women could continue practising midwifery albeit under male control.

During the sixteenth century, midwifery manuals began to appear in several European countries. Previously, works on the subject of obstetrics had been published, but not midwifery manuals. The first known obstetric work in print was Albertus Magnus's *Secreta Mulierum* published in 1476. The new manuals were written primarily by physicians and their purpose was to instruct and educate the midwife in her craft. Many physicians held a low opinion of the midwife and thus felt that education was necessary to eliminate problems and deaths associated with the birthing process. However, these manuals often contained more information on sexuality than on midwifery.[26] As Helen King states, most midwives' manuals provide little specific information on childbirth.[27] Neither were they particularly useful as most rural midwives were illiterate. Those midwives who could read sometimes took exception to these books as they felt they would lose their special status if anyone who read the book could become a midwife. In other words, they felt their profession to be under threat by physicians.[28]

The first Early Modern midwifery manual was written by the German Eucharius Roesslin the Elder, a physician who lived and worked in Frankfurt. He was also the city examiner of midwives. He found them to be careless and incompetent and the cause of many unnecessary deaths.[29] Roesslin's *Der Swangern frawen und he bammen Roszengarten* or *The Rose Garden for Pregnant Women and Midwives*, was published in 1513.[30] Roesslin was clearly unhappy with the state of midwifery, writing that: 'I'm talking about the midwives all. Whose heads are empty as a hall, And through their dreadful negligence, cause babies' deaths devoid of sense. So thus we see far and about official murder, there's no doubt.'[31] Roesslin covered every aspect of pregnancy and childbirth in his book. The subjects he discussed were difficult labours, medicines to aid delivery, miscarriages, stillborn births, how to handle new babies, how to nurse and how to treat the illnesses of the newborn.[32] His book was translated into French in 1539 as *Divers Travaux* and into English from the Latin by Richard Jonas in 1540 with the title, *The Byrth of Mankynde or the Woman's Book*, and by Dr Thomas Raynalde in 1545 as *The Byrth of Mankynde, Otherwise known as the Woman's Book*. Raynalde, in his Prologue, echoed Roesslin's criticism, stating that most midwives learned their craft 'by haunting women in their labours'.[33]

As well as being a skilled practitioner, whose practical work is discussed below, royal midwife Louise Bourgeois was the author of several treatises and texts on childbirth. She became the accepted authority on the matter. Her obstetric text, *Observations diverses sur la sterilité perte de fruict foecondité accouchements et maladies des femmes et enfants nouveauz naiz,*[34] was first published in 1608 and reprinted in 1617, 1626 and 1634, with additions to each edition. The first edition is approximately two hundred pages with fifty chapters. Sections included 'General advice on midwifery', 'Advice on normal births', 'Why many women cannot carry children', 'Why the conceived infant does not last until full term', and 'Positions during childbirth', in which she advised 'standing with legs apart or sitting on a low stool with a pillow on it and put her arms on the table'.[35] Attention to birthing positions and the use of the birthing chair, and changing designs in the chair became more common in the later sixteenth and seventeenth centuries. Bourgeois paid attention to this subject in detail stating that Marie de Médicis gave birth on a red velvet birthing chair in a green walled room with the king in attendance. Bourgeois promoted the use of the chair except in difficult births.[36] Other subjects covered in the text included sterility, leucorrhea, amenorrhea and spontaneous abortion. Bourgeois examined the causes of infertility, how to determine whether or not a woman was pregnant, how to deal with premature births, and related subjects. As far as problem births were concerned, she suggested inducing premature labour in cases of contracted pelvis. For haemorrhaging problems, she recommended manual extraction, advice which she probably obtained from obstetrician Ambroise Paré or her husband, who had been Paré's student.[37] This significant contribution to midwifery literature helped to make midwifery a profession that physicians and surgeons respected rather than condemned.

The additions to the second edition of *Observations* include a 'description of the births and baptisms of the children of France', a biographical summary of what made Bourgeios become a midwife, and a section entitled, 'Advice to my daughter'. Later editions contained more sections, such as an appendix called 'A Collection of Secrets of Louyse Bourgeois' found in the sixth edition of 1634. In 'Secrets', Bourgeois recommended treatments for general illnesses including headaches, hydrophobia and catarrh and eye problems, deafness, problems with teeth, coughs, pleurisy, fevers and the plague, diseases of the liver, kidneys, bladder and intestines, and haemorrhoids.[38]

English, German and Dutch editions were also published in the course of the seventeenth century. Bourgeois's book is the first obstetric treatise written by a woman and it established her international reputation. Even by today's medical standards, the work provided sound practical advice to midwives, although the contemporary remedies would be rejected. Bourgeois stressed certain qualities as being necessary for a good midwife. These were patience, sympathy, calmness and non-intervention unless necessary: 'You should wait for the time which God has ordained and especially in normal births where there is no accident.' For relief after a difficult birth she advised wrapping the patient in the skin of a black sheep and the abdomen with hare skin.[39]

In Spain, the first handbook for midwives was written by Damián Carbón.[40] Entitled, *Libro del arte de las comadres o madrinas: del regimiento de las preñadas y paridas, y de los niños*, it was published in 1541. Carbón was born in Palma de Mallorca at the end of the fifteenth century, the seventh son of Andres Carbón and Ascenda Malferit. He was a doctor in arts and medicine. Carbón's treatise was the second of the obstetric works published in Early Modern Europe. He stated that the first part of his book was written in 1528, which pre-dated Roesslin's book. Carbón did not cite Roesslin's work.[41]

Carbón's instructions for the midwife are strikingly similar to those of Louise Bourgeois: midwives were to be experts in their art, they were to be efficient, moderate, of good character, caring and considerate of the mother, good Catholics, devoted to the Virgin Mary and all the saints and to 'have a good complexion'. They should avoid 'superstition and sorcery for it hates the church'.[42] The last characteristic was not one mentioned by Bourgeois. Interestingly, Carbón believed that women were best qualified to deliver babies because of their 'honesty'. He favoured women over men for women could 'see things' men could not. These 'secrets' should be kept to themselves 'for shame and damage that would result' if they were told to others. A physician should only be called in cases of extreme emergency.[43]

Carbón's manual was not the only text to be published in Spain during the Early Modern period, although it is the best known. Physicians Francisco Nunez and Juan Alonso Ruizes de Fontecha published texts intended for midwives. The lengthy sections in Latin demonstrate that they were also aimed at the better educated physicians.[44] In the seventeenth century, Juan Gallego Benítez de la Serna described the moral qualities of a midwife in addition to offering medical instructions.[45]

In Florence, Jacobi Tronconi published his work, an instruction manual for midwives, *De custodienda puerorum sanitate ante partum, in partu et post-partum* in 1593. He dedicated it to the grand duchess.[46] However, it was not until the mid-eighteenth century, when the Italian government was preoccupied with a declining population, that safer birthing techniques became a serious concern. In 1755, in Verona, G. Verardo Zeviani published a dissertation, *Dissertazione medica sulle numerose morti di bambini* in which he argued that 'public welfare' and an increase in the population could not be ensured as long as so many babies were dying at birth or as newborns. He blamed this on midwives' lack of education.[47] Unlike in other parts of Europe, in Italy, new manuals of instruction were often authored by priests, such as Girolamo Baruffaldi's book of instruction entitled, *Mammana istruita per validamente amministrare il Santo Sacramento del Battesimo in caso di necessitá alle creature nascenti* (The Midwife Instructed in Administering the Holy Sacrament of Baptism in Cases of Necessity in Children during Birth).[48]

In some countries, midwifery was regulated by municipal authorities in the later Middle Ages, in others such regulation was not imposed until as late as the early twentieth century.[49] Before this, the Church tended to regulate midwives through various rulings such as the Trier Synod of 1277, which stated that priests were to teach midwives how to baptize infants in danger of death.[50] Changes in the fifteenth century were the result of various factors, including the development in knowledge about the human body, the printing press, the increasing control of the state in everyday life and the concern of the Church that each infant be baptized.[51]

In the sixteenth century, in many parts of Europe and for a variety of reasons, licensing was introduced for midwives. These reasons included the secularization of medicine, which led to a more scientific approach, and the rise of the medical profession, in particular surgery, and eventually, the obstetrician-surgeon who would displace the midwife as the primary caregiver. The regulation of midwives also coincided with the witch-hunts.

The first known midwifery ordinance was made in the German town of Regensburg in Bavaria in 1452. The regulation did not stipulate any special training for midwives, only that they be examined and supervised by 'honourable, sworn women'.[52]

During the Counter-Reformation, the Council of Trent stipulated that midwives swear an oath before the local bishop – which included promising not to practise witchcraft nor to perform abortions – so they could baptize sickly infants who might die before having a Church baptism.[53]

With respect to single pregnant women, a law was passed in 1556 by Henry II of France, declaring that the midwife was responsible for discovering the identity of the father. This reversed an earlier decree in which the midwife was sworn to secrecy concerning family information. The French government was determined that an illegitimate child would not be baptized as a Protestant so Henry II passed a law decreeing that all unwed women must declare their pregnancy (the *Déclaration de grossesse*), a law renewed by Henry III in 1586 and Louis XIV in 1708.[54]

According to Edward Shorter, those midwives who went through an apprenticeship and who were organized into guilds in towns and cities were as skilled as surgeons; however, the typical rural midwife was not, and often women died in childbirth.[55] This view is echoed by another scholar who argued that 'medical men had no advantages to offer parturient women over the services of a mid-wife'.[56] During the Middle Ages some midwives, such as those who worked under Guy de Chauliac, were permitted to carry out quite complex and serious operations including embryotomies.[57] In smaller urban centres, such as Lille, midwives could learn their trade through an apprenticeship. Records exist documenting the experiences of several women from 1460 to 1696. These included Catherine Lemersne, who was the wife of a baker, Agnès Leclerc, wife of an old-clothes man, and Claire Vaas, wife of Jehan Cuvielle, all of whom spent a period of apprenticeship and then passed examinations set by doctors and received their licences from the city officials in 1460, 1472 and 1473.[58] Until the eighteenth century in Lille, training for midwifery was private. Experienced 'matrons' would provide practical training for their successors. From the late seventeenth century, we have evidence that local doctors from the medical college wrote midwifery and surgical manuals which were used for training. One of these, written by Michel Renaurt, physician of Lille, and published in 1689, is entitled, *Le chemin frayé et infaillible aux accouchements*. In Paris, before the eighteenth century, midwives were required to pass an examination at either the Châtelet or Saint-Côme which was usually a simple formality in which they were received 'otherwise for money'. The questions that they were asked were intended to discover whether or not 'they learned their trade by parroting others'.[59] In provincial cities, such as Nancy, local town officials would nominate midwives. The postulants would provide a certificate delivered by the local priest, indicating that they were of good moral standing, and practitioners of Roman Catholicism. Once 'elected', the midwives would swear an oath before the town officials.[60]

Before the 1560 law, which regulated midwives in the countryside, the only regulation to which midwives were subjected was from the Church: the local parish priest would issue them with a certificate of morality which would authorize them to practise. They received no formal training whatsoever.[61] In the larger centres, such as Paris, midwives learned certain rudimentary practices from a *matrone-jurée*. There were four in Paris. As long as all went well, the midwife performed the birth. If the birth was complicated or something went wrong, a barber-surgeon was called in, but usually too late to save either life. In France, nationwide midwifery regulations date from 1726 and 1730, although these laws were rarely followed until a national training system was established during the French Revolution.[62]

Paid or unpaid, until the eighteenth century when they were replaced by surgeons, midwifery was one of the most important occupations for women in Spain.[63] Most Spanish midwives were illiterate and Christian midwives had complete control and autonomy over the supervision of birth. They learned their trade from mothers, sisters and neighbours, who were the local midwives. Men were not involved at all until the seventeenth century except in cases of emergency or stillbirth.[64]

During the sixteenth century, secular officials demanded closer scrutiny of midwives in Spain. There were regional differences in Spain because of the various kingdoms, but one can make some generalizations. After 1523, the *Protomedicos* (the king's doctors who were the chief medical officers), no longer granted licences to midwives for whose examinations they had been responsible since 1477.[65] Midwives fell under the jurisdiction of local physicians who would examine them before the city would grant them a licence.[66] Requests were made to the *Cortes* in 1538 and 1558 for formal examinations of midwives by physicians.[67] Authorities wished to ensure safer deliveries, but they also feared that midwives were practising witchcraft.[68]

The case of one Spanish midwife who tried to overstep the line by practising medicine as well as midwifery provides an insight into the extent to which the medical community protected their monopoly. Luisa Rosado[69] was no ordinary midwife. She was midwife to the Royal House for the Abandoned and resided at Court. She was an empirically trained (we know nothing of her education), literate and licensed midwife who challenged the medical-surgical world by prescribing a remedy for miscarriages and other problems associated with difficult births such as failure to expel the afterbirth. Retention of the afterbirth was a serious problem in births at this time in Europe.[70] Rosado was licensed in 1765 by the Royal *Protomedicato* as a midwife, but this did not license her to treat difficult births. She was a fully qualified and experienced midwife who had been successful in her craft for many years when she advertised her poultice as the most effective treatment in 1770. 'The Public is informed that any woman accustomed to aborting for 15 to 20 years is offered a poultice ... The poultice keeps the baby in the womb for nine months and also strengthen bones.' In addition, Rosado claimed that she was capable of expelling the afterbirth or placenta 'within six minutes without causing discomfort or injury ...'[71] It is this latter claim that led to her problems with the medical profession, as her midwifery licence stated that she was required to have a 'physician or surgeon at difficult births and that she may not send a pregnant woman for bloodletting nor purging without a physician's order'.[72] Physicians from the *Protomedicato* rejected her petition to carry out the above procedure as they argued that surgeons were more qualified to deal with difficult births than midwives.[73] Rosado next sought approval from King Charles III in 1770 and 1771. The king approved her right to advertise. Nevertheless, her battle continued with the *Protomedicato* which maintained that her poultice did not bring about the promised results and that her medical knowledge of the placenta was incorrect.

The Spanish situation is further complicated because of the religious and cultural mix of Christian, Muslim and Jews. The Muslim minority in Spain lived in the countryside, unlike the Spanish Jews. The Muslims remained an unassimilated group on the margins of Spanish society. They kept their own culture and language especially in Granada and Valencia. Conversion to Christianity was for the most part considered to be a failure. Spain's Arabs also practised medicine according to Islamic standards. Few of their practitioners attended university although there were exceptions, such as Alonso del Castillo. They retained their own administrative apparatus to regulate medicine. In this system, doctors were examined by experienced experts before being allowed to practise medicine.[74] As with Christian medical practice, women remained outside this world. However, the prestige attached to the knowledge of the Muslim minority, including Muslim women, extended over medicine, contraception, magical practices and the occult.[75]

In 1484, the Council of Burgos banned Muslim women from practising midwifery and any form of healing.[76] Further regulations were passed in other cities throughout the sixteenth century. One of these regulations dealt with 'new Christians' practising midwifery. Spanish officials were particularly suspicious of recent converts to Christianity from Judaism or Islam. A 1565 ordinance passed by the city of Granada decreed that 'Old Christians' should avoid 'New Christian' midwives. Some Morisca[77] midwives were prosecuted by the Inquisition, which feared midwives and other female healers because it believed they were heretics practising witchcraft. However, in Valencia a list of professions dating from the sixteenth century based upon documents from the Inquisition indicated that these women continued to practise.[78] One of these was a woman named María Tubarri, a resident of Xea, who was fifty years old in 1607. She would deliver babies and then give them an Islamic baptism which involved a bathing ritual and the recitation of several sayings of Mohammed.[79] There are other cases recorded, among them that of a woman from Boset, which are similar in nature to cases of female Muslim midwives baptizing babies in the Islamic faith.[80] According to the midwife Xuxa, in the event of a male birth, a barber would sometimes circumcise the infant.[81]

Inquisitional trials in Saragossa provide further examples of female Muslim healers and midwives who would work from their homes. One such woman was Esperanza Alquezí of Aytona, a midwife who was also permitted to give the newborns the 'fadas' which marked their adherence to Islam.[82]

Jewish women also had trouble with the Inquisition. The Jewish *conversa* Béatriz Rodríguez worked as a paid midwife from 1511 until she was imprisoned by the Inquisition in 1536 and again from 1550 when she was seventy years of age. Her work included more than delivery of babies – she relieved menstrual cramps by applying herbs to the patient's abdomen. She also prepared painkillers with herbs and spices, provided post-partum care and may have baptized infants.[83]

Conversely, Christian midwives were given complete freedom of practice with an arrangement from 1567 which freed them from being examined before the licensing board as they had been from 1498. Their duties were to assist with the birth and to treat illnesses associated with childbirth and in infants.[84]

In Italy, the midwife was an essential member of the community. As with Spain, the midwife dominated birth and all aspects of obstetrics in the Early Modern period and also in common with Spain, regulations varied throughout the peninsula. In the later Middle Ages, licences were often dispensed by the king or his representatives, as in the case of Naples. These licences clearly indicate the right of women to 'exercise the profession of physician' and treat female patients and women's diseases.[85] Changes did not take place until the second half of the eighteenth century when the state began to intervene, largely as the result of pressure from obstetric surgeons.

The lack of a unified nation-state complicated matters. The typical midwife in Italy was an older woman, and age was a qualification for the job. Skills were passed on from one generation to the next. In addition to their traditional duties, Italian midwives carried out other functions. They took the babies of unwed mothers to the local hospice, in common with other European rural midwives they gave advice about contraception and provided herbs, and they carried out abortions. If the church discovered they were discussing contraception and were abortion providers, they would be excommunicated in public and punished.[86]

Throughout Catholic Europe, the Church paid special attention to midwives at the time of the Counter-Reformation for fear of heresy and witchcraft. In 1614, Pope Paul V issued a cyclical, *Rituale Romanorum*, which demanded closer supervision of midwives by the local church authorities. By the eighteenth century, parish priests were in charge of choosing the local midwife. As a rule, this would be the oldest woman who was most experienced and who no longer had family obligations.[87] The state built on the policies of the Church but was motivated by Enlightenment ideology and hoped to reduce infant mortality. The midwife took the brunt of the blame for this and thus she was subject to better training and more control. As in Spain, midwifery schools were founded and midwives were taught to read and write and were given lessons in anatomy. In Venice and the Duchies, thirteen midwifery schools were established between 1757 and 1779.[88]

The Church was also involved in the regulation of midwifery in England where local bishops were authorized in 1512 to examine midwives in addition to other medical practitioners. Before receiving their licence, midwives were required to swear an oath before the bishop or his chancellor. The midwife had to be recommended by experienced matrons and be a member of the Church of England. The oath contained several dos and don'ts: naturally the health and lives of mother and baby were primary, but it was also clear that midwifery was the province of women. No man should be in the birthing room: 'You shall be secret and not open in any matter appertaining to your office in the presence of any man, unless necessity or great urgent causes do constrain you so to do.' If the child was stillborn, it was the midwife's responsibility to 'see it buried in such secret place as neither hog nor dog nor any other beast many come unto it...' Witchcraft was clearly considered to be a threat or potential problem and midwives were prohibited from dabbling in herbal medicine as is clear from these 'items': 'You shall not in any wise use or exercise any manner of witchcraft, charm or sorcery, invocation or other prayers that may stand with God's laws and the King's. You should not give any counsel or minister any herb, medicine, or potion, or any other thing, to any woman being with child whereby she should destroy or cast out that she goeth withal before her time.' During the eighteenth century, after taking this oath, the midwife would pay up to eighteen shillings.[89] Some midwives paid high fees to obtain a licence, as high as two pounds to practise.[90] But many remained unlicensed until the early twentieth century. It was only in 1872 that the British obstetric society granted diplomas to midwives, by which time there were a few London maternity hospitals which trained midwives.[91] In the countryside, the local women themselves were in control of their profession. A meeting would be held in the parish to decide who the most capable midwives were, based on criteria such as who had delivered the greatest number and the healthiest babies.[92] For the most part, English women were untrained during the period under consideration here. The only courses available were privately run by surgeons such as John Maubry of Bond Street, London.[93] His courses were directed towards man midwives and were theoretical rather than practical in content. In 1739, Robert Manningham, a London practitioner, opened an infirmary in the Saint James area for poor women to give birth and as a training place for male and female midwives. William Smellie, a famous obstetrician, started a similar course, and in 1741 he claimed to have given over 280 classes to more than 900 surgery students, excluding the numbers of midwives.[94]

In France, Louise Bourgeois (1563–1636), midwife to Queen Marie de Médicis, wife of Henry IV, dedicated to her life to the improvement of midwifery. She set new standards for the profession and contributed to France's reputation as the leading European country in the field of midwifery. Important changes took place in midwifery during the sixteenth century, which are crucial to understanding the role of female midwives such as Bourgeois, her contemporaries and those who followed her. These changes are summarized below.

Born in 1563, Louise Bourgeois Boursier[95] came from a wealthy and influential family. Her father Charles Bourgeois, was the owner of several properties in the wealthy Saint-Germain section of Paris. Louise received a good education and was one of the first graduates of the school for midwives established at the Hôtel Dieu hospital in the late sixteenth century. She passed the official test giving her a licence to practise in 1598. The Hôtel Dieu school for midwives was the most prestigious in Europe and offered the most skilled training. The hospital itself dated from the seventh century. Its maternity hospital existed from the fourteenth century with a record of midwives (mistress of births or *maîtresse des accouchées*) from 1385.[96] In 1560, midwifery was attached to the College of Surgery. In 1630, an 'Office of births' was created which took in about three to four students every trimester. They practised their birthing skills on the poor of the city. They did not receive any theoretical training and the course lasted for three weeks.[97]

Bourgeois married Martin Boursier, one of the king's surgeons, and a former student of Ambroise Paré in 1584. They had five children, including one daughter to whom Louise dedicated one of her many treatises, *L'Instruction*.[98] She dedicated her major work, *Observations diverses sur la sterilité* to Marie de Médicis in addition to a number of royal physicians. Bourgeois founded a monastery as a school for midwives and was chief midwife at the Hôtel Dieu by 1626.[99] In addition, she had a thriving practice in the Latin Quarter of Paris.[100] Like many physicians and surgeons at this time, Bourgeois was critical of unskilled midwives and their practice. She referred to them as 'so presumptuous as to think that if after a few efforts they could not deliver a woman then, for better or worse, all is lost'.[101]

However, not all of Bourgeois's own deliveries were successful. She had an unfortunate case in 1627, near the end of her career, when the Duchess of Orleans died in childbirth, apparently from puerperal peritonitis. Louise was attacked by several doctors in their report of the death and to all intents and purposes was blamed for it. Bourgeois felt compelled to defend herself and responded with a pamphlet, *Apologie de Louyse Bourgeois, dite Bourcier, sage-femme de la reine mère du roi, et de feue Madame; contre le Rapport des médecins* (Paris, 1627). According to Bourgeois, the duchess did not die as a result of part of the placenta being retained in the body. Rather, Marie de Bourbon-Montpensier had died from an 'inflammation of the tissues in the lower abdomen'.[102] In addition to a discussion of the causes of the duchess's death, this work provides a defence of Bourgeois's career as a midwife. She wrote that she had,

> practiced my profession now for fully thirty-four years, faithfully, diligently, and honorably, and acquired not only good certificate, after various examinations, but have also written books treating on this subject, which has been printed and published in several editions and were translated into foreign languages, for which trouble many noted physicians have rendered me thanks and have gladly confessed that they were of great use to humanity.

Bourgeois's most recent biographer argues that this treatise is also a strong defence of the midwifery profession. Bourgeois maintained that in certain cases, such as the one described here, doctors should defer to midwives who had the practical experience which medical men lacked.[103]

Bourgeois's knowledge influenced other practitioners, such as François Mauriceau (1637–1709), a seventeenth-century surgeon and obstetrician who also trained at the Hôtel Dieu. He became the head of the faculty of the Collegium of Paris Surgeons at the Saint-Côme. He was the author of several obstetric treatises, the most significant of which was *Traité des maladies des femmes grosses et accouchées* (Paris, 1668), which helped to lay the foundation for the science of obstetrics.[104] It was ironic that Bourgeois could be seen to prepare the way for men like Mauriceau, who would come to replace competent and educated midwives such as herself. Bourgeois is considered to be 'the principal link between the Renaissance development of midwifery and the pre-modern phase of obstetrics' in the sense that she was educated by and consulted with the surgeons who would replace midwives.[105]

During the Renaissance period, a number of medical men and scientists concerned themselves with the state of midwifery. Cultural factors account for this change at this point in history. One of these was the scientific revolution which would demand the 'displacement of the intuitive model of knowledge acquisition by a scientific or rational model of acquisition'. This new ideology of rationality dominated male-only institutions: universities, academies and hospitals. Midwives stressed intuition and knowledge based on practical experience, while university trained physicians stressed theoretical knowledge, and not only mistrusted practical knowledge but believed it to be inferior.[106] An additional reason for this change was the fact that midwives, although experienced, often received no formal training and before the foundation of the school for midwives at the Hôtel Dieu hospital in 1530 were largely ignorant of the basics of hygiene and anatomy. By the sixteenth century, it was clear to the medical men that many midwives were ill-equipped for their important role. Surgeons in particular were concerned for the health of the mother and baby. One of these physicians who wrote about the poor quality of midwifery was François Rabelais who expressed his concern over the incompetence of many midwives. This was made plain in his description of the midwives in his novel *Gargantua*:

> A little while after she began to groan, lament and cry. Then suddenly came the midwives from all quarters, who groping her below, found some peloderies, which was a certain filthy stuff, and of a taste truly bad enough. This they thought had been the child, but it was her fundament, that was slipped out with the mollification of her straight entrail, which you call the bum-gut, and that merely by eating of too many tripes, as we have showed you before. Whereupon an old ugly trot in the company, who had the repute of an expert she-physician, and was come from Brisepaille, near to Saint Genou, three score years before, made her so horrible a restrictive and binding medicine, and whereby all her larris, arse-pipes, and conduits were so oppilated, stopped, obstructed, and contracted, that you could hardly have opened and enlarged them with your teeth...[107]

Ambroise Paré, the physician who 'restored obstetrics in France', was also critical of the 'impudence of the matrons'.[108] Others – apart from Bourgeois and Mauriceau whom we have mentioned above – who helped to make great progress in midwifery in this period were Jacques Guillemeau (1550–1613), Paul Mortel (d. 1703) and Guillaume Mauquest de la Motte (1665–1737).[109] Guillemeau's *De l'Heureux Accouchement des femmes...* (Paris, 1609), contains two chapters directed to midwives delineating their skills and duties. It is clear that Guillemeau believed that the surgeon or physician was the primary care-giver, while the midwife was a mere assistant in the birthing process.[110]

No discussion of sixteenth-century French obstetrics would be complete without mentioning Laurent Joubert (1529–83), who was a professor of medicine at Montpellier. His *Traités des erreurs populaires et propos vulgaires touchant la medicine et le regime de santé*, first published in 1570, was one of the most significant works condemning the practice of many midwives. His major criticism against midwives was their lack of understanding of ailments and diseases peculiar to women. These diseases included the suffocation of the child in the womb, miscarriage and the process of giving birth. In addition, he attacked them for not calling upon the assistance of a physician in difficult births.[111] He dedicated his work to Marguerite de Navarre whom he treated for infertility, which was one of his major concerns.[112] The treatise was published many times during the later years of the sixteenth century and translated into Italian in 1592.[113] Joubert was not opposed to women practising midwifery and he even praised the good midwives such as 'donne Gervaise, matron at Montpellier, a true midwife, well instructed...',[114] he merely advocated their proper education and regulation. Texts similar to Joubert's led to the Paris ordinance of 1560, *Statuts et reiglements ordonnez par toutes les matrons ou saiges femmes de la ville, prevosté et vicomté de Paris*. It was reprinted with some additions in 1587. This regulation stipulated that every midwife would follow a prescribed course taught by surgeons for a certain term and would then be required to sit an examination. She would be subject to strict regulations. These included baptizing the baby and informing the authorities of secret births, abortions, infanticides and other transgressions.[115]

During the latter years of the sixteenth century, there were conflicts between male practitioners and midwives over the monopoly of the profession, but for the most part, male midwifery practice in France remained limited until the middle of the eighteenth century. The respect for tradition, and taboos – in particular female modesty with respect to nudity – meant that men remained out of the birthing room. Nevertheless, the period between the mid-seventeenth and mid-eighteenth centuries was one of great change in the history of French obstetrics.

Yet another French physician who wrote on midwifery and birth was Philippe Hecquet (1661–1737), who was doctor to the nuns at Port Royal and Dean of the Faculty of Medicine of Paris. Hecquet was the author of a tract in which he defended female midwives and opposed the entry of men into this area of medicine. In his treatise, *De l'indécence aux hommes d'accoucher les femmes* (Paris: Etienne, 1708) Hecquet inveighed strongly against the attempt by surgeons and male midwives to replace female midwives. He maintained that it was the natural order of things for women to deliver babies. The profession of midwifery was a natural right of woman.[116]

Hecquet argued that birthing had been performed by women since the beginning of time, and in *De L'indécence*, he provided a historical overview of the role of midwives in history beginning with the Hebrews. What is interesting in this sketch is his praise for the quality of female doctors in the ancient societies of Egypt, Israel, Greece and Rome. He indicated that the Greeks even had female doctors who served their queens.[117]

Unlike most medical men of his age, Hecquet did not believe in the natural inferiority of women. His treatise was not only a plea for midwives but a defence of women. Hecquet insisted that women possessed equal intelligence to men, that they were created by the same hand, and were of the same material and organization.[118] Moreover, women were better designed to deliver babies than men and were more adroit. Hecquet also believed that midwives should extend their practice of medicine to include the treatment of diseases of women and children in the manner of the midwife Louise Bourgeois.[119]

In order to discourage surgeons from delivering babies, Hecquet felt that he had to prove that midwives' knowledge of medicine was superior to that of surgeons. If some midwives were lacking in education and knowledge of the science of their subject, they should spend a period of apprenticeship at the Hôtel Dieu in Paris.[120]

However, Hecquet was primarily opposed to the presence of men at the birth of children, regardless of whether or not they were medical practitioners, on grounds of modesty. His Christian faith underpinned this belief, and he thought that women lost their innocence and purity if men were present at a birth. According to Hecquet, who based his beliefs on those of the Church fathers, the practice of having men present was 'repugnant to nature itself as well it is contrary to the modesty which is natural to women'.[121]

In England, as in other parts of Europe, midwifery or obstetrics was one aspect of medicine which for a long time was exclusively female. However, changes began to occur during the seventeenth century, and it was in the British Isles – primarily in England – that the most heated controversy around midwives occurred.[122] The debate over midwifery was the outcome of the increasing professionalization of medicine and the secularization of society. At the heart of the issue was the application of monopolistic privileges designed to exclude women. Examples of the attitude come from prominent men of science. The physician and scientist William Harvey in his 1651 pamphlet condemned midwives for their ignorance. Dr James MacMath in *The Expert Mid-wife: a treatise of the diseases of women with child and in child-bed* (Edinburgh: G. Mosman, 1694) argued that midwives were in league with the devil.[123]

The debate focused on the question of whether or not a male midwife or doctor rather than a female midwife should be employed in cases of difficult delivery. As MacMath commented, 'Natural labour, where all goes right and naturally, is the proper work of the Midwife, and which she alone most easily performs aright, being only to sit and attend Nature's pace and progress ... and perform some other things of smaller moment, which Physicians gave midwives to do, as unnecessary and indecent for them...'[124]

Key players in the debate were the Chamberlen family. William Chamberlen and his two sons were members of the Barber-Surgeon's Company and practising obstetricians. Peter Chamberlen was the queen's surgeon. What made them unusual and ahead of their time was their use of forceps, which they tried to keep secret. They attempted to dominate the profession of midwifery by incorporating it into the College of Physicians, which was opposed by the college in 1616 and by the House of Lords in 1634.[125] Midwives had petitioned Charles I in 1634 to grant them a charter for their incorporation into a society to control the standards of their practice. This was opposed by the physicians of the time. In England, midwives were still under the control of the Church, which was not the case in continental Europe where municipal councils granted licences. A charter would allow for a general standard of practice and regulation of their trade. It would also end the Church's control of midwifery. The Chamberlens did not support the midwives' cause per se, but only wanted to further their own position as the men who would control the distribution of licences.[126] The 1634 petition to the House of Lords originated with Chamberlen's nephew, Peter, and was opposed by a number of midwives who did not trust the Chamberlens and saw that they wanted to control them. This group was led by a Mrs Shaw and Mrs Whipp.[127]

Support for female midwives came from physician and herbalist Nicholas Culpeper who wrote *A Directory for Midwives*. He opposed men becoming midwives because of the elitism and exclusiveness of the medical profession. Culpeper's book was designed to teach midwives how to upgrade their skills so they could deal with difficult births and it was dedicated to them. He complained about the seriousness of not allowing the proper education of midwives: 'What an insufferable injury it is, that men and women should be trained up in such ignorance...' He stated that he would write his book in English so all could understand it. And the book would be short and simple: 'If you please to make experience of my Rules, they are very plain and easy enough; neither are they so many, that they will burden your brain, nor so few that they will be insufficient for your necessity. If you make use of them, you not need call for the help of a man-midwife, which is a disparagement not only to yourselves but also to your profession.' He closed with the words: 'All the perfections that can be in a woman, ought to be in a midwife; the first step which is, You know your ignorance in that part of Physick which is the basis of your Act. When you know what you want, then you know what to crave ... Grave Matrons, be diligent in your Office, and be as careful as diligent...' [128] The chapters in his book provide the details of subjects of which he felt the midwives were ignorant: details of the female anatomy, the conception of a child and its 'furthering', miscarriage, labour, the lying in and the nursing of children.

Jane Sharp and Elizabeth Cellier,[129] both English midwives, also worked to defend and organize female midwives. Sharp was the author of the first educational textbook on midwifery by a woman, *The Midwives Book, or the Whole Art of Midwifery Improved* (1671), which was reprinted four times by 1725. She was a successful midwife who had been practising for thirty or more years when she wrote her manual. *The Midwives Book* is 418 pages in length and is structured in a similar fashion to other midwifery manuals at this time. She combines 'Galenic, humoural theory, renaissance speculations about reproductive anatomy' with birthing techniques and remedies.[130] Sharp feared the threat by men, who had an educational advantage, to female midwives:

> Some perhaps think, that then it is not proper for women to be of this profession, because they cannot attain so rarely to the knowledge of things as men may, who are bred up in Universities, Schools of Learning or serve their Apprenticeship for that end and purpose, where Anatomy Lectures being frequently read the situation of the parts both of men and women ... are often made plain to them. But that objection is easily answered, by the former example of the Midwives amongst the Israelites, for, though we women cannot deny that men in some things may come to a greater perfection of knowledge than women ordinarily can, by reason of the former helps that women want; yet the Holy Scriptures hath recorded Midwives to the perpetual honour of the female sex ... It is commendable for men to employ their spare time in some things of deeper Speculation than is required of the female sex; but the art of Midwifery chiefly concerns us.[131]

The lack of education and of language skills required to read many medical texts still in Latin, were not the only disadvantages of female midwives as is demonstrated in the career of midwife Elizabeth Cellier.[132] Cellier's aim was to improve the lot of midwives to which end she tried to unite them into a corporation. She did get the government to establish a corporation, but that was as far as it was taken. She was arrested on a number of occasions for her activities, most notably for libel in a pamphlet entitled *Malice Defeated*.[133]

Cellier also wrote a treatise, *A Scheme for the Foundation of a Royal Hospital* (1687), in which she envisioned a proper college for midwives. She proposed that only 1000 midwives should be admitted in the first instance, that they should pay a fee of five pounds sterling upon being admitted and for each year in attendance. The money from the fees would be employed for the purpose of building 'one good, large and convenient House, or Hospital'. There would be 'twelve lesser convenient houses, in twelve of the great parishes, each to be governed by one of the twelve Matrons, Assistants to the Corporation of Midwives, which Houses may be for the taking in, delivery and month's Maintenance, at a price certain of any woman...'

The children born to these women would be provided an education in the 'Arts and Sciences, according to their several Capacities...'[134] All children would learn to read and male children would be separated from their female counterparts. The sexes would learn gender-oriented skills: the boys learning crafts such as watch-making, painting, engraving and carving, while the girls would be instructed in sewing, plain-work and lace-making.[135] James II welcomed her plan and promised to incorporate the midwives. Her pamphlet *To Dr.— An Answer to his Queries, concerning the Colledg of Midwives,* written a year later, was a response to a critique of her plan for the school and incorporation of midwives. Her proposal for a college called for female governors and instructors with periodic visits from a physician at Oxford or Cambridge who would be appointed by the king.[136] We do not know the author of the critique, but it was likely another Chamberlen, Dr Hugh Chamberlen, a male midwife and grandson of Dr Peter Chamberlen. Cellier defended midwives by stating that women were the first physicians going back to the ancients. This is not unlike the tactics employed by Sophia Jex-Blake in the nineteenth century when putting forward a case for women attending medical schools in the United Kingdom.

Throughout the eighteenth century, women continued to lose ground. The number of male midwives increased dramatically and they began to take over routine cases. They became responsible for everything related to childbirth and children: pregnancy, delivery, postpartum care and even childhood diseases. Thomas Young (1726?–83), first professor of midwifery at Edinburgh University, described the establishment of his chair of midwifery at the University of Edinburgh in the following terms: 'Disturbed by the many fatal consequences that have happened to women in childbirth, and to their children, through the ignorance and unskilfulness of midwives in this country and city, who enter upon that difficult sphere at their own hand, without the knowledge of the principles upon which they are to practice that art, the town council added a chair of midwifery to those of anatomy, chemistry, institutes of medicine, practice of medicine and botany in the formation of its new medical faculty.'[137]

As has been argued by one expert on the history of gynaecology, the whole movement away from midwives was really 'an attempt to substitute women's customs for new medical rites masquerading as scientific practices founded in "objective knowledge"'.[138] Among the reasons for this change, which resulted in the marginalization of the female midwife, were the use of forceps by doctors, fashion, formal education and secularization as the Church lost its role in licensing midwives. The Industrial Revolution also played a part as governments encouraged larger populations and focused more closely on infant deaths. Male midwives, it was thought, had the expertise females did not possess. The upper classes felt that it was more fashionable and socially acceptable to have a man deliver a baby. The old question of education appeared once again. Female midwives were considered to be ill-educated and unprofessional. Some midwives, like Sarah Stone author of the *Complete Practice of Midwifery* (1737), entered the debate and tried to protect midwifery as a female profession. She wrote that a 'midwife's business' was 'only to be well instructed in her Profession'.[139] Stone wanted to improve the education of midwives by teaching them the basics of female anatomy and disease.[140] In this she foreshadowed the work of William Smellie. Both wanted to 'keep instruments and violent methods to a minimum'. Smellie however, was partial to male practitioners, believing that the female midwife should always consult a doctor when in difficulty.[141]

Elizabeth Nihell (b. 1723), a leading London midwife, led the fight against the use of forceps. In 1760, she published a pamphlet opposing the use of forceps and other instruments and the incursion of the male midwife into the female practice.[142] She claimed, in her preface, not to be attacking any individual, but she specifically addressed her pamphlet to the male practitioners, 'who in these later times have ... added new and worse errors of their own to those bequeathed to us by the ancients'.[143] What particularly angered her was the arrogance of the male midwife whose 'subtleties of theory, which, when reduced to practice, are infinitely worse than any deficiency in some particular female practitioners'. Men midwives were no better at the practice of their craft than women. In fact, she argued, 'the surgeons, in form of men midwives, have been the death of more children with their speculum matrices, their crotchets, their extractors or forceps, their tire-têtes, than they have preserved'.[144]

At the time it seemed as if these women were fighting a losing battle in the sense that male practitioners had taken over the birthing process. However, history seems to have come full circle. Today, midwives are licensed practitioners in many countries, participating fully in pre-natal, birth and post-natal care.

6
The Healing Care of Nurses

Throughout history, nurses have played a significant yet often overlooked role within the healing community,[1] either ignored or disparaged by historians of medicine. Gender has unquestionably played a role in the historiography of nurses. The historical fact that women have dominated the nursing profession and men the medical profession has contributed both to the paucity of sources and the often negative view of nurses and nursing. The reality is that nurses have always provided the majority of the hands-on care given to sick people and that the nursing and medical professions share a long history of similar functions and tasks.

Written records of women nurses date as far back as Hammurabi's Code.[2] The Greek Hippocratic Corpus contains instructions for physicians' apprentices to perform what would be considered nursing duties: 'Let one of your pupils be left in charge, to carry out instructions without unpleasantness, and to administer the treatment ... Never put a layman in charge of anything, or otherwise, if a mischance occur, the blame will fall on you.'[3]

This chapter surveys the significant contribution made by nurses to the care of the sick, often the poor sick, from the Middle Ages to the late Renaissance. In addition to chronicling the important but neglected role of nurses in the history of medicine, this chapter aims to redress the often negative image of the nurse as incompetent and uneducated.[4] Vern Bullough and Bonnie Bullough have suggested that the negative image of nurses derives from the time when women came to dominate what had been a primarily male profession in Greek and Roman cultures. At this time, the status of nurses started to decline. As the occupation developed, two types of nurses emerged: those in religious orders, who were respected for their devotion, and those who were grouped with the lowest class of cooks and servants.[5] Some nurses were reformed prostitutes, hence the use of terminology such as *filles repenties* and *péniteuses* for nurses in France. Single women and widows – women who did not fit the acceptable norms of society – also became nurses, working both inside hospital institutions and in the community, ministering to the sick poor. Hospital administrators preferred older women as they were less tempted to become engaged in immoral behaviour with patients.[6] Hospitals were originally either 'houses or hostels for the reception and entertainment of pilgrims, travellers, and strangers; a hospice', or 'charitable institutions for the housing and maintenance of the needy; an asylum for the destitute and infirm'.[7] The medieval hospital was a church-run facility and since the focus of patient care was the soul rather than the body, mortality rates were high. Physical treatment involved the feeding and cleaning of the patient. Medical remedies were limited and basic. Blood-letting and the use of leeches were common. Minor surgery was also performed.[8]

It is important to be aware of the fact that nurses, like most other women, were denied any formal education. During the twelfth and thirteenth centuries with the creation of universities, knowledge was distributed between major and minor faculties. Nursing was not recognized in these faculties. Nurses were under the direction of physicians[9] who taught the nurses what they needed to know in terms of new remedies and the administration of medicines so that they could best assist the doctors.[10]

With the establishment of universities, licensing for medical practitioners became the norm throughout Europe. Thus, from the twelfth century onwards, nurses, like all other female medical practitioners, were practising without a licence. Nevertheless, as recent scholarship has observed, nurses performed many functions which could not be differentiated from those carried out by university trained doctors, and often 'nursing healing activities were superior to those of physicians', presumably because the university trained practitioner received more of a theoretical than a practical education.[11]

The etymological origin of the term nurse is from the Latin *nutricius* or *nutritius* meaning nourishing. This word developed into the old French *norrice* or *nurice* and the Middle English *norse* and *nurice*.[12] One of the earliest citations of 'nurse' dates from 1425. It describes a person 'who takes care of, looks after another or advises another'.[13] Another early reference to the term nurse is from Shakespeare's *A Comedy of Errors* (1590). Adriana explains her role as a nurse: 'I will attend my husband, be his nurse, Diet his sickness, for it is my office, And will have no attorney but myself; And therefore let me have him home with me.'[14] The 1989 edition of the *OED* defines a nurse as a 'person, generally a woman, who attends or waits upon the sick; now especially one properly trained for this purpose'.[15]

Historically, the care of the sick was closely connected with religion and acts of charity. The rise of Christianity changed the understanding of illness from a naturalistic to a supernatural phenomenon. The Gospels and early Christian writings call on Christians to take care of the sick.[16] James's Epistle echoes Matthew when he calls upon Christians to take care of their brethren's 'physical needs'.[17] The principal motive in caring for the sick became Christian charity and this led to the establishment of places where people could be cared for. Infirmaries were attached to monasteries where elementary medical care was provided for the sick for religious as well as medical reasons. Patients were given food and warmth. This was the beginning of the hospital.[18]

Bishops were placed in charge of the sick and poor and hospitals began to be built. Basil, bishop of Caesaria, built one of the earliest, the Basiliade, in 370 AD. This was a hospital for the poor sick.[19] In Rome, the earliest hospital was founded in 390 by Fabiola, a wealthy widow who had converted to Christianity and desired to do good works.[20] Priests, sisters and deacons gave alms to the poor and practised empirical medicine.[21] In France, hospitals were often private and religious establishments. The Hôtel Dieu in Lyon was founded in 542 and the Hôtel Dieu in Paris in 651.[22] These establishments provided medical care as well as charitable assistance in the form of alms. They often also provided hostel accommodation, a place for people in need to stay. The Hôtel Dieu in Lyon was founded by the archbishop of Lyon with Childebert I, the son of Clovis, and his wife.[23] The archives refer to the nurses as '*servantes chambrières*', '*filles repenties*', '*pénitentes*', and in fact, many of them were former prostitutes, initially admitted as patients. Others were widows.[24] Regulations were adopted in the mid-sixteenth century when aspiring nurses were required to make formal applications to the Mother Superior and were placed on probation for a year. In common with most hospitals, the Hôtel Dieu in Lyon was understaffed and the nurses were overworked.[25]

The Council of Aix of 817 re-affirmed that the most important role of monasteries was to care for the poor. Even before this declaration, Benedict had stated in his Rule that: 'Before all things and above all things care must be taken of the sick.'[26]

The Crusades inaugurated a new era in health-care by bringing to Europe the higher standards of the Arab hospitals through the various military orders of nurses. Arab hospitals had been constructed from the eighth to the tenth centuries. According to recent scholarship, the first Islamic hospital dates from 707 CE and was founded by the Umayyad caliph al-Walid (705–15 CE) in Damascus to care for lepers.[27] These hospitals, which were well funded institutions and massive buildings, displayed the wealth and power of the princes. They were far superior in medical care and hygiene to their western counterparts. Suggested reasons for the superiority of the Islamic hospital are their secular nature and emphasis on Galenic medicine,[28] but Arab medical knowledge also superseded that of the West at this time, not least because Arabs had retained Greek knowledge during the early Middle Ages. The three major hospitals of the Muslim world were the Adudi Hospital in Baghdad, the Nuri Hospital in Damascus and the al-Mansuri Hospital in Cairo. The hospital in Baghdad was staffed by twenty-four physicians. Orderlies and female nurses cared for the patients.[29] Like the Byzantine hospitals, in the al-Mansuri Hospital there were separate wards for male and female patients. The hospital also served as a teaching institution complete with a library and a lecture theatre.[30]

The wounded and sick crusaders required medical care, and out of this need, the military nursing orders evolved. They were composed of monks, nuns and lay people. International standards were established for nurses, who visited the sick every morning and evening. They controlled the supplies and changed bed linen. Since contact with a physician was minimal, the nurses were the primary medical care-givers.[31]

One of the most important of the military orders of nurses was that of the Knights Hospitallers of St John of Jerusalem.[32] The order began with two hospitals that were founded in Jerusalem by Italian merchants from Amalfi in 1050. There were separate orders for men and women; the female order was founded by Agnes of Rome and dedicated to St Mary Magdalene – initially as a purely nursing order which only later developed into a military order – and the men's order was dedicated to St John the Almoner. The knights opened a 1000-bed hospital directed by the monk Peter Gerhard. Many of the practices in this hospital were modern by comparison with other European hospitals: these included the keeping of records in the form of patient charts and patient prescriptions. The women carried out nursing duties, which included feeding, medicating and caring for the patients when the men were away. After the capture of Jerusalem, the order moved to Malta and the women gave up nursing.[33] There is no evidence that this order nursed in Spain.[34]

The Hospitaller order of the Holy Spirit was founded by Guy de Montpellier in 1075. He established in his native town a lay community for the care of the sick under the patronage of the Holy Spirit.[35] This order, which had its own statutes, consisted of religious brothers and sisters in addition to the lay members of the community, who were called oblates, meaning that they accepted a life of dedication and religious sacrifice. All workers lived in the same hospital. The order was approved by Innocent III in 1198. Guy de Montpellier's hospital was controlled by Rome. The oblates of Florence have nursed in hospitals from the thirteenth century to the present day. The oblate order spread throughout Europe with eighty-seven houses by the fifteenth century.[36]

The 'third order' Franciscan Hospitallers originated in the fourteenth century.[37] The group was composed of associations of women whose aim was to care for the poor and sick. These associations came together under the auspices of the Franciscans in 1388. They were first and foremost nursing sisters who were primarily located in France and the Low Countries. By 1500, they had about one hundred houses. They established their own hospitals, but often nursed the sick in their homes.[38] They were different from the Béguines (who are discussed below) in the sense that they were officially sanctioned by the Church and thus thrived.

Early nurses were nuns, and were called nursing sisters, but the oldest order founded specifically as a nursing order was that of the Augustinian sisters, who provided nursing care at the Hôtel Dieu[39] hospital in Paris. Founded in the Middle Ages, the Hôtel Dieu hospitals in France served as hospices, orphanages, homes for the aged, maternity centres for pregnant girls and accommodation for pilgrims. They also provided medical care, particularly for the poor.[40] The Augustinian sisters nursed at these institutions for 1200 years. They spent twelve years on probation and were permitted to leave the hospital only in order to carry out hospital duties. Wards in the hospital were named after saints. Regulations for French hospitals were passed in 1212 for the first time by the bishops in council. The bishops passed statutes ordering that all nurses take vows of poverty, chastity and obedience and wear a religious outfit, a white robe. The number of nurses should be kept to a minimum as these hospitals relied on charity. The consequence of this decree for the nurses was an even heavier work load. Nurses were under the control of the brothers or male nurses.[41]

The nursing sisters were given great responsibilities, including the administration of medicines.[42] An experienced sister was placed in charge of the drug department and delivered the medicines to the wards accompanied by a younger sister and a boy assistant.[43] Drugs were plant-based and mainly consisted of enemas and lotions.[44] At times there were problems with sisters not following the physicians' orders in making up the medicines. The hospital attempted to solve this problem by employing an apothecary to teach the nuns the basics of pharmacy. A few of the nuns abused this power by selling drugs off hospital premises.[45]

Nursing care in hospitals during the Middle Ages covered the patients' basic physical needs: food, drink, cleanliness, dressing ulcers and wounds. Hygiene was not an important consideration, and plumbing, heating and lighting were primitive or non-existent. Nurses in Paris would take the dirty linen to the Seine for washing.[46] Moreover, because these women were nuns, the priests forbade them from assisting doctors with gynaecological examinations, from caring for those patients suffering from venereal diseases, from assisting in births, from diapering male infants and from administering enemas to men.[47]

Since the Church would not properly fund the hospital, it was understaffed and the nurses were neither properly trained nor fed and they were terribly overworked. Their day began at 4 a.m. and they were still working after 9 p.m. They had prayers and religious duties ten times per day in addition to their nursing work. They endured difficult and often life-threatening conditions as depicted by Cardinal de Vitry in the thirteenth century:

> The sisters endured with cheerfulness and without repugnance the stench, the filth and infections of the sick so insupportable to others that no other form of penitence could be compared to this species of

> martyrdom. No one who saw the religious sisters of the Hôtel-Dieu not only do dressings, make beds and bathe patients, but also in cold winter break the ice in river Seine and stand knee deep in the water to wash the filthy clothes, could regard them as other than holy victims, who from excess of love and charity for their neighbors hastened willingly to the death which they courted amidst the stenches and infections.[48]

The nun with the most responsibility in the hospital was the prioress, who supervised the day to day operations of the hospital, which meant supervising the sisters, novices and servants under her control. Overall control of the hospitals was in the hands of the monks. The prioress was also in charge of the patients and their well-being, including their food and the provision of clean linen. Finally, it was the prioress who decided when patients would be discharged from the hospital.[49]

The Augustinian sisters' philosophy of nursing may be found in their constitution of 1652, revised in 1724. Although the constitution is primarily a list of rules, it provides a insight into the nuns' belief that nursing was indeed a religious vocation: 'The hospital religious ... have a particular obligation to honor Our Lord because He must be the sole and unique object of their charity and mercy, and the assistance and service they render the sick and all the charitable duties of hospitality must have for their end and principal purpose not at all the person of the sick man but the sacred person of Jesus.'[50]

The priests, who had their own views on healing, often overruled physicians' instructions. Religious persons were often more concerned with saving souls than with healing the body and thus they subordinated the sisters' nursing duties to their religious practice, often to the detriment of the patients. The sisters were often praying when they should have been tending to the sick. However, the concept of curing disease was unknown to them. Their aim was to care for the sick, but they believed that illness was sent by God to punish people for their sins.[51]

Although the Church was in charge of the hospital, this did not prevent the state from interfering in its administration, which it did on numerous occasions. As a result of the poor quality of care, several investigations were made, beginning as early as the fourteenth century but also in the seventeenth and eighteenth centuries. There were two major complaints made against the sisters by the state: first, that the sisters were disobedient and resisted administrators' orders and second, that they were neglectful in their duties. The hospital was not kept clean and there were rumours of bed bugs.[52] These complaints were made not only about the sisters at the Hôtel Dieu in Paris, but also about those in the provinces. At the Hôtel Dieu in Provins, the sisters 'had turned the establishment into a house of pleasure...' There were also serious problems at the Hôtel Dieu in Orléans where investigation of a complaint led to the discovery of many more irregularities. The initial scandal involved Sister Marie-Françoise Berthelin who was indicted for having her mother sell hospital linen for five to six years. She was arrested and sent to Salpêtrière prison. This event attracted the magistrate's attention to the internal administration of the institution. An investigation revealed some serious further charges against the sisters. They stole the patients' food, they did not administer medicines to the sick when they were gravely ill, and they did not account for the money they spent. Medicines were not taken by the patients in the sisters' presence. Sisters sold drugs, they substituted water for herbal teas, falsified the records, and demanded thirty *sous* a week from anyone who wanted a bed and a night wash basin.[53] The Hôtel Dieu of Notre-Dame du Puy also experienced problems with nuns failing to feed patients properly, with serious results, sometimes even the death of patients. Other sisters would leave the convent for extended periods. Eventually, the Bureau of Administration had these sisters replaced with nuns from Moulins and later by brothers of charity.[54]

The Hôtel Dieu hospital system was controlled entirely by the Church until the sixteenth century when a series of measures were taken by the kings of France to encroach on the Church's jurisdiction. This extension of secular authority was connected to the general growth in royal authority at the expense of the Church. At the same time, there was a growth in the influence of municipal authorities in the towns of France, which were usually dominated by the bourgeoisie. News of problems within the hospitals reached the Parlement which, in 1505, ruled that the chapter of Notre Dame was deposed of its temporal authority and replaced by members of the bourgeoisie commissioned by the Court. In addition, royal judges would now keep a watch on the administration of the hospital and would have the right to review the accounts and those in charge of them.[55]

At the beginning of the sixteenth century, there was such disorder in the administration of the Paris Hôtel Dieu, which was at the time in the hands of the Chapter of Notre Dame, that Louis XII, by a patent letter of 11 April 1505, ordered the removal of the temporal administration of the canons, entrusting it instead to lay administrators. The edict of the Parlement of 2 May 1505 provided for the first lay administrators and inaugurated the temporal administration of the Hôtel Dieu after having noted that 'the Hôtel Dieu of Paris, was in a terrible state, spiritual as well as temporal'. These revolutionary reforms were never accepted by the nursing sisters nor by the canons, who never ceased to fight against the temporal authority. The Church made it clear that its power was superior to that of the state: 'The Hôtel Dieu of Paris is governed by two administrations very distinct, one purely spiritual, one temporal. The chapter of the church of Paris is superior. The temporal administration is presided over by M. the archbishop and by the first magistrates and composed to the citizens of the first order presented by the city of Paris – exercise of charitable functions.' The Church passed two constitutions, in 1652 and 1725, governing the sisters,[56] and several reforms were introduced in the seventeenth century by Geneviève Bouquet.[57] These constitutions constantly reminded the sisters of their religious service to the poor and 'to remove any idea of ownership, they declared that it was permanent and well known that to everyone that the Hôtel Dieu was founded as an institution to serve the poor invalids ... Sisters are not only subordinate to their spiritual superiors for their personal conduct and service to the poor but they are also to the temporal administration for all things that are not spiritual.'[58]

On the eve of the French Revolution in the late 1780s, a series of more extensive reforms were instituted by the French government. The man in charge of these changes was Jean Colombier (1736–89), a military physician and Royal Inspector of Civil Hospitals and Prisons. In July 1787, he drafted a new code consisting of fifty-two articles, which was designed to modernize and improve the state of the hospital.[59] Effectively, from the end of the eighteenth century, the hospital came under the control of physicians and surgeons. The nuns were permitted to continue working during the French Revolution but as lay workers. It was not until 1908, after the separation of church and state in France, that the nuns ceased to be the nursing sisters at the hospital. Henceforth, nurses received outside training at proper state-run training schools.[60]

The earliest hospitals in England were founded during the Roman occupation and were similar to those on the continent in that they provided basic care, consisting of shelter, food and warmth. Also in common with continental Europe, the next hospitals were founded by the Church. Athelstan founded St Leonard's hospital in York in 936. There were eight nursing sisters at St Leonard's hospital and it appears that these nurses possessed sufficient knowledge of medicine, based on herbal remedies, to be able to treat patients when physicians were not available. There is even evidence that the nurses at this hospital carried out minor surgery.[61] Two hospitals were founded in the eleventh century by Lanfranc, Archbishop of Canterbury.

Four types of hospitals existed in the Middle Ages: leper houses, almshouses, hospices for pilgrims and the poor and institutions that took care of the poor sick. According to existing records, medical care for those in the medieval hospital was exceptional.[62]

The Augustinian sisters and brothers staffed the two oldest London hospitals, St Bartholomew's and St Thomas's. St Bartholomew's was founded in 1123 by a monk by the name of Rahere. Rahere's mandate was 'to create a hostel or hospital where the sick poor could be succoured or the destitute given refuge'.[63] Initially, it was staffed by four sisters and seven brothers. The sisters provided food and rest and religious consultation, in addition to nursing care. Some information about the exact nature of the medical care they provided is available from the hospital records. The sisters provided care for women in childbirth (which contrasted to the situation in France) and for orphans. In addition, rudimentary physiotherapy and psychotherapeutic services were provided.[64] When patients recovered, the cure was usually attributed to supernatural rather than medical intervention.[65]

St Thomas's Hospital was founded as the Priory of St Mary Overie. Its actual foundation date is not known, but is often given as around 1106.[66] The hospital's functions were similar to other hospitals of the Middle Ages: the provision of hospitality to travellers, a home for the destitute and a place where the 'sick were nursed'.[67]

Monarchs in England were also responsible for the founding of hospitals. Du Mans hospital was founded in 1180 by Henry II. It was administered by a magister or preceptor at the choice of the bishop and lay brothers. The sisters, of whom there were six by 1329, served as nurses.[68] The hospital of St Giles in the Field was founded by Queen Mathilda, wife of Henry I, as was St Katharine's in 1148. These hospitals were founded without consulting physicians and at St Giles, the Poor Clares cared for lepers. At St Katharine's hospital, many noblewomen were employed in nursing duties. Queen Mathilda herself took care of lepers in her home in an age when they were banned from cities.[69]

The Protestant Reformation in England meant the closing of the church hospitals as Henry VIII dissolved the monasteries. There were no state institutions to replace the closed church hospitals. During the Reformation, nursing and hospital care deteriorated to their lowest point. Stories of women about to give birth being turned away from hospitals were common. In order to redress this dire situation, Henry VIII reconstituted some of the former church hospitals, including St Bartholomew's in 1544, while in 1547 his son Edward VI gave the city of London control over St Thomas's, St Bartholomew's, Bethlehem and smaller hospitals. Unfortunately, the state of health-care did not improve with the new secular authorities. Nursing care, without its religious basis, became little more than domestic work. A matron was put in charge of the nurses and instructed them in care of the linen, food and drink. They were also responsible for distributing medicines and special foods or drinks as prescribed by the doctor. The monastic term 'sister' was retained and remains in use to this day in England. Health-care in hospitals did not become the standard until the twentieth century. Moreover, hospitals in the Early Modern period were multi-purpose institutions: they also provided shelter for the poor and homeless, and orphans.[70]

In 1585, Abruzzese Camillo de Lellis (1550–1614),[71] a noble soldier turned Franciscan friar, founded an order of nursing priests, the Camillians, 'Ministers of the Sick', and a second order, the Daughters of Camillus in Rome. The brothers and sisters worked at the hospital of Santo Spirito. Each day they would serve the sick in their homes, in hospitals and on the battlefields. The order spread throughout continental Europe and into South America. Unfortunately, the Daughters of Camillus, as they were called, nursed during the last great plague of Barcelona. This Spanish branch became extinct, as all perished. The French abolished their wing at the time of the French Revolution.[72]

Nursing care in Florentine hospitals, with the exception of two or three special institutions reserved for men, was under the control of a secular order of women, the Florentine oblates, 'Donne Oblate di Santa Maria Nuova'. The order of Santa Maria Nova dates from 1296 and was founded by Mona Tessa, sometimes known as Tancia. Nurses were originally attached to the convent, but later were free to leave after three years. Their nursing duties consisted of administering medicines and care to the sick, and undertaking housekeeping chores. They also employed the equivalent of modern nursing aides, who performed the more menial tasks. Apparently, these nurses learned more of the science of medicine than their counterparts in religious nursing orders.[73]

In Catholic countries, the Counter-Reformation strengthened Church control over hospitals. At the Council of Trent, various acts were passed to provide more supervision and new orders were founded. Caroli Barromei (Charles Borromeo, 1538–84), who was involved in hospital reform, founded a hospital and a nursing order in Milan. The Sisters of Nancy, later the Sisters of St Caroli Barromei, were established to conduct his work.[74]

In Spain, nursing did not possess sufficient value to aspire to a body of knowledge. Nurses did not write about their work. They were not discussed in medical literature until recently, when physicians, authors of medical manuals, discussed the practical application of medicine. Most of the nurses in Spain were male and any instruction manuals that there were, were intended for male nurses. Only on a rare occasion does one find mention of a woman in the manuals. These manuals were first published in the sixteenth century and they were designed to provide sufficient guidelines for practitioners to exercise a useful function in the community.[75]

During the fifteenth and sixteenth centuries, a number of hospitals were founded by the Catholic Monarchs, Ferdinand and Isabella. These included the Kings' Hospital in Granada (1504) and the Royal Hospital of Santiago which opened in 1509.[76] The Santa Creu hospital in Barcelona, dating from the early 1400s, had a separate ward for women and children and this ward was administered by a woman. However, there is no evidence that there were female nurses caring for the patients.[77]

In Madrid, during the last decade of the fifteenth century, Beatriz de Galindo (1474–1534) founded La Latina hospital in Madrid. Contrary to Beatriz's mandate, the hospital was staffed entirely by men, with a minor exception. Five 'honest women', who were to be at least forty-five or fifty years of age, called 'Dueñas de la Caridad', worked as nurses, watched over the interns, and cleaned the hospital.[78]

Galindo was an exceptional woman for her time. She had attended the University of Salerno in Italy where she studied philosophy, medicine and Latin. Here she received a degree in Latin and philosophy.[79] She returned to Spain and took up a post as a professor at the prestigious University of Salamanca. She was even hired to teach Isabella's daughter Juana.

In the sixteenth century, there is some evidence of females nursing in Spanish hospitals. The main hospital of San Sebastían in Córdoba had a 'service' staff of five people: three men and two women. The women were called 'housekeepers'; they were assigned to washing the patients' bedding, feeding and cleaning the patients. Two of the three men were employed as nurses and the third as a custodian.[80]

During the seventeenth century, female nurses could be found in the female wards of Spanish hospitals. Such was the case in the hospital of the city of Pamplona. The male nurses were brothers of the Congregation of Bernardino de Obregón (1608–1727). The female nurses formed the same functions as the male nurses: they visited patients and decided who required special care, they accompanied the doctors on their rounds, noted special diets and gave the patients their food, wine and medicines. An additional function of the female nurses was to prevent male nurses from entering the female wards.[81]

The Béguines[82] was an organization of religious women who did not take vows and often supported themselves by nursing in addition to other occupations such as textile work. They were founded in the late twelfth century, the first group forming in 1180 in Flanders. In 1215, they received a papal dispensation obtained by Jacques de Vitry from Honorius III for women living together in chastity and poverty doing works of Christian charity.[83] De Vitry, cardinal of Champagne, was a promoter of the group. A number of experts have suggested that the name Béguine is derived from Lambert le Bégue, a Liège priest who died in 1180, and his name is sometimes taken as an indication that he was either a heretic or had a stammer.[84]

The Béguines lived in groups of three and four, and even though they had taken vows of chastity, they were still free to marry. They did not possess many attributes commonly associated with religious groups: they lacked a leader, a mother house, a rule, a centralized authority.[85] They were not enclosed like other religious women but lived and worked in the community. They did take a vow of poverty. Béguine houses were founded by philanthropic members of the nobility such as the countess of Flanders. Ordinary members of the community also founded Béguine houses. Agnes de Corbie in 1265 founded a house for 'poor *Béguines*, women and the elderly'.[86]

Béguines were found mainly in the Low Countries, Germany, parts of Italy and Switzerland and northern France. The earliest *Béguinage* in France was in Cambrai and dates from 1236. The local bishop, Godfrey of Fontaines, supported the women. In 1239, a Béguine hospital opened in Valenciennes. The largest house was in Paris with 400 women.[87] They were very successful and had some 200,000 adherents by 1300.[88]

The Béguines are relevant to the history of female medical practitioners because they worked extensively in the medical field, treating the poor sick in their homes as well as in hospitals such as St Thomas, founded by Gauthier de Bellair in 1378. The most important Béguine hospital was the Hôtel de Beaume founded in France in 1493.

They tended to care for elderly women. Their 'medical villages', known as *Béguinages*, were composed of small houses, a chapel, an infirmary or small hospital and a cemetery. The infirmary was a central part of the village. Physical and spiritual care for the sick, particularly the elderly was the primary function of the infirmary. The infirmary also served as a hospice for men, usually religious brothers, as well as relatives of the Béguines. Some *Béguinages* charged patients for their medical care. This was the case in Louvain.[89]

Béguines are particularly associated with leper hospitals. Here, they cared for male and female patients, usually for charity but sometimes for a modest fee to support themselves. We know of their work in a leper house at Mont-Cornillon in Liège and as nurses in hospitals in Cambrai and Antwerp as well as in other cities in northern France.[90] One of the earliest Béguines was Mary of Oignies (1177–1213). She was married but lived in chastity with her husband before joining the Béguines. Mary and her husband both worked in hospitals taking care of lepers and later they converted their own home into a leper hospital.[91] Other notable medical women were Mechtilde of Magdeburg (1212–82), Beatrice of Nazareth (1200–68), Hadewijch of Brabant (1221–40) and Marguerite Porete (fl. c. 1310). Marguerite was burned at the stake for heresy.[92]

Since medical care was of utmost importance to the Béguines, we can assume that they received some sort of medical training, in particular in order to be qualified to treat diseases like leprosy, but there is no documented evidence for this. In addition to their work with lepers and the sick poor, the Béguines also performed tasks associated with death: the laying out of the body, accompanying the dead to their graves and conducting wakes.[93]

The first documentation for hospital care of the sick in Spain dates from the end of the thirteenth century or even later.[94] In Valencia, Beatas – the Spanish version or equivalent of the Béguines – were involved in nursing work at the Hospital of Santa María, founded in 1334 by Ramón Guillem Catalá, a healer from Valencia.[95] The term beata means 'blessed one'.[96] These women dedicated their lives to serving God through assisting the sick poor. They were similar to third orders like Béguines and Beghards, Franciscans and Dominicans and often Beatas were members of these various third orders.[97] They were found in the larger cities of Madrid, Toledo, Seville and Granada, and at one point, constituted up to 30 per cent of the population.[98] They took a 'private vow' of chastity, and devoted themselves to good works and charity.[99] Beatas had a considerable amount of freedom. Some worked in city prisons as spiritual and physical healers – one example is that of Augustina de la Cruz of Seville – who was paid 12,000 *maravedís* in salary in 1636 and 1639.[100]

The papacy looked upon Béguines and Beatas with suspicion – they were pious women, yet they did not live in convents. They were often older and unmarried. Their 'awkward, middling posture produced a constant and finally destructive tension between themselves and the thirteenth century, which had little sympathy for anomalous persons'.[101] They were condemned for heresy by the Council of Vienne in 1312,[102] and while the Béguines did not completely disappear their numbers were significantly reduced after this accusation. Beatas such as Isabel de la Cruz, who were often mystics, had visions, made prophesies and were believed to have power to contact the deity directly, were hunted down by the Inquisition. Isabel was publicly flogged and condemned to life imprisonment on 22 July 1529 for her mysticism.[103] These women represented a significant challenge to the authority of the Church.

A further implication or ramification of the Counter-Reformation was the foundation of many new religious orders in countries such as France and Italy at the end of the sixteenth and start of the seventeenth centuries. In addition, existing religious orders brought in reforms. The goal of the new orders was piety and spiritual renewal, but their focus was the welfare of the poor sick. The seventeenth century in particular saw considerable growth in associations whose goal was to help the sick and poor. The creation and growth of hospital orders occurred throughout the Catholic nations of Europe, but France was distinguished by the fact that many of the new orders were composed of women.[104]

The Ursuline order was founded in Italy in 1535 by Angela de Merici to educate girls. Originally, the Ursulines were not enclosed and did not take vows. However, this changed after Merici stepped down from the position of Mother Superior. The nuns now took vows and wore a habit. The reforming bishop of Milan, Carlo Borromeo was responsible for changing the Ursulines from a comparatively independent and female-run order to one under the control of men. He re-wrote the rule, stressing obedience, and instituted control by the Catholic hierarchy.[105] From the sixteenth to eighteenth centuries, the order expanded throughout Italy and France. There were 10,000 Ursuline sisters in France by 1789. The French Ursulines were originally not enclosed, but this changed by the seventeenth century.[106] Although primarily dedicated to education, the Ursulines also took care of the sick. Some Ursuline sisters staffed hospitals.[107]

In Grenoble, a pioneering hospital was founded in 1676. This was the hospital of Grenoble Providence, an institution intended for local people. Its founders were primarily lay women and patients were cared for by the Soeurs de Saint Joseph, a female nursing order founded in 1650 in Puy by Bishop Monsignor Maupas du Tour.[108] This hospital and the nurses of Saint Joseph represent the 'renewal of nursing during the Counter-Reformation as the most effective way of imparting to the sick and poor within the hospital routine, a concept of illness that is revalued by the Counter-Reformation and as a spiritual imprint'.[109]

One of these new charitable orders was the Order of the *Visitandines* founded by Jeanne Françoise de Chantal (1572–1641), a widow, and friend of François de Sales (1567–1622), bishop of Geneva. This order was a precursor to Vincent de Paul's Daughters or Sisters of Charity. In fact, Jeanne later met Vincent de Paul in 1619 when she founded a house in Paris. With the assistance of François de Sales, Jeanne instituted the *Visitandines* in 1610. The mandate of the order was to visit the sick poor in their homes to which end they would work outside the cloister. However, they soon became a cloistered order at Annecy. The convent was dedicated to the sick and Jeanne attempted to influence secular local authorities to improve health-care.[110] However, among the charitable groups, the most significant was the organization founded by Vincent de Paul.

In France, charitable organizations such as the Ladies of Charity and Ladies Bountiful and the Daughters of Charity were founded in the seventeenth century to take care of the sick poor in homes and hospitals. The Co-fraternities of Charity (the Ladies of Charity and the Ladies Bountiful) were associations of laywomen while the Daughters (or Sisters – the terms are used interchangeably because of the English translation of 'filles'; they are 'Les Filles' in French) of Charity were an association patterned after the co-fraternities. The Daughters of Charity of Vincent de Paul, founded in 1630, were the first group to care for the poor sick at home.[111] They were young women, usually from peasant stock, who assisted the Ladies of Charity and worked on their own as nurses.[112] Vincent de Paul and Louise de Marillac (Mademoiselle Le Gras) organized these young women into a community of which she took charge. They had met in 1624 and 1625.[113]

Vincent de Paul (1581–1660),[114] came from a French peasant family. He received an education from the Franciscans at Dax and graduated from the University of Toulouse in 1604. He was ordained at the age of nineteen and received a parish at Chatillon-les-Dombes in the diocese of Lyon in 1617. He founded a congregation of priests in 1625.[115] It was during his time as a parish priest that he brought together the *Confrérie de la Charité* or Ladies of Charity. They were women of the nobility who devoted themselves to helping the poor and sick. Initially there were about twenty of them.

Louise de Marillac (1591–1660)[116] was a member of an influential noble family who had served at the courts of Marie de Médici and Louis XIII. She was educated by her father and at the royal monastery of Poissy, near Paris. De Marillac was married to Antoine le Gras, a secretary to Marie de Médici, and had one son. While raising her son, she still worked outside the home in service of the poor. When her husband died in 1625, she devoted herself full time to charity.[117]

The purpose of the Daughters is as follows:

> The Co-fraternity of Charity is instituted for the honor of our Lord Jesus Christ and His Holy Mother, and to assist the sick poor of the places where it is established both in body and soul: in body, by administering to them their food and drink, and the necessary medicines during the

> time of their illnesses: in soul, by obtaining for them the administration of the Sacraments of Penance, the Eucharist, and Extreme Unction; and by taking care that those who are dying shall leave this world in a right condition; and that those who are cured shall make a resolution to live well for the future.[118]

The sisters could be married or single and were required to obtain the consent of their husbands or parents.[119] They were admitted without a dowry.[120] They were to be at least eighteen or twenty years old and to bring their own clothing with them. Vincent de Paul recruited simple village girls who were usually poor themselves: 'You have the happiness to be the first who have been called to this holy work, you, poor village girls and daughters of working men.'[121] The Sisters of Charity did not take vows but renewed their commitment each year. They were permitted to wear civilian clothing, but many donned the renowned grey uniform, hence the name the Grey Sisters.[122]

Initially, the Sisters of Charity nursed people in their homes but they soon began to run hospitals. The organization was revolutionary for the time, as it was the first successful congregation of non-cloistered women devoted to helping the poor in their homes. Vincent de Paul did not insist that his sisters be enclosed, for he believed this to be incompatible with their mandate of nursing, nor did they take vows. He called his sisters 'Daughters' and told them that they were 'not nuns ... for whoever says the word nun says cloister and the Sisters should go everywhere'.[123]

The Sisters of Charity have been called precursors to the modern public health nurse, the visiting nurse and the social worked all rolled into one. They provided staff at a number of hospitals including the Hôpital des Petites-Maisons, the Hôpital des Invalides, where most of the patients were elderly, the Hôpital des Incurables, where the chronically ill predominated, and the Hospice de Vaugirard, which was for those suffering from venereal disease. The Sisters of Charity also worked at institutions for the poor, the criminal and the insane, such as the Pitié, the Salpêtrière (which housed females) and Bîcetre (which housed males) as well as in orphanages and foundling homes. They also nursed wounded soldiers. Vincent de Paul issued special instructions for dealing with soldiers who may become insolent. The sisters were told to 'reprehend him in a severe manner...' If this tactic did not work, they had the authority to 'register a complaint against him...'[124]

Vincent instructed his daughters to treat patients with 'compassion, kindness, cordiality, respect, and devotion...' He stressed the maternal role of the nurse. They should listen to 'their little complaints as a good mother would do, for they look upon you as their foster mothers, as persons sent to assist them'.[125]

Physical healing as well as comforting the sick were vital aspects of the sisters' work. De Paul instructed the sisters that their 'care extends not only to the body but principally to the soul'.[126] They were to be pure in their motives: 'What would be the use of your carrying soup or medicines to the poor if the motive for such an action was not love?'[127] Sisters were to be focused and devoted to their tasks. They were told not to 'waste time in conversation with one sick person while others suffer because their food and medicines were not brought to them at a proper time, they should take great care to observe moderation and proportion in this respect'.[128]

The sisters performed important medical tasks which today would be carried out by physicians. They took the patients' medical histories and made simple diagnoses – in de Marillac's words, 'the sisters shall then find out how long they have been ill…' They would then 'begin administering remedies by means of cold sponges or bloodletting when the sick are adverse to the sponges'. The sisters would decide when to start and end medical treatment. As de Marillac wrote, describing the treatment of blood-letting: 'When the fever persists, they shall let blood from the patient's foot, then begin once again to let blood from the arm until the fever goes down.'[129] The sisters would know enough 'not to administer any remedies while a patient is shivering or sweating'.[130] They carried medical instruments including syringes and ligatures for the purpose of carrying out minor surgery. Since physicians were few in number and often not available in hospitals, the sisters conducted most medical care.[131] In addition to general care, they managed and distributed drugs[132] and were responsible for undertaking the necessary procedures following the death of a patient.[133]

The sisters made a difference to medical treatment through the stress they put on cleanliness. They were convinced that contagious diseases and moral contamination were intimately connected. Hygiene and godliness were of supreme spiritual importance. Thus, a new crusade against dirt was launched.[134]

Training was in the hands of the co-founder of the order, Louise de Marillac, who instructed the sisters in basic nursing. They were told to obey doctors' orders, as stipulated in their rules: 'You should act my sisters, with great respect and obedience toward the doctors, taking great care never to condemn or contradict their orders. Endeavour, on the contrary, to fulfil them with great exactitude and without ever presuming to prepare the medicines according to your own way of thinking. Punctually follow what they have prescribed, both with regard to quantity of dose and the ingredients of which it is composed…'[135] The rules indicate that the sisters must follow prescriptions to the letter as the life of the patient depended on accuracy. There must have been a temptation for the sisters to follow their own instincts with respect to medicines as they spent a great deal more time with the patients that did the doctors, but de Paul insisted that the doctors were more learned and that the nurses 'were ignorant of the reasons they have for pursuing different methods in the treatment of maladies which seem to you to be the same'.[136] In other words, they were not simply women who took care of bedpans, nourished, watched over and prayed for the sick. They actually engaged in medical care and were well trained in it. In addition to caring for the sick, they assisted with the burial of the sick poor.[137]

One of the most important mandates of the sisters was to care for the sick in their homes in rural villages. In many cases, doctors were simply unavailable in such remote locations. The sisters would be on their own and thus would need to understand basic medical methods of treatment. The medical instructions to the sisters were made clear by de Paul:

> You must endeavor particularly to remember and observe their [the doctor's] method of treating the sick, so that when you will be in the villages; or any other place in which there is no doctor, you may render yourself useful by applying their method. You ought therefore to instruct yourselves, so as to know in what case it is necessary to bleed in the arm or in the foot; what quantity of blood you should take on each occasion; when to apply the cupping glasses. Learn also the different remedies necessary to be used in the various kinds of diseases and the proper time and manner of administering them.[138]

When the sisters worked with physicians, they were clearly in subordinate positions and were instructed by de Paul to obey the physicians' orders at all times. 'They shall make it a matter of conscience not to fail in the slightest service which they ought to render to the sick, particularly as regards the remedies which they ought to give to them in the manner and at the hour prescribed by the physician ... Thus, my Sisters, you ought to be exact in doing all that physicians prescribe, because if any accident happened to a sick person, you would be responsible...' By obeying the physicians' instructions, Vincent told his daughters that they were doing God's will: 'You ought, then, to obey them in all that concerns the service of the sick and think that you are doing the will of God in doing theirs.' Sisters were also ordered to respect the doctors.[139] It appears from the writings of de Paul that his daughters did not always follow doctors' instructions and show them the respect he believed they were owed. He asks the sisters why they 'refuse to show them the honor and respect you owe them?'[140]

The sisters were also instructed to obey the Ladies of Charity, who were in charge of the parishes, and not to 'undertake the care of any sick or to give anything to any poor person contrary to the prescribed order or against the intention of the lady officers'.[141] They were also supposed to provide the Ladies of Charity with an account of patients' progress.

Vincent de Paul and Louise de Marillac both died in 1660. At the time of their deaths, the movement had expanded beyond France to Poland with some 350 sisters in 70 establishments. By 1789, the sisters numbered 2500 in France.[142] In the seventeenth century, the Sisters of Charity were nursing in hospitals in Spain, such as the hospital of Santa Cruz in Barcelona and the hospital of the Catholic Kings of Santiago and Compostela.[143] The Sisters of Charity founded a house in Spain in 1703.[144]

In Italy, Virginia Centurione Bracelli (1587–1651) founded a congregation devoted to healing children and the poor, which was known as the Brignolines, or the Daughters of Our Lady of Mount Cavalry. They were named after Cardinal Brignole, who became their protector in 1650. Bracelli was the daughter of Giorgio Centurione, the Doge of Genoa, and Lelia Spinola. She was married young and had two children. Virginia was a pious individual, who devoted herself to helping others after she was widowed at the age of twenty. After raising her children with the help of her family, Virginia founded her order in Genoa during the plague of 1629 to 1631. She brought orphans to her home and when her home was too small, she rented the Convent of Monte Calvario, otherwise known as the Bregara, which was no longer in use. The former convent served as a hospital for 300 patients and received government recognition in 1635. However, the convent proved to be too expensive to run and Virginia moved her hospital to two villas, also ordering that a church be built. Her sisters wore the robe of the Franciscan Tertiaries. These women were knowledgeable in many medical fields, including pharmacy and worked in a similar manner to de Paul's Sisters of Charity, healing the sick and educating the poor. Their rule was virtually indistinguishable from that of the Sisters of Charity.[145]

During an outbreak of syphilis in Italy, a number of noblewomen were involved in founding hospitals for the sick poor. Women like Caterina Fieschi Adorno (1447–1510), later Saint Catherine of Genoa, who founded a 'charitable fraternity', which in turn founded a hospital to care for those suffering from the 'Great Pox', later known as syphilis. Other hospitals would not treat those suffering from this disease. Caterina came from the Ligurian noble family of Fieschi; her father was Viceroy of Naples and the nephew of Pope Innocent IV. At the age of sixteen, she married the Genoese nobleman Giuliano Adorno. She spent ten years in this unhappy union, spending most of her time pursuing pleasure. In 1473, she had a mystical experience which changed her life. From the time of her conversion, she devoted herself to the patients in the hospital Pammatone in Genoa, and she became its administrator or matron in 1491. During two plague epidemics she worked untiringly for the sick and dying. She combined her hospital work with prayer, writing a treatise on Purgatory and a dialogue between the soul and the body. She did not join a third order for the laity. In 1493 she nearly died of the plague, in 1496 her health broke down again and in 1497 her husband, who had become a Franciscan tertiary, died. Catherine was beatified in 1737 and canonized by Pope Benedict XIV a few years later. Appropriately, she is the patron saint of Genoa and of Italian hospitals.[146] Catherine's unselfish behaviour set an example for others. She had a particular influence over Ettore Vernazza who is believed to have co-founded, with Maria Lorenzo Longo, the hospital for the poor incurables in Naples.[147] Two noblewomen,

Maria Malipiero and Marina Grimani, with the assistance of the Church, men from prominent families and the state, were involved in hospitals for a similar purpose in Venice in 1522.[148]

What this sketch of the history of nursing has endeavored to demonstrate is the integral role that nurses have performed in health-care since the time of the foundation of monasteries and the hospitals that were established within their domains. Primary care inside and outside the hospital setting was most often performed by the nuns or nursing sisters, whose perception of their Christian duty underlay their particular dedication to the care of the poor sick. Central to the further development of the nursing profession was the foundation of new hospital orders during the Counter-Reformation.

7

The 'Irregular' Female Healer in Early Modern Europe: A Variety of Practitioners

In this chapter, we will consider the role and activities of the irregular or unlicensed female practitioner outside the realm of nursing and midwifery in the Early Modern period, including the function of female healers after the rise of universities and the professionalization of medicine. What role could women play if they were not university trained and were unable to obtain local licences to practise medicine other than midwifery? And what part did they play in Italy where they could hold chairs of anatomy? Sources of information on the unlicensed women healers who are the subject of this chapter are often difficult to find. Diaries and correspondence, private papers, trial records, advertisements, newspapers and published pamphlets all contribute and have been utilized here. Official sources such as records of licences, lists of physicians, surgeons, barber-surgeons and apothecaries compiled by their guilds or corporations are of necessity of limited use in this context.

As we saw in Chapter 2, the general trend in the Early Modern period was to force women out of the practice of 'official' medicine, which category came to comprise university trained and state licensed practitioners, usually male and Christian.[1] This led women to work 'underground' and 'illegally'. In short, women were marginalized by the medical profession. As the skills and knowledge of the university trained physician became more valuable, the practical experience of the female practitioner tended to become increasingly devalued by the established medical community. Licensed medical professionals regarded women practitioners as 'quacks' or 'charlatans' who did more harm than good. Many men, including the Northamptonshire doctor John Cotta, and Robert Pitt, a prominent fellow of the Royal Society, were concerned about the ubiquity of the so-called quack.

More recently, medical historians have questioned the stark division between licensed physicians and the irregular or unlicensed medical practitioners.[2] Historian of medicine Roy Porter has emphasized that so-called 'quacks' were 'mostly medically proficient', and a few were even 'well trained'. Perhaps most importantly, quacks could be characterized as those who did not fit 'the approved mould'. Porter argues that women were the most important of these healers.[3] Women often provided care that the trained physicians – for a myriad of reasons – did not. Physicians were expensive and they were few in number compared with the local healers. Rural dwellers often felt more comfortable with a non-licensed healer. While orthodox practitioners bled and purged and often gave the patient drugs which did not work, the 'fringe' or 'quack' female practitioners attempted to 'treat sickness in the context of individual life experiences'. These practitioners stressed the cooperation of patient and practitioner in the healing process.[4] It is safe to argue that women were 'amateur' healers, but this did not mean that their services were not important to the community. In fact, these women, whether they were paid or unpaid, provided a vital service. Porter has demonstrated that in England from the late seventeenth into the eighteenth century, the numbers of female healers increased rather than decreased.[5] In addition, academically trained doctors borrowed from their remedies. Lucinda McCray Beier in her work on illness in seventeenth-century England pointed out that 'there was a spectrum of medical knowledge shared by a population as a whole. Licensed physicians sometimes used popular therapies; lay-people were acquainted with learned medical theories and prescribed officially endorsed remedies for themselves and their friends.'[6] Beier maintained that licensed practitioners competed with the unlicensed for patients, and that amongst the public there was no consensus that the licensed were any better at healing people.[7]

Margaret Pelling has also stressed the diversity in medical practice in her studies of medicine in London and Norwich between 1550 and 1640. Perhaps more importantly, she argues that particular legislation, regulation and licensing 'had a limited effect' on medical services. According to Pelling, regular practitioners are not well represented in such official sources as parish registers. Pelling has scrutinized the Annals of the London College of Physicians. Through meticulous research, she has discovered that the college pursued action against some 110 female practitioners in the London area over a 90-year period. Since the college only hunted down those practising 'physic' without a licence, Pelling has estimated that this total comprises only about one-third of the women practising some form of medicine in the London area. In addition, she posited that the college did not chiefly go after 'women practisers of physic ... Cases involving women have been cited by the College's apologists chiefly as a way of ridiculing the pretensions of empirics in general.'[8] Helen Rix of London and Jane Clarke of Southwark, both practised medicine without a licence. Rix practised for over twenty years. With other women, Clarke comprised a network of practitioners who performed phlebotomies.[9] Another Londoner, Avis Murrey, was the wife of a surgeon, Robert Murrey, who secured her entrance into surgery.

In Norwich, Pelling found 37 female practitioners, including midwives, who had formal qualifications, which for women, meant an apprenticeship. Like female medical practitioners of the Middle Ages and as was the case across Europe, these women tended to join their husband's practice.[10] Apart from the inadequate supply of professional medical practitioners and the fact that ordinary people often trusted female healers above and beyond the university educated, their views on health and illness often took a more religious view. Ordinary people were actually much more likely to believe in faith healing than in the 'scientific' medicine practised by the university educated doctor.[11] Further, in pre-industrial Europe, it is difficult, if not impossible to draw a clear line between those using professional and those using popular medicine.[12]

Licensed male practitioners regularly competed against non-licensees. A case in point was the situation in Norwich in 1561 when the physicians and barber-surgeons drafted new rules for the control of their guild, citing 'sondrye women' among others practising medicine without a licence.[13] Similar comments were made by physicians and barber-surgeons in Salisbury in 1614, the year in which the barber-surgeons received their charter. To practise, one was required to be examined by the Bishop of London. The charter stated that: 'No surgeon or barber is to practice any surgery or barbery, unless first made a free citizen, and then a free brother of the company. Whereas, also, there are divers women and others within this city, altogether unskillful in the art of chirurgery; who oftentimes take cures on them, to the great danger of the patient ... no such woman, or any other, shall take or meddle with any cure of Chirurgery...'[14]

Nonetheless, as well as being self-employed, women were also regularly employed by institutions such as hospitals.[15] William Clowes, who became the chief surgeon at Christ Church Hospital in 1576, reported that a certain Mrs Cook was the resident surgeon-apothecary.[16] It was also reported that one Goody Peckham was paid twelve shillings for 'nursing Wickham's boy with the small pox'. She treated him for six weeks as doctor as well as nurse because his family could not afford the fees of a physician.[17]

Women were also employed for particular skills, as was the case with Frances Holcombe who was hired by St Bartholomew's hospital for her talent in curing scald head.[18] The Hôtel Dieu in Lyon hired women after the 1576 ordinances, which were passed by the College of Physicians and stipulated that empirics, charlatans and others would be fined 25 *livres tournois* for the first offence, for the second they would be put out of the city ignominiously and for the third offence, they would receive corporal punishment.[19] Françoise Page was hired by the Hôtel Dieu specifically to treat syphilis.[20] Her husband, from whom she learned her trade, was a surgeon at the same hospital in the same outpatient ward. She claimed not only to have an effective cure for the pox, but also effective treatments for herpes through special diets of her own devising. She and her husband practised together and after his death she was allowed, as was the case for female healers in other parts of Europe, to continue working in the outpatient ward.[21] Page provides historians with one example of a husband-and-wife team of practitioners where the widow continued practising after the husband's death. Another case in point is Lavinia Olimpi and her husband who had a licence to treat external diseases. Lavinia could treat patients on her own when her husband was away, and unlike midwives, she could legally administer medications.[22]

Women surgeons also continued their deceased husbands' practices. French women surgeons belonged to the 'Corporation of Surgeons', or surgical guilds. Members undertook an apprenticeship where they learned their craft. Dame Léonard Pachaude of Avignon, widow of Master Mangin Guérin, 'was given legal authority to inherit her husband's boutique de barbier et de Chirurgien, with its equipment and to carry on his business'.[23] According to official statistics, women composed approximately 1.5 per cent of medical practitioners from 1100 to 1500, and one-third of these were midwives. This is certainly a much lower percentage than the reality.[24] However, in 1484, Charles VII passed a law preventing women from practising as surgeons under threat of imprisonment. There were women who continued to practise, but their numbers declined as time went on. Until 1694, widows of surgeons were still permitted to take over their husbands' practices, although the right was soon withdrawn except in cases of extreme poverty.[25] Women could practise as apothecaries as long as they inherited their husbands' businesses, although this too became more difficult during the late sixteenth and seventeenth centuries.[26] The Paris statutes of 1699 introduced a special examination and licence for *bandagistes*, a group which included dentists, hernia surgeons, oculists, lithotomists and bone-setters.[27]

As we have seen, female medical practitioners have often been characterized by both historians and contemporaries as quacks, charlatans and irregulars. Many writers have understood quacks to mean those who practised without 'academic or guild credentials', and thus were 'ignorant and incompetent' and motivated by greed, usually possessing 'secret' remedies. On the other hand, the medical professional was 'knowledgeable, prudent, honest, concerned with patients' welfare'.[28] Contemporary definitions described female quacks as 'tatling old wives, chattering char-women, long-tongued midwives...'[29] Charlatans were understood to lack the theoretical knowledge possessed by university trained physicians.[30]

The assumption that the quack or charlatan had no medical knowledge and was motivated solely by greed was not necessarily true, neither were the assumptions made in favour of regular practitioners. Porter has demonstrated that many so-called quacks did possess medical knowledge and some male quacks even had a diploma or a degree and a licence. Physicians, he argues, 'have often been the heroes of historians...' Although healers who worked on the margins, women included, have their supporters, 'few scholars have chosen to champion the quacks and the result is that we know very little about them'.[31] Many quacks had practical experience and empirical knowledge. Some women, particularly surgeons, had been through a formal training in the form of an apprenticeship or had learned from their husbands or brothers who were also surgeons. Among these were Mary Buberville, who continued her brother's oculist practice after his death, and Margaret Searl, who carried on with her deceased husband's ear surgery.[32] Further, Porter has shown in his work that many 'regulars' were not as ethical as they claimed to be, sometimes selling cures to gain money and or fame.[33]

Unlicensed practitioners, male and female alike, often advertised their skills in contemporary newspapers and journals. Mrs Plunkett Edgcumbe of Bath advertised as a cancer-curer in the *Bath Journal*.[34] The *Gentleman's Magazine*, a publication read by the educated lay person, advertised the services of the renowned bone-setter Sarah Mapp of Epsom and testimonies provided for Joanna Stephens's famous medicine for the stone.[35] Mapp, also known as 'Crazy Sally', was the daughter of a bone-setter from Hindon, Wiltshire. She learned her trade from her father.[36] 'Mrs Mabbs', as she was sometimes called, practised her trade in Epsom where the town provided her with a retaining fee to entice her to stay.[37] In one advertisement, Mapp called herself the 'doctress of Epsom'.[38] In addition to her practice in Epsom, Mapp also took her skills on the road, treating patients in various parts of London. One of her cases was a man 'of Wardour Street, whose back had been broken nine years and stuck out two inches, a niece of Sir Hans Sloane in the like condition and a gentleman who went with one shoe heel six inches high having been lame twenty years, of his hip and knee whom she set straight and brought his leg down even with the other'.[39] She 'performed surprising cures before Sir Hans Sloane at the Grecian Coffee House where she comes once a week from Epsom in her Chariot with four horses and four liveried footmen'.[40] Mapp was successful in 'reducing dislocations and setting of fractured bones wonderful [sic]'.[41]

Mrs Joanna Stephens, the daughter 'of a gentleman of good estate and family of Berkshire', discovered, unexpectedly, a remedy for dissolving stones.[42] The discovery, which had been made some twenty years before it became widely known, brought her great success with several people suffering from stones in the bladder.[43] Patients whose testimonies appeared in the *Gentleman's Magazine* included the Right Reverend, the Bishop of Bath and Wells, Mr Botton of Newcastle upon Tyne who was cured after five months of taking the medicine, and the Postmaster General, the Hon. Edward Carteret, Esq, who in 1735, 'received great benefit' from Mrs Stephens's medicines and 'this engaged the attention of the Public'.[44] By 1738, her cure was well known, and in that year, Parliament awarded her a sum of £5000 sterling on the condition that she would reveal the ingredients of her medicine: a pill or powder of dried eggshells and soap.[45]

Stephens's case is interesting for although she has been categorized by modern critics as a charlatan who tricked Parliament into giving her £5000, there is no proof that she was motivated solely by monetary compensation.[46] Contemporaries took her remedy for urinary lithiasis very seriously and she was held in the greatest respect by eminent physicians of the day. Whether or not Mrs Stephens was a quack is not the question here, what is important is that her case demonstrates that there was often a very fine line between official and unofficial medicine and that her drug was considered to be effective by many of the most prestigious physicians of the day.

Mrs Stephens received support from several eminent physicians, including two members of the French Academy of Sciences, Saveur François Morand[47] and C.J. Geoffroy. Geoffroy, a chemist, undertook a chemical analysis of the medicine, passing his results to Morand who tested the medicine on patients suffering from various diseases of the bladder and kidney. Both physicians published their findings in scientific papers. Geoffroy read his results to the French Academy of Sciences on 23 December 1739, while Morand read his finding to the same body on 12 November 1740. Geoffroy argued that the medicine could be prepared by sufferers at home if the ingredients were changed slightly. Morand's tests were carried out on 40 people and the results were broadly favourable, although he reported an increase in pain initially and that the medicine was only effective in certain types of stone. However, he recommended the drug as, 'it caused no inconvenience; would not hinder lithotomy, if surgical removal of the stone was still thought to be necessary; would lengthen the lives of older patients', who often died from unnecessary surgery.[48] He concluded that the drug was 'efficacious in curing the stone in the bladder'.[49]

French physicians were not the only investigators of Mrs Stephens's medicine. Dr David Hartley, fellow of the Royal Society, was her greatest advocate in England and it was he who recommended her for an award of £5000 from Parliament.[50] Hartley who suffered from vesical calculi, was reported to have been cured by Mrs Stephens's drug.[51] He published the medicinal receipt in Latin. He not only testified to his own cure, but to one 155 other successful cases. Hartley also cited chemical experiments on the drug.[52]

This phenomenon was not exclusive to female practitioners in England. In France, during the reign of Louis XIV, women advertised their medical skills in newspapers such as the cultural gazette, *Le Mercure Galant*,[53] where we find advertisements for the bone-setter Mlle de Remirand from the Bourbonnais and Madame de Vaux's cures for hernia.[54] In the first case, the writer reported the story of a woman who broke her arm and was treated by Mlle de Remirand, who had a 'remarkable talent for bone-setting'. The woman's arm functioned normally after de Remirand's treatment. She had operated successfully in this way many times. Her method of treatment depended on the case. She did not always re-break bones but merely re-set them. Madame de Vaux's cures were applauded by none other than the king's first physician, Monsieur Fagon. Although Monsieur Fagon warned against popular remedies and 'secrets', he witnessed the healing powers of 'la demoiselle de Vaux', who was the widow of M de Vaux, master surgeon of Paris and a practitioner of medicine, in their Paris apartment. Apparently, Miss Vaux, whose 'secret' was performed in the presence of Fagon by order of the king, was accorded a considerable sum of money to disclose the ingredients in her remedy. This case demonstrates that official medical practitioners of the highest rank did, in some instances, support female healers.

Conversely, women could be prosecuted for treating patients illegally. A case in point was Madeleine Colombier, a Parisian widow who in 1704 was briefly imprisoned in the Bastille for healing without a licence. Evidently, she treated her poor patients without charge and claimed to have cured numbers of them of the flux, venereal disease and the head-cold. She possessed only a rudimentary education. Her skills included reading, writing with some effort, and preparing medicines on a daily basis in her home. She was encouraged by local physicians and surgeons. Apparently she kept excellent records of her patients' diseases, and the treatments she administered. An apothecary who testified at her trial reported that some of the drugs found in her medicine cabinet were standard medicines, but others were questionable in that they were harmful to the patient. He described the powders and salts as dangerous because they contained the chemical nitre or saltpetre. She was set free after her trial.[55]

As far as physicians were concerned, they were university trained and medical faculties throughout the country controlled access to the profession. The Parlement of Toulouse confirmed by a ruling of 3 July 1558, a judgement given by the governor of Montpellier against a woman who 'embroiled herself in Medicine and Surgery, was held prisoner in the Conciergerie of Toulouse, was given the death sentence and executed'.[56]

In spite of the various regulations and licensing laws, women continued to practise medicine of all sorts. Women's names appear in the works of many seventeenth-century writers, both their own and others. They often treated the poor who could not afford a regular physician. Indeed, as medicine became more professionalized, only the very wealthy could procure the services of a university trained physician. Women were constantly at the bedside of the sick. The seventeenth-century medical marketplace was eclectic and the sick had plenty of choice when seeking cures for their illnesses. One example of a female French physician was Jeanne Biscot (1601–64). She founded a hospital at Arras to care for children and wounded soldiers at a time of the plague.[57] The surgeon Babeau, who was active in the early 1600s, provides another illustration of a female practitioner working with plague victims with the advice of the local doctors and surgeons. She lived and worked in Troyes and Champagne.[58]

The practice of community medicine was common among women in rural England. Elizabeth Bedell (1571–1624) was a local surgeon in Black Notley in Essex. William Bedell, Elizabeth's son, and Lord Bishop of Kilmore, praised his mother as a 'person of superior mental endowments'. As far as her medical skills were concerned, she was 'very famous and expert in Chirurgery, which she continually practiced upon multitudes that flocked to her, and gratis, without respect of persons, poor or rich'.[59]

Women such as Elizabeth Dunton combined their works of charity with virtuous lives and medical practice. In a eulogy delivered at her funeral the Reverend Timothy Rogers remarked that 'she takes care that her dependants had plenty ... she distributes among the indigent, money, and books, and clothes and physic, as their several circumstances may require. She will visit and discourse with them.' Her closet contained 'several medicines to relieve her poorer neighbors in sudden distress, when a doctor is not at hand, or when they have no money to buy what may be necessary for them.' She was very successful in her healing practice: 'the charitableness of her physic is often attended by some cure, or other that is remarkable.'[60] In a similar way, Lady Margaret Mainard was remembered by Thomas Ken, Bishop of Bath, in his speech at her funeral. He eulogized: 'Her charity made her sympathize with all in misery...' She was a 'common physician to her sick neighbors, and would often with her own hands dress their most loathsome sores, and sometimes keep them in her family, and would give them both diet and lodging until they were cured.'[61] Similarly, the Reverend Ralph Josselin wrote in his diary about his friend, the physician Lady Honeywood, 'I stayed to March 10, in which time my Lady was my nurse and physician ... they considered scurvy. I took purge and other things for it.'[62] The Presbyterian minister Adam Martindale, who had consulted three physicians each of whom differed in their prognosis, was cured from impetigo by a poor woman who applied to his sores a salve of moss from an ash-root and celandine, shredded and boiled in 'May-butter'.[63] Thomas Hobbes preferred to consult with 'an experienced old woman' to the 'most learned physician' when he was ill. Henry Fielding contacted a female dentist to cure his wife's toothache.[64]

Often women of medicine were the wives of clergymen. Both husbands and wives were convinced that medical care for the poor was their religious duty. This was the case for Elizabeth Walker (1623–90) whose father was a London pharmacist who also traded in tobacco.[65] Her husband was the Reverend Anthony Walker of Fyfield, Essex, and her brother-in-law was a doctor of the London College and was the owner of a 'well-stocked pharmacy, the usual medicines and also surgical dressings'.[66] Walker learned her medicine from her brother-in-law who 'wrote her many receipts and directed her as to what methods to proceed in most diseases into which her poor neighbors might be incident'. She had read the works of the doctors and herbalists Culpeper, Riverius and Bonettus and wrote her own medical recipes.[67]

Anthony Walker described his wife's skills in his diary: she 'had a competent good measure of Knowledge both in Physick and Chirurgery, which she attained with no small Industry and Labour and increased by Experience'. Anthony Walker characterized Elizabeth as devoted to her patients, visiting them daily and travelling two miles to take care of a sick minister, staying with him until he recovered.[68] She delivered babies at any time of day or night, taking with her 'skill and stock of medicines always ready by her for such occasions'.[69]

After her child-bearing and rearing years were over – she gave birth to eleven children – Elizabeth devoted herself to visiting her sick neighbours and preparing medicines to treat their illnesses. She 'distilled waters, syrups, oils, ointments, salves and would distribute them, or apply them to those who needed...'[70] Interestingly, when she and her husband were ill, they called in a physician whose chief remedy was blood-letting.[71]

Elizabeth Walker provided detailed descriptions of two daughters' illnesses and her treatment of them. They read like case studies written by a physician. She narrated the type of illness, 'quartane ague' (a type of epilepsy), the medicines which she administered, and the one which cured her daughter, 'Matthew's Pill'. She received the advice from a friend to give her daughter 20 grams of this drug. To her other daughter, Elizabeth, who was near death, she administered oil of sweet almonds which brought on a purge and her daughter was cured. In both cases, Elizabeth Walker recognized the importance of not only natural medicines in the healing process but also the power of prayer. After her daughter Margaret had recovered she wrote in her diary that she believed 'the benefit was more from the Prayers ... than from the Medicines'.[72]

The Italian peninsula seems to have been the exception throughout Europe during the Early Modern era. In this region, between the fourteenth and eighteenth centuries, there were a number of female practitioners: Beatrice di Candia was a doctor-surgeon in Florence; Alessandra Giliani was an anatomist at the University of Bologna; Dorotea Bucca held a chair of medicine at the University of Bologna; Laurea Constantia Calenda (Constanza Calenda) succeeded her father as professor of medicine and moral philosophy at Naples University and taught there for forty years during the fifteenth century.[73] Thomasia de Mattio of Castro Isiae and Maria Incarnata of Naples possessed diplomas for surgery. Marie-Angèle Ardingheli (1730–1825) was a physician and naturalist in Naples who translated the works of the Reverend Stephen Hales, the English botanist and chemist whose works influenced William Harvey. She was honoured by the Paris Academy of Sciences.[74]

During the seventeenth century, Nichola Salvaggia of Sienna and Margareta Sarrochi of Naples were graduates of the medical school at Padua. Elena Lucrezia Cornaro Piscopia (1646–84) was born in Venice, the daughter of Giovanni Battista Cornaro, the Procurator of St Mark's, and taught at the University of Padua.[75] As a child, she studied Latin and Greek under distinguished tutors. She also mastered Hebrew, Spanish, French and Arabic, and later studied mathematics, philosophy and theology.[76] Elena was the first woman to earn a doctorate, which was in philosophy from the University of Padua.[77]

As far as medical practitioners outside the university system are concerned, the medical system in Italy, particularly in Bologna, was predominantly male from the end of the sixteenth century to the middle of the eighteenth century.[78] Women could practise legally as midwives and as merchants of patented medicines. The drug business tended to run in families. The Grimaldi family received its patent in 1614 from the city of Bologna. It was granted to Martino Grimaldi who passed it down to his brother-in-law who then passed it on to his widow.[79] As in other parts of Europe, women were excluded from the guilds of barbers and apothecaries. In 1556, the barber guilds specifically stated that only masters' sons and grandsons could take over a business, but four years later, women were included. The clause read that in addition to male members, 'female heirs could inherit the right to keep shop open' but only if a man was in charge of the business.[80]

In France, the situation was similar. Women could produce and sell medicines. A case in point is the widow of Joseph Garrus. He was a doctor in Montpellier who had produced a drug, 'the elixir of Garrus'. After his death in 1723, his widow and her heirs 'enjoyed the production and distribution of the drug'.[81]

Women were often permitted to practise medicine when male personnel were in short supply during outbreaks of plague. In Spain, the fourteenth-century plague had important consequences for female and other minority healers, such as Muslims and Jews. In the years before the plague, the numbers of medical practitioners, particularly apothecaries and surgeons, had grown considerably.[82] With the plague, their numbers declined significantly and the result was a severe shortage of medical personnel. The main duties of healing fell upon women, who nursed the sick and administered first aid, grew herbs, dispensed remedies, healed the wounded and performed minor surgical operations.

Female practitioners were also in demand in Italy when there was a shortage of men, such as during the plague and perhaps in wartime. There were unlicensed female practitioners who specialized in female ailments and worked alongside the licensed midwives.[83] Nuns were involved in the preparation of drugs which they would sell to the sick outside the convent. The involvement of this group in the drug trade was resented by the apothecaries but tolerated by the Church. The apothecaries protested against 'the monasteries both of friars and nuns who sell internal and external remedies'.[84]

In addition to practising various types of medicine, European women contributed to the development of medicine through their work as anatomists. Two important anatomists were Anna Morandi Manzolini (1716–71) of Bologna and Marie Cathérine Biheron (1719–86)[85] of Paris. Morandi Manzolini[86] was not a medical practitioner in the traditional sense in that she was not a healer; however, she is worth noting for the contribution that she made to our understanding of the functioning of the human body.

Morandi Manzolini was the first female practitioner of anatomy to make models of internal organs, especially of the uterus and abdominal cavity and the ear, which could be dissected to teach medical students. One of her models demonstrated the stages which the foetus passes through in the womb and how it is nourished.[87] Her models demonstrate a marked improvement over other models at this time in terms of the understanding of the functioning of parts of the human body, the sense organs, and cardiovascular and reproductive systems. Previous ceroplasticists such as Ercole Lelli had focused on osteology and mycology.

Manzolini was the daughter of Rose Giovanni and Charles Morandi. At the age of twenty, she married Giovanni Manzolini. They would have six children in five years.[88] Manzolini began her career by serving as assistant to her husband who was a professor of anatomy at the University of Bologna. Giovanni Manzolini had been assistant to Ercole Lelli, a famous anatomical wax modeller 'whose wax sculptures of a horse and a human kidney had inspired Archbishop Lambertini to propose to the Bolognese Senate the establishment of an anatomical museum in the Institute of Science'.[89] Giovanni, who was frequently unwell, gave Anna lessons in the art of ceroplastics. She learned how to perform dissections, and initially dissected animals as a way of perfecting her modelling skills. She also helped her husband with his dissections and lectured in his place when he was ill. In order to supplement their income, the couple constructed life-size models of the human body. They used a mixture of clay and wax to reproduce the illusion of human tissue. Anna was soon selling her models and supplementing the family income.

Following the death of her husband from tuberculosis at the age of forty-eight, Morandi Manzolini swiftly built a considerable reputation. By 1750, the famous anatomy professor and surgeon, Dr Giovanni Galli, having opened in his own house a school of obstetrics for surgeons and midwives, had commissioned her to give a series of private lessons.[90] Ten years later, she was appointed to the chair of anatomy, with the additional title of 'modellatrice' in wax, with a salary of 300 liras per year. She could teach classes in anatomy and wax-modelling, in private and public. In addition, she was elected to the Academy Clementina (or Arts Academy) in 1755. The Academy Clementina was part of the Institute of Sciences. She was not, however, made a member of the Academy of Sciences. Nevertheless, her fame spread throughout Europe. She was elected to the British Royal Society and the Russian Royal Scientific Association. Joseph II, Emperor of Austria, purchased some of her models as did the King of Sardinia, the Royal Society of London and the procurator of Venice.[91]

Morandi died in 1774 at the age of fifty-eight. The senate of Bologna had her models placed in the Anatomical Museum of the Institute of Sciences which also housed Lelli and Galli's work. Luigi Galvani (1737–98), a professor of anatomy at the Institute of Sciences, and a possible collaborator of Morandi's made use of her sculptures in his human anatomy courses.[92] She is today represented by statues in the Pantheon in Rome and in the University of Bologna medical museum.[93]

Morandi's birth coincided with the start of the century of Enlightenment, in which the climate of intellectual fervour made it possible for women to participate more meaningfully in science. Marie Cathérine Biheron, Morandi's contemporary and fellow anatomist, also profited from Enlightenment attitudes. Her models were important in the sense that they prepared the way for extensive changes in surgery which took place at the close of the eighteenth century. Biheron's father was a Parisian apothecary. She studied with Madeleine Basseport, an illustrator at the Jardin Royal des Herbes Médicinales, and the Parisian surgeon, François Morand who, in 1759, presented one of her models to the Academy of Sciences.[94]

Biheron made wax models of interest to those in medicine and midwifery, including the famous Madame de Coudray. Her models were of both sexes and demonstrated a sophisticated knowledge of human anatomy. Biheron displayed her models at the French Royal Academy of Sciences, even in the presence of foreign royalty. In March 1771, Gustav III of Sweden hosted an evening of scientific presentations by such Enlightenment luminaries as the chemist Lavoisier. The last presentation was by Biheron. Baron Grimm, a friend of Diderot, who was present, remarked 'In effect, I believe that the marvelous work of Mlle. Biheron is something unique in Europe.' However, Mlle Biheron was not given a pension by the Academy nor made a member for her work.[95]

Biheron gave anatomy lessons in her home and counted many of the *philosophes*, including Diderot, among her friends. Indeed, Diderot was one of her greatest supporters. His daughter took three courses in anatomy and sex education before her marriage, which his brother, a priest, did not support.[96] Girls were supposed to remain innocent and ignorant of sex until their wedding night. Biheron's extensive knowledge and understanding of the female reproductive system led Diderot to recommend her to the English politician John Wilkes for instruction to his daughter.[97]

In spite of these triumphs, contemporary physicians and surgeons were less admiring of her endeavours. She did, however, have supporters at the Jardin Royal, the botanist Jussieu and the classical scholar Villoison. She travelled to London but received little encouragement there except from anatomist William Hunter and his student William Hewson who appreciated her work.[98] Like Anna Morandi Manzolini, Biheron's models brought her renown across Europe. Catherine the Great purchased some of her models.[99]

General Luigi Ferdinando Marsili (1680–1730) and archbishop of Bologna Prospero Lambertini (1675–1758), who in 1742 became Pope Benedict XIV, were partially responsible for making this climate of scientific excellence possible in Bologna.[100] They desired to return Bologna to its previous status as a leader in academic excellence and they both had a great interest in and devotion to the new science. Thus, from the middle of the seventeenth century, changes were made to the university curriculum which involved the introduction of the new experimental science and philosophies of the Enlightenment era. However, the curriculum was still dominated by medieval Aristotelian philosophy. In 1711, an Institute of Science was founded to facilitate these demands. Students could study experimental science at the Institute, but it was run by the senate which was distinct from the university and considered inferior. Women, however, found the Institute along with its Academy of Sciences much more welcoming to them than the university.[101]

Laura Maria Caterina Bassi (1711–78),[102] perhaps better known for her work in physics than in the medical field – she was the first woman to hold a chair of physics at a university – was also an anatomist and lectured on anatomy at the University of Bologna.[103] The daughter of a legal specialist, Giuseppe Bassi, and Rosa Cesari, Bassi's family was well connected in Bolognese society, and she had been educated at home by her family doctor, Gaetano Tacconi.[104] A contemporary of Manzolini, she was awarded a doctorate in philosophy in 1732 from the University of Bologna. She also had the support of Cardinal Lambertini.[105] She was married to a physician, Giuseppe Verati in 1738 and had five children.[106]

Bassi did most of her teaching and research at home because of the reluctance of the university professors to let women lecture at the university. She was not happy with this situation as her letters to Dr Flaminio Scarselli reveal. Since her classes were so large, her home was too small to accommodate the numbers. In addition, she spent a great deal of her own money buying equipment. She asked Scarselli to speak on her behalf to the 'Principe supreme' about receiving some recompense, but we do not know the outcome.[107] There was resistance among her male colleagues to her presence at the university. They would not inform her of organizational meetings such as one established by Benedictine academies.[108]

Bologna's reputation as an intellectual centre also attracted English women of noble birth who travelled to Italy to study. One such woman was Elizabeth Bury (1644–1720), a scholar of anatomy, 'who never neglected the wretch on the sick-bed'. Bury was the daughter of Captain Adam Lawrence and Elizabeth Cutts and the wife of the Reverend Sam Bury.[109] Her major interests were anatomy and medicine, partly because she herself suffered from ill-health and partly because she desired to help her neighbours. According to her memoirs, she had 'studied almost everything, including anatomy and medicine'. Bury wrote that she had 'acquired considerable skill in diagnosis and she impressed 'many of the great men of the Faculty ... by her stating the most difficult cases in such proper terms, which could have been expected only from men of their own profession...' Apparently, she understood the 'human carcass and the Materia Medica much better than most of her sex which ever they had been acquainted with'. She visited the sick, not only to practise medicine, but also to preach to them.[110] She left behind her papers containing her 'critical observations' in anatomy, medicine, mathematics and music.[111]

The important role played by upper-class English women from the late sixteenth and mid-seventeenth centuries in practising medicine has been largely overlooked by scholars. Only recently have these women's diaries and letters begun to be published and their lives explored. Practising medicine within the home and village was an acceptable form of behaviour for women as it was often considered a form of charity and an extension of the mothering role. Indeed, it was a societal expectation that women treated their sick relatives and neighbours.[112] Women were often appointed by the town to take care of those suffering from smallpox and during the turbulent years of the English Civil War, as in times of plague when male medical practitioners were in short supply, the services of women were in particular demand. Many treated wounded soldiers at this time.

Charity was often a motivation for women performing medical service within their community and beyond and this was particularly the case with aristocratic women, from whom competence in basic medical skills was expected.

Lady Grace Mildmay, née Sheridan, was such a woman. She was raised by her father's niece, Mistress Hamblyn, who 'had a Good knowledge in medicine and surgery'.[113] Fortunately for historians, she left behind her a journal or autobiography for her children and her grandchildren. Her journal provides researchers with a great deal of information concerning her medical skills. She wrote the journal in 1617, three years before her death, when she was already a widow. In common with other written pieces of this era, Mildmay's journal was spiritual in nature.[114] It is composed of two volumes, the first dealing with symptoms and causes of diseases, the second with home remedies.[115] Like other upper-class women, Lady Mildmay administered medicines and treated sores and syphilis, but unlike Margaret Hoby (see below) she did not perform surgery. Neither did she bleed or cut patients. She worked regularly and did not charge her patients. She followed the instructions of university trained physicians, as she wrote: 'Now followeth several courses of physic practiced by the advice of several physicians upon several patients for the headache.'[116] She had read Dr William Turner's *A New Herball* published in 1551 and John de Vigo's, *The Most Excellent Worke of Chirurgery* (translated from Latin in 1543 by Bartholomew Traheson) to educate herself on herbal substances and medicine.[117]

Lady Margaret Hoby also left behind a diary[118] which provides interesting insights into a woman who practised community medicine during the first half of the seventeenth century. She is thought to be one of the first English women to write a diary.[119] Lady Margaret Hoby lived during the late Tudor period, from 1599 to 1605, and received a religious education in the household of Henry Hastings, third Earl of Huntington. This had a determining influence on her life and work. She believed that God was the true healer, 'I may truly conclude that it is the Lord and not the physician, who both ordains the medicine for our health and ordereth the ministering of it for the good of his children.'[120] Like Mildmay, as part of her education, Hoby had read Turner's *Herball* and Vigo's book on surgery and thus had some knowledge of plants, medicines and surgical methods.[121]

Margaret Hoby, née Dakins, was the only child of a wealthy Yorkshire landowner, an heiress and thus a much sought after bride. She was married three times: her first husband Walter Devereux, was killed in battle in Rouen, France, in 1591. From this marriage, she gained an estate in north Yorkshire. Later the same year she was married to Thomas Sidney. He died four years later and she married Sir Thomas Posthumous Hoby, a JP and MP, in 1596. They lived on her estate.[122]

Margaret Hoby's diary was written between 1599 and 1605. It is a record of her daily activities, her very active prayer life, and an account of her medical practice. She was engaged in healing all sorts of sick people and animals on her estate. Primarily, she treated servants and she extended this care to the nearby village. Her medical care included dressing wounds and sores and dispensing medicines from her own herb garden. She also performed midwifery functions and minor surgery.[123] Her diary contains thirty-two reports of 'dressing patients'. Medical care was as much a part of her daily routine as praying. She used the term 'patient' for those under her care. She indicated that she 'dressed the sores that came to me' and those she had 'undertaken'. Presumably, she worked from her home and visited patients in their homes.[124] This entry is typical: 'After private prayer I saw a man's leg dressed.'[125] Hoby, in common with other gentry ladies, often treated the poor: 'After I had prayed privately I dressed a poor boy's leg that came to me ... after I dressed the hand of one of our servants that was very sore cut...'[126] Apparently, this injury was to a man named Jarden, one of Hoby's principal servants.[127] Based on her diary entries, it appears that her practice of medicine primarily involved the dressing of wounds; however, on one occasion, she refers to performing anal surgery on a child: 'This day, in the afternoon, I had had a child brought to see that was born at Silpho ... who had no fundament, and had no passage for excrements but at the Mouth: I was earnestly entreated to cut the place to see if any passage could be made, but, although I cut deep and searched, there was none to be found.'[128]

Another titled woman, Anne Dacres, Countess of Arundel and Surrey,[129] treated 'all kinds of people who either wanting will, or means to go to Doctors and Chirugeons'. They came to her for 'the curing of their wounds and distempers'. Anne Dacres not only cured people in her village of various ailments, but 'several out of other shires, 20, 40 and more miles distant...'[130] Apparently she could cure those who had released from hospitals as incurables. Dacres would take these people into her own home out of compassion. She had her own medicines, including salves, which she purchased or made herself. She used sheepskins to make her plasters.[131]

Presumably, there were many other upper-class women who practised medicine and surgery without a licence, thereby performing a valuable service to their communities. Sources for this sort of information are difficult to obtain as few of these practitioners left diaries or other records behind them.

A number of women practised a basic form of military medicine during the English Civil War. One of these women was Lady (Apsley) Hutchinson (1620–75), who was best known for the biography of her husband, *Memoirs of the Life of Colonel Hutchinson by his widow, Lucy*, first published in 1808. Born Lucy Apsley, daughter of Sir Allen Apsley, Lieutenant Governor of the Tower, she learned the art of medicine from her mother – she was one of nine children, five of whom survived. Her mother had patronized and assisted Sir Walter Raleigh with his chemical experiments when he was a prisoner in the Tower of London. Mrs Apsley passed the knowledge she had acquired to her daughter.[132]

Lucy received her education at home and was literate by the age of four. She had several tutors who taught her languages, including Latin, music, dancing, writing and needlework.[133] She was afflicted with smallpox as a child which left her face permanently scarred. In spite of her lack of physical attractiveness, she married Colonel Hutchinson at the age of eighteen in 1638. She had several pregnancies, most of which resulted in miscarriages, but she did give birth to twin sons in 1640, and two further sons, neither of whom survived childhood.[134] Colonel Hutchinson was a regicide and was imprisoned in Nottingham in 1643. His family joined him in prison and it is here that Lucy performed her medical work. She cared for the sick and wounded prisoners. Her memoirs describe some of her cases, such as a Derby captain, 'and five of our men hurt, who for want of another surgeon, were brought to the governor's wife, and she having some excellent balsams and plasters in her closet, with the assistance of a gentleman that has some skill, dressed all their wounds, whereof some were dangerous, being all shots, with good success, they were well cured in convenient time.'[135] She made 'broths and restoratives with her own hand, visited and took care of them, and provided them all necessaries'.[136]

In Scotland, Lady Anne Halkett (1622–99) served as a surgeon in the royal army at various battles, including the Battle of Dunfermline. She recalled taking care of wounded soldiers:

> I cannot omit to insert here the opportunity I had of serving many poor wounded soldiers; for as we were riding to Kinrose [her lodging where she established a dressing station] I saw that two looked desperately ill, who were so weak they were hardly able to go along the high way; and inquiring what ailed them, they told me they had been soldiers at Dunbar and were going towards Kinrose, if their wounds would suffer them. I bid them when they came there inquire for the Countess of D.'s lodging and there would be one there would dress them… They came, attended with twenty more. And betwixt that time and Monday that we left that

> place, I believe threescore was the least that was dressed by me and my woman and Ar. Ro, who I employed to such as was unfit for me to dress; and besides the plasters or balsam I applied, I gave every one of them as much with them as might dress them 3 or 4 times, for I had provided myself very well of things necessary for that employment, expecting they might be useful.

She goes on to describe in detail the various types of wounds which she dressed: 'one was a man whose head was cut so that the [?] was very visibly seen and the water came bubbling up, which when Ar. R. saw he cried out, "Lord have mercy upon thee for thou art but a dead man."' She told him not to be discouraged 'and the man's wound did heal'.[137]

Lady Halkett received tremendous praise from her contemporaries and her fame continued into the next century. After the Battle of Dunbar, when he heard of her good work, the king thanked her in person.[138] George Ballard, writing in the mid-eighteenth century, observed that: 'Next to the studies of divinity, she seems to have taken most delight in those of physik and surgery, in which she was no mean proficient.'[139]

The circumstances in Spain were more complex than in the other European countries under consideration here. Spain had a considerable Muslim as well as Jewish minority population. Many women in these communities practised medicine in some form although the training necessary to obtain a licence was closed to Muslim healers. Both Muslim men and women treated the sick in their own communities.[140]

In general, medicine and law were almost exclusively in the hands of Christians (not including converts, who were treated with a fair measure of distrust). Muslims worked primarily in the trades. However, as we have seen, Spanish women were also effectively banned from the front line or official practice of medicine except in times of shortages of regular male physicians.[141] The Cortes of Monzón (1363) provided an alternative licensing procedure for Jews and Muslims who, like women, were barred from Christian universities. Female Muslim women practitioners or *metgesses* practised midwifery, surgery and general medicine. As noted in Chapter 1, Çahud practised medicine in the royal household of Valencia while other Muslim women performed surgery in Barcelona. The king ruled that these women could sit an examination set by licensed surgeons, and if they passed it, they were permitted to practise.[142] Experts in the history of Spanish medical licensing argue that the *furs* which banned women from medical practice may have been directed against Muslims only.[143] However, with the shortage of male Christian physicians, these minorities, including women, were permitted to practise until the end of the fifteenth century.[144] Although Christian Spain rejected Muslim culture, Morisco medicine – that of the Moriscos and Moriscas, former Muslims who had been forced to convert to Catholicism between 1502 and 1526[145] – was held in high regard and both male and female medical practitioners treated members of the Spanish upper class, including King Philip II.

What made the situation even more complex were the views held by Christian clergymen on Moriscas (female converts to Christianity) whom they perceived as sexual, exotic and as demonstrating a refusal to assimilate.[146] In 1609, Philip III ordered the expulsion of Moriscas from Spain and directed those who were going to non-Christian lands to leave behind children aged seven and younger.[147] It is estimated that about 300,000 people left Spain at this time, about 5 per cent of the total population.[148]

As time progressed, Morisco medicine became increasingly marginalized. Mary Elizabeth Perry has maintained that the 'invisibility' is 'especially remarkable in early modern Spain, where Jews, Muslims and Christians had made their homes for centuries…'[149] But however invisible they were, unofficial female Muslim healers remained part and parcel of the Spanish countryside. Women worked as healers and seers. As a rule, their patients were female and healing was often a second job. One example was the innkeeper María de Ubecar. Another was the butcher, Gerónima de Muza from Belchite. These women did not necessarily practise for monetary remuneration. They would stop their activities on Thursday evenings just before the Muslim Sabbath.[150] In Valencia, a list of professions dating from the sixteenth century based upon documents from the Inquisition includes some male Muslim barbers (11), healers (11) and physicians (6) but no women.[151]

Jews also treated members of their own community. Those who had been in practice before the 1329 *furs* were permitted to continue practising medicine and surgery after an examination.[152] Until the start of the Spanish Inquisition in 1478, Jews were not marginalized in the same way as Muslims and male surgeons and physicians achieved a great deal of success among the Christian majority in Castile and Aragón.[153] There is little evidence for Jewish women practising medicine during the Early Modern period, although there is evidence dating from the fourteenth century for women doctors who were licensed by the crown of Aragón.[154] However, in the Early Modern period, the situation for Jews deteriorated. They were forced to live in ghettos in the towns and were brought under the direct control of the king. Generally speaking, the crown did its best to protect Jews from hostile municipalities but arbitrary laws were passed by hostile Christian municipalities including laws preventing Jews from practising medicine and surgery.[155] The Jews were expelled from Spain in 1492. As with the Muslim minority, women remained invisible and outside the official records including those from the Spanish Inquisition. Jews were much more likely to be tried for heresy than for healing.

Despite the concerted efforts of constituted authorities in Early Modern Europe to prevent women from practising medicine, they continued to relieve the suffering of very many people, utilizing skills from herbalism to surgery. Middle and upper-class women often treated patients unofficially in the community and in general women's skills were sought after, whether they were in medicine, surgery, bone-setting or any other area of medicine, because they charged much lower fees than the professionals if they charged at all. At a more academic level, women anatomists such as Morandi Manzolini and Biheron contributed substantially to the development of modern medicine.

8
Motherly Medicine: Domestic Healers and Apothecaries

'Medicine began at home', aptly wrote historian Keith Thomas,[1] and 'Lay medical practice was centred on the family.' Indeed, self-medication and healing were commonplace in the Early Modern period: 'Patients often treated themselves, and the women members of the family especially were the sources of medical knowledge and treatment.'[2] One could add to these statements that medicine was practised by mothers and handed down through the ages by their mothers, grandmothers and great-grandmothers.[3] The influential and innovative sixteenth-century French agronomist Olivier de Serres, Seigneur du Pradel,[4] believed that women were better suited for family or domestic medicine than men because they were naturally 'officious and charitable'. 'Mothers', he wrote, 'opened their hearts to understanding apothecary, healing minor cuts, wounds, and many other ailments.' From books, 'they take several salutory remedies which come to them easily. They also used many remedies they have learned from their experiences.'[5] Likewise, Juan Vives, the Spanish humanist, instructed wives to look after their husbands when they were unwell. Wives should, 'treat his wounds, cover his limbs to keep them from the cold'. Wives 'should look after their husbands themselves, rather than employing their domestics'.[6]

The focus of this chapter is domestic or household medicine as practised by women. The archives of the Wellcome Library for the History and Understanding of Medicine possess a significant collection of medical receipts compiled by women, and much of the material for this chapter is based on a sample of some thirty-three manuscript collections, which date from 1621 to the mid-eighteenth century.[7]

In addition to an examination of a selection of cures found in English receipt books, this chapter will present the domestic cures suggested by a seventeenth-century French noblewoman, Marie de Rabutin-Chantal, Madame de Sévigné. Although de Sévigné did not put together a book of medicinal recipes, she wrote a great deal about domestic medicine in her letters, which were mainly addressed to her often unwell daughter,

Françoise-Marguerite de Sévigné, who became Madame de Grignan.[8] Madame de Sévigné was a great believer in self-healing, and healing by amateurs, and was very wary of the medicine practised by physicians. Her writings provide researchers with a window onto the world of unofficial and domestic medicine in seventeenth-century France. As was the case with so many women healers in England, the de Sévignés belonged to the aristocracy. They acquired at least a minimal amount of informal education, either through tutors or relatives. For many of these women, recipe collection and swapping was a leisure activity, a necessity of rural life (the vast majority lived in the country) and part of the responsibility of a lady.

One of the principal objectives of this chapter is to introduce the reader to the nature of the ailments from which people suffered in the Early Modern period, and their proposed cures in the household. At a time when few people could afford access to a physician, when physicians were often mistrusted and very low in number, especially in the countryside, we will explore how people attempted to treat minor afflictions and even more serious diseases.

The vast majority of medical recipe books were penned by upper-class Englishwomen although there are also a number written by French women. Although women in Spain played a pivotal role in domestic medicine, there is no evidence that they compiled recipe books. Mary Elizabeth Perry's research on Spain shows that during the sixteenth and seventeenth centuries, Sevillian women played a large role in the work of curing illness, primarily in their own homes, cooking up various recipes with which to treat their children, husbands and neighbours,[9] but we do not know a great deal about their work, because as domestic work it has not been documented. As Perry has noted, 'Their healing is neither visible nor official. It is unpaid, and unnoted. Medicine appeared to pertain only to the masculine world, a science that had to be controlled and studied in books, protecting all from female superstition.'[10] It has not been easy to uncover their work. Inquisitorial cases, local regulations, hagiographies and the contemporary literature have shed some light on domestic medicine, but documents provide evidence through the male voice and not that of women themselves.[11]

During the fifteenth century, the Spanish physician Juan de Avignon (fl. c. 1418) compiled information on the health of the city of Seville and its environs.[12] Avignon's book, *Sevilla medicina*, was published in 1545 by another physician, Nicolás Monardes, when Seville was experiencing health problems associated with population growth. The book analysed the air quality of the city and its relation to good health, in addition to recording symptoms and treatments for diseases afflicting the city. The majority of the recipes in Avignon's book were based on remedies prepared in the home from domestic ingredients, such as sugar and eggs. Although both Avignon and Monardes, who contributed a preface to the book, stressed the importance of diet for health, neither referred to the fact that it was mothers in the home who were at the forefront of the provision of diet and medicine.[13]

The sort of medicine that these women practised is often referred to by scholars as domestic or household medicine.[14] Women healers in the home played a crucial medical role, not only because of the cost and limited availability of physicians, but also because many people preferred to consult local women. In the case of the wealthier classes, they might do both.[15] Domestic medicine can be characterized as an Early Modern type of 'folk medicine', which had been around since ancient times. Folk medicine can be distinguished from 'scientific' medicine in that it lacks a theory of disease, and it does not follow logical testing based on observation. Folk medicine tends to be practised in rural areas. In the Middle Ages and into the Early Modern period, it was often performed by monks and nuns. Hildegard of Bingen practised this sort of medicine, ministering not only to the nuns in her monastery, but also to lay people.[16]

Women of the upper classes, such as the Paston women in England, practised as healers in their homes. Margaret Paston, for example, treated family members, including her husband, for a number of ailments including a sore eye, and a bad leg, with various herbal medicines in addition to household items such as treacle and white wine. She made plasters and relieved the pain in a friend's bad knee. In a letter to Margaret, John urged his wife to send 'by the next sure messenger that you can get, a large plaster of your floes, ungwentorum for the King's Attorney James Hobart, for all his disease is but an ache in his knee'.[17] Margaret also refers to mint and milfoil essence for a sick cousin who was unable to keep down food.[18] As was frequently the case, trained physicians were only consulted when it was considered absolutely necessary. When Margaret's husband was sick while in London, she wanted him to be at home where she could treat him.[19] She warned him to 'beware what medicines you take of any physicians of London: I shall never trust to them because of you[r] father and my uncle…'[20]

Jennifer K. Stine's unpublished doctoral dissertation is one of the few detailed studies of domestic medicine. Stine observed the importance of family medical recipes: 'Household medicinal recipe collections are among the most common of 17th century medical manuscripts and the least analyzed.'[21] Stine argued that the Early Modern period in England is important because it was during the first half of the seventeenth century that women began to collect and organize these recipes and put them into books.[22] Linda Pollock's study of Lady Grace Mildmay's recipe book, Raymond A. Anselment's examination of Elizabeth Freke's diary, and Leonard Guthrie's article analysing Lady Sedley's receipt book,[23] are among the small number of published modern studies on this subject.[24]

One suggestion for the paucity of studies of medical recipe books authored by women is that there is a great deal of basic information missing from these books, particularly in comparison with doctors' case books, such as to whom were these medicines administered, how often and in what dosages. Nor do we know to what extent these remedies were effective. In many cases, we know nothing about the author or authors except their names. Further complicating such research is the fact that the books are largely unpublished and only accessible in specialized libraries such as the Wellcome Library in London.

There is, in fact, little evidence that these women cured diseases, but they did relieve symptoms, and in doing so, apparently, they were as successful as the regulars.[25] Adam Martindale, who suffered from 'a vehement fermentation in my body ... ugly, dry, scurvy, eating deep and spreading broad', preferred to be treated by a 'poor woman' rather than the 'skilful men' who 'differed much in their opinions'. The woman, who made a salve from celandine and ash root, was successful in healing the ailment.[26]

Practising medicine within the home and village was an acceptable form of behaviour for women, as it was often considered a form of charity and an extension of the mothering role.[27] This view was articulated at the time by English poet, playwright and writer on country life, Gervase Markham,[28] author of *The English Housewife*, first published in 1615 and reprinted sixteen times by 1683. Markham, in sketching the duties of the housewife, specifically mentions her duty in 'the preservation and care of the family touching their health and soundness of body'. In terms of caring for her family's welfare, she should 'have a physical kind of knowledge, how to administer many wholesome receipts or medicines for the good of their health, as well to prevent sickness, as to take away the effects and evil of the same'.[29] Markham published his collection of recipes in order to assist the housewife with her medical duties, which involved 'the curing of those ordinary sicknesses' using 'approved medicines',[30] although he made it clear that the housewife should not consider herself to be a physician or a professional in any sense of the word. Markham was not alone in affirming the housewife's medical duties. The Reverend Timothy Rogers wrote that one of the duties of the 'Good Woman' was to practise medicine when a 'Doctor is not at Hand' or when there is not enough money to pay for his services.[31] Indeed, 'Housewives were expected to grow herbs and use them for healing purposes.'[32]

Two British women who practised domestic medicine as prescribed by Markham and Rogers were Lady Anne Clifford (1590–1676), Countess of Dorset and Countess of Pembroke and Montgomery, and Lady Brilliana Harley (1600–43). Anne Clifford was a 'distiller of medicinal waters, a dabbler in alchemy, an expert in the property of plants, flowers and herbs'.[33] She treated her mother when she was ill as she recorded in her diary: 'Upon the 9th, I received a letter from Mr. Bellasis how extreme ill my mother had been...& as they thought in some danger of Death so as I sent Rivers presently to London with letters to be sent to her & certain Cordials & conserves.'[34]

Lady Brilliana Harley was renowned for her defence of Brampton Bryan Castle near Hereford during the English Civil War. She was the third wife of Sir Robert Harley, a Puritan Member of Parliament.[35] Evidence for Lady Harley's medical care may be found in the letter she wrote to her son while he was away at Oxford and unwell: 'I have sent some bessor stone, which you take at night when you go to bed; and the Lord bless all means to you. I have sent you 2 grains of orampotabely, which I would have you take in 2 spoonfuls of cordus water, when you find yourself not well.'[36] In addition to sending remedies to her son, she told him that his illness could be a result of his reckless behaviour, that God was teaching him a moral lesson. She encouraged him to seek help from God in healing his illness: 'My dear Ned, if it pleases God that you are still not well, look up to your God; consider why He corrects; it is better us, that we may see the evil of our ways, and find how bitter sin is, that had brought such bitter things upon us…'[37]

'Family' medicine involved mothers teaching their daughters what was considered to be a domestic art. Both family receipt books and published guides, such as Leonard Sowerby's *The Ladies Dispensatory*(1651),[38] were used as instruction manuals. Sowerby claimed in the preface to his book that he based his recipes on remedies by Dioscorides, Gerard, Goraeus and Fuchsius.[39] In addition, he maintained that his remedies had never been published before in English. Sarah Fell wrote in her *Household Accounts* on 5 July 1674 that a Thomas Lawson had instructed her sister 'in the knowledge of herbs'. He was paid for his services.[40]

The term 'domestic medicine' was popularized by Scottish physician Dr William Buchan (1729–1805) in his book, *Domestic Medicine, or the family physician*, which was published in Edinburgh in 1769 and printed by William Smellie.[41] According to Robert Kerr, whose biography of William Smellie was published in 1811, Smellie was also among a number of contributors to the book.[42] Like the earlier books written by women, Buchan's work focused on ailments and their cures. Lawrence argues that what distinguished Buchan's book from earlier receipt books were his clinical knowledge and his emphasis on hygiene.[43]

Another printed book written by a man for women is John Ball's (1704–79), *The female physician: or, every woman her own doctor. Wherein is summarily comprised, all that is necessary to be known in the cure of the several disorders to which the fair sex are liable. Together with prescriptions in English* (London, 1770; reprinted Edinburgh, 1771). Ball, a medical doctor, was already known as the author of a number of other medical treatises.[44] His *Female physician* is organized by illness, symptoms and cure for minor disorders, many of which are common or female in nature, and include back pain, menstrual problems, abortion and miscarriage, breast and womb cancer. He included recipes from other physicians, including Dr Whytt, and he quoted from Smellie in his chapter concerning 'Of the Menses, and their Suppression'.[45]

Similar types of books were published in Spain. One work on domestic medicine, *Tesoro de los pobres* (1519) by Pedro Hispano was reprinted several times. Girolamo de Manfredi's text on domestic medicine, *Liber de homine*

(1497), was published in Castilian, and Gregorio López's *Tesoro de medicinas* was published in 1708 in Madrid (Imprenta de Música). These recipe books went hand in hand with prescriptive books from the sixteenth century such as Vives's *Instruction*, in which he wrote that it is the wife's duty to take care of her sick husband and children.[46]

Lord Ruthven, who described himself as a 'chemist', collected the recipes for *The Ladies Cabinet, Enlarged, and Opened containing many rare Secrets and Rich Ornaments of several kinds and different uses*, first published in 1639. It was organized under three general headings: (1) Preserving, conserving, candying; (2) Physick and Chirurgerie; (3) Cookery. It was a model for the *Queen's Closet Opened*, a cookery book containing medical receipts first published in 1655, with nine editions to follow, and written by 'WM'.[47] The queen of this title is Charles I's wife Henrietta Maria, from whose royal kitchen the book apparently originated. It guaranteed 'incomparable Secrets in Physick, Chyryrgery, preserving and candying'.[48] The book is divided into three sections: 'The Pearl of Practice' which covers medical remedies; 'A Queen's Delight', which examines confectionery; and 'The Compleat Cook', which looks at general culinary recipes. The *Queen's Closet Opened* is one of the few published books containing medical recipes to have been compiled by a woman. The majority of women's receipt books remain unprinted. Consequently, substantial work has been conducted on published books of domestic medicine written by men for women, but very little on books written by women for women. Lynette Hunter underscores this point in the introduction to her discussion of three published receipt books by women. 'There is a curious gap that confronts anyone interested in the history of women in England in the early modern period.'[49] However, there are two printed books of cookery and medical recipes in addition to that allegedly by Henrietta Maria which should be discussed. One of these is Elizabeth (Talbot) Grey's (1581–1651), *A choice Manual of rare and select Secrets in Physick and Chirurgerie, Collected and practiced by the Countess of Kent*, which is probably based on a manuscript book in her collection, and the other is Aletheia Talbot Howard's, *Natura Exenterata* (1655). Elizabeth Grey, Countess of Kent, and Aletheia Talbot Howard, the Countess of Arundel, were sisters and their two texts have been described as 'the first printed books of technical and scientific material in England' by women.[50] The earliest extant copy of Grey's book is a second edition published in 1653, a year after her death, which is housed in the British Library. Grey's book went through some twenty-two editions. Grey was known for her expertise in herbal medicine and one of her recipes for a diuretic, 'The Countess of Kent's Powder', 'Pulvis Cantianus' or 'Testacious powder', was recommended by John Quincy, MD, author of the eighteenth-century *Dispensatory*.[51] Quincy maintained that 'this is vastly a better Composition than that of Gascoign's Powder for the Purpose of a diaphoretic; this will in reality promote sweating and drive out powerfully by the Skin, which makes it a very good medicine in all fevers whatsoever, as they are always affected by such discharges.' Quincy recommended the powder for diseases such as measles and smallpox. The 'Countess of Kent's Powder' was made from crab claws, pearl, red and white coral and crabs' eyes with lemon juice.[52] Aletheia Talbot's *Natura Exenterata*, was published in 1655.[53] Unlike the queen's book and Elizabeth Grey's manual it does not use a three-part division, but is comprised primarily of medicinal and pharmaceutical receipts.[54]

Henrietta Maria and the Talbot sisters formed part of an elite group of women who received an adequate education, albeit informal, which enabled them to read and to understand basic chemistry. They were part of the new scientific milieu of the seventeenth century which included men such as the mathematician John Pell and the naturalist and botanist John Evelyn. Henrietta Maria's chamberlain, Sir Kenneth Digby, was a chemist. The women presumably picked up scientific information from these men, all of whom were caught up in Paracelsian or experimental science.[55]

Most of the receipt books compiled by women were intended for family and close friends; they were never intended for publication and remain comparatively inaccessible. Perhaps more importantly, historians have not considered female medical practices to be valid or important. The practice of domestic medicine by women has been called 'dabbling', 'well meaning' but 'crude'.[56] Ministering to the sick was considered either to be part of a housewife's duty or to be a form of charity, both of which were belittled by contemporary writers. Many historians' views may well be based on negative contemporary commentary about women and medicine, filtered through the work of physicians who viewed only themselves, licensed surgeons and apothecaries as capable of practising medicine. And even within this group, physicians still looked down on apothecaries and surgeons.[57] Comments such as that of Sir William D'Avenant do not paint a positive picture:

> I choose
> None of your dull country madams, that spend
> Their time in studying receipts to make
> Marchpane and preserve plums, that talk
> Of painful childbirth, servants' wages, and
> Their husband's good complexion and his leg.[58]

Dr Walter Harris's comments were hardly complimentary, writing in 1689 that 'country people, who lying at a considerable distance from physicians, are supported by my Lady's Cordials out of Charity, which her Ladyship exhibits promiscuously in every disease with very great applause; for be the event what it will, the Cordial, to be sure, must never be blamed'.[59] Dr James Primrose wrote on the subject of medicinal remedies and the women who applied them; their motives may have been pure in wanting to take care of their men folk, but 'All which things, seeing they cannot be known but by a skilful Physician, women ought not to rashly and adventurously intermeddle with them. Again they usually take their remedies out of English books, or else make use of such as are communicated to them by others, and then they think they have rare remedies for all diseases.'[60] A better-known physician, Thomas Sydenham (1624–89) remarked that 'Nowadays every house has its old woman, or practitioner, in an art that she has never learnt, to the killing of mankind.'[61]

There were a few dissenting voices. One of these was the famous seventeenth-century herbalist Dr Nicholas Culpeper, an expert on domestic medicine, who wrote that, 'All the nation are already physicians ... If you ail anything, every one you meet, whether a man or woman, will prescribe you a medicine for it.'[62] Undoubtedly, the publication of Culpeper's *The English Physician*, later known as *Culpeper's Herbal: Culpeper's complete herbal: consisting of a comprehensive description of nearly all herbs with their medicinal properties and directions for compounding the medicines extracted from them*, had some impact on the practice of domestic medicine. It definitely had a great influence in medical publishing, going through some one hundred editions.[63] The clergyman Robert Burton also dissented from the dominant view of domestic practitioners, writing that, 'Many an old wife or country woman doth often more good with a few known and common garden herbs than our bombast Physicians with all their prodigious, sumptuous, far-fetched, rare, conjectural medicines.'[64]

Historians Roy and Dorothy Porter have portrayed women's practise of domestic medicine in a more positive light. They proposed that it was part and parcel of the movement of 'self-help' or 'self-treatment' which was popular after the Protestant Reformation.[65] Keith Thomas has also stressed the significance of self-help, which grew out of the Protestant worldview. Thomas proposed that after the Reformation, 'people were now taught that their practical difficulties could only be solved by a combination of self-help and prayer to God'.[66] However, evidence demonstrates that female domestic treatment of ailments had existed long before the Reformation. European medical manuals authored by men were in existence as early as the 1300s.[67] Certainly, during the Elizabethan era in England, medical books of every type, ranging from cookery manuals interspersed with medical recipes to simple books of herbal remedies, were being printed and reprinted. These books were often geared toward the lay person for use 'in time of necessity when no learned Physician is at hand'.[68]

Treating illness outside the home in an institutional setting is a very modern practice.[69] Treatment of minor ailments and the preparation of drugs were considered to be the housewife's duty and compilations of traditional remedies date from approximately the 1400s. As with those works that were published, these receipts are often mixed in with cooking recipes and provide an important source for the practice of unofficial medicine. These traditional medicines provide evidence that women were practising medicine from the home, taking care of the sick, and that they understood the use of herbal and other medicines.

Women treated family ailments with potions and powders they composed themselves from garden ingredients of herbs, roots and flowers. Their concoctions were probably as effective as the medicines prescribed by official physicians and licensed apothecaries, and relief from symptoms alone was considered a 'success' in Early Modern times[70] when the majority of people would have well recognized the lack of curative potential of contemporary medicines. The most important answer they sought from their physician was 'is this illness fatal'.[71] Regular medical recipes devised by doctors were often found in ladies' books of receipts,[72] which were an assortment of remedies derived from a multitude of sources. Some recipes were taken from newspapers, others were passed down through the generations, others came from neighbours, nursemaids and others.[73] Gentlewomen had access to medical information from their family, friends, acquaintances in their villages and local medical personnel. Their knowledge of particular illnesses and diseases was surprisingly sophisticated given the fact that they had no formal education. They would generally learn the properties of herbs and how to prepare medicines from their mothers.[74]

The Reverend Ralph Josselin – as noted in Chapter 7 – evidences the fact that women were prescribing medicines when he acknowledges in his diary that Lady L. Honeywood was his 'nurse and Physician' at the time that he thought he was suffering from scurvy. She gave him 'a purge'.[75] Josselin was the vicar of Earls Colne, and like many others he preferred to consult women, including his wife, rather than physicians.[76] Lady Honeywood's role in medical care typifies the importance of aristocratic women to the practice of household medicine. Their role as wives and mothers burdened them with responsibility for the well-being of household members and gave them access to both the knowledge and materials needed to practise medicine. Since they were literate, they were able to assemble and even author collections of recipes and to acquire a good knowledge of plants and herbs, shared and augmented by neighbours and local physicians.[77] A few, such as Lady Catherine Sedley,[78] included medicinal recipes passed onto them by local physicians who were in turn passing on formulae developed by renowned physicians such as Sir Thomas Witherley, Dr King, Richard Lower and Thomas Sydenham. Witherley, King and Lower were Charles II's physicians.[79]

Contemporaries such as John Evelyn remarked that compiling recipe books was part and parcel of the life of an upper-class woman. These women worked in the 'distillatory', they had considerable 'knowledge of plants' and they used this knowledge 'for the comfort of their poor neighbours and the use of their family'. Evelyn's wife and mother-in-law were such women. Lady Brown (his mother-in-law) took in many sick and needy people while Evelyn may well have acquired the receipts found in his *Acetaria: A Discourse of Sallets* from his wife.[80]

The recipes are contained within bound but unpublished books, often as 'commonplace' books,[81] which could contain 'an encyclopaedic array of topics' and comprise compendia of knowledge on the 'arts and sciences'.[82] Commonplace books under consideration here contained primarily medical recipes, although a good number contained cookery recipes as well, such as Letitia Owen's (afterwards Mytton) cookery book (MS 3730, c. 1715) which provided recipes for purges and minor complaints such as dropsy and rickets. Her recipe for curing dropsy used 'penny royal' water, caster sugar, syrup of 'ringwort', lemon water and liquorice, while she prescribed figs, raisins, aniseed, coriander seeds and various roots for the alleviation of rickets (MS 1180).

These books were found in the homes of upper-class or 'gentle' women who were at least semi-literate. Most receipt books were written by individual women, although some were family productions with script in more than one hand. An example of a family collection of medicines is the Boyle Family archive (MS 1340) which dates from the 1670s to 1710. The volume contains 712 medical receipts written by both Lady Ranelagh (Katherine Boyle) and her secretary.

There are many similarities in manuscript collections. They used ingredients and equipment employed by physicians and apothecaries. Indeed, many medical cures prescribed by women were identical to those recommended by physicians.[83] Dr John Symcotts, who held a medical degree from Cambridge University, and practised medicine in Huntington and Bedfordshire, accepted remedies from gentlewomen and he also happily received medical tips from his brother, who was not an MD, on healing ailments such as gout.[84] John Ward praised the treatment that women had recommended for an ague or fever: 'I have heard some women say that nothing cures an ague so certainly as a spoonful of Alum in sack.'[85] Richard Napier, 'an astrological healer and Anglican clergyman who ministered to more than 60,000 clients from his home in Great Linford',[86] also consulted unlicensed healers, and gentlewomen in particular, when looking for recipes. He specifically refers to Elisabeth Clarke, a patient, who 'told me of a very rare pultish ...; An excellent and Approved water distilled for the stone & wynd cholick whc I had of my Lady dormer the older of Wing; The Lady Tyrrles receipt of spitting blood by fault of the longues.'[87]

The recipes used by these women imply a fairly sophisticated knowledge of herbs and their properties. Ingredients used in medicinal recipes were common foodstuffs, such as bread, ale, sugar and water and common herbs and plants that were either grown specifically in gardens or foraged from nearby fields. The most regularly employed substances were chamomile, rue, penny royal, wormwood, fennel, liquorice, rhubarb in powder form, onions and violets. Many of these herbs and plants are still believed to have medicinal properties. Other ingredients were milk, cow's dung for plasters, certain alcohols, wine, usually white, less often red (claret), and occasionally brandy, eggs, barley, turpentine, sugar, garlic and honey. Some imported and exotic ingredients such as pepper, oranges, anise, cloves, almond oil, frankincense, myrrh and musk had to be purchased from the local apothecary. During the course of the seventeenth century, new drugs began to enter the medical marketplace, over time replacing the use of traditional garden herbs by both physicians and laywomen.[88]

Since these women were effectively practising pharmacy, some comment on the contemporary regulation of apothecaries seems apposite.[89] Women practising domestic medicine worked within the law of the time with respect to apothecaries, and there is no evidence that they sold their concoctions, which would have been illegal. Women who practised medicine in the home, as well as midwives, wise women and herbalists, in essence, 'those with knowledge of the nature, kind and operation of certain herbs, roots and waters', were protected in law by an Act of Parliament in 1542. To avoid prosecution, they could not accept payment for their services which were described for the purpose of 'the ease and comfort, succour, help, relief and health of the King's poor subjects'.[90] However, in 1617 in London, another law was passed which separated apothecaries from grocers. The Apothecaries' Charter read:

> No persons or person whatsoever may have, hold, or keep an Apothecaries Shop or Warehouse, or that they may exercise or use the Art or Mystery of Apothecaries, or make, mingle, work, compound, prepare, give, apply, or administer, any Medicines, or that may sell on sale, utter, set forth, or lend any Compound or Composition to any person or persons whatsoever.

Finally anyone wishing to become an apothecary would be examined.[91] Although banned from medicine and surgery, women could be admitted to the profession of apothecary by marriage or apprenticeship and there is some evidence of widows of apothecaries practising, but since the majority of the women under consideration here were treating patients in the home and not as professionals, contemporary laws did not apply. In addition, the law was not often vigorously enforced.[92]

The medical problems described in these recipe books, and for which cures were sought, were common ailments from the sixteenth to the eighteenth centuries. They were illnesses and diseases that tended not to be life threatening, but that were often painful and an impediment to the conduct of people's daily lives. Dropsy, pox, worms, rickets, scurvy, numerous skin problems and gout were the most frequently cited illnesses. Equipment used in the preparation of these home remedies involved cooking utensils: skillets, kettles, pots, jugs, saucers, various spoons. Remedies were measured in spoonfuls, pints and ounces.[93]

The earliest English book in the Wellcome collection is a collection dating from 1606, compiled by Aletheia Talbot Howard, Countess of Arundel (nearly 50 years before the publication of her *Natura Exenterata*). The full title is 'A Booke of diuers Medecines, Broothes, Salues, Waters, Syroppes and Oyntementes of which many or the most part haue been experienced and tryed by the speciall practize of Mrs Corlyon'. It is in an original gilt-stamped calf binding, with central arabesque ornament stamped 'A[letheia] A[rundel]' (MS 213).

This book was put together by the Countess of Arundel and her family, and is one of three existing copies. Aletheia (née Talbot, 1584–1654) was the Countess of Arundel and Surrey and wife of Thomas Howard, second Earl of Arundel (1586–1646). The reason historians know that this book belonged to Arundel is because of the inscription 'Liber Comitissae Arundeliae' (child of the countess) and the frontispiece of the book which contains a portrait of the countess by Hollar. In addition, there is a copy of the Wellcome manuscript in the Arundel Castle library.[94] A third copy of the manuscript is in the Folger Library in Washington, DC. The connection between the Corlyon (or Carlyon) family whose name is in the title of the book and the Arundel family is that they were Catholic families in the same community. Apparently, with Arundel patronage, the Carlyon manuscript was 'copied and distributed ... to encourage traditional charitable activities by recusant Catholic women'.[95] This book is composed of 397 recipes arranged according to ailment, from minor aches and pains, bruises, dog bites and gunshot wounds to scurvy, consumption and kidney problems. In over 200 pages, the countess's book provides insight into the most common ailments of the period and their treatments. While most of the illnesses she writes about are minor in nature, more serious diseases such as pleurisy, kidney stone, liver problems, consumption and cataracts are also included. The first part of the book is in the same hand as the title page, but there are different hands in the latter sections. Possibly, the countess acquired her extensive knowledge of herbs from the books she purchased on trips to the continent with her husband. One of these was Fabio Colonna's *Fabi Columnae Lyncei Minus Congitarum Plantarum Pars Prima & Secunda Pars* (Rome, 1616). Colonna was a renowned naturalist and member of the Italian scientific Academia dei Lincei.[96]

Thorough and well-organized, ailments follow a division of the book according to bodily parts: eyes, head, ears, face, teeth and mouth, throat, breasts, lungs, liver and spleen, stomach. An extensive table 'of all medicines contained in the book according to the several parts and members of the body, disease, infirmities...' is provided at the back of the book. In Chapter One, Talbot Howard provides various remedies to relieve eye problems from minor ailments including 'bruise in the eye, redness in the eye (two), weak eye, clearing of the eye and preserving sight to a condition as serious as cataracts'. For cataract, she recommends a plaster of 'botany leaves, egg yolk and honey'. For sore eyes, grass, wild daisy roots, water and honey, and a powder for pearl in the eye. Chapter Two deals with head problems, from recipes to 'cleanse the brain and lungs of corrupt matter' to headaches, ear problems, cosmetic improvements to the face (acne, red face) canker sores and toothache.

Three books dating from the 1620s are written in a similar fashion to that of the Countess of Arundel. The first is Grace Acton's book (MS 1), 'Herbes to season, herbes to cure', dating from 1621. We know nothing about Grace Acton, as is the case with the majority of these women. Although most of her book deals with cookery, there are some medical receipts included for minor ailments such as a wen on the neck, stye on the eye and cough. Some of these receipts are child-oriented. One is a cure for bed-wetting and another deals with childbirth. The ingredients used in the receipts are regular house and garden products: lard, honey, lemon, acorns and fish oils. Acton seemed to write the book entirely herself. All recipes are by the same hand, as is the title.

Jane Barber and Lady Frances Catchmay authored receipt and cookery books circa 1625. Barber's manuscript, 'A Booke of Receipts' (MS 108), contains primarily cooking recipes, although there are some home remedies to alleviate the symptoms of eye problems and various recipes for pastes and syrups. Catchmay's work, 'A Booke of Medicens' (MS 184a), contains recipes for almost every common ailment as well as for some more serious diseases, such as the plague. There are numerous recipes for expulsions and purges using rose water, white and black pepper, ginger; there are cures for the bloody flux, haemorrhoids, pleurisy and worms, and ointments for eye ailments. Common afflictions were migraines, earaches, toothaches, gout, colds and coughs, 'falling sickness' and general aches and pains. Ginger is cited quite frequently as are sage, salt and pepper, vinegar, white wine, wormwood seeds, garlic and rose buds. More exotic spices including cinnamon, nutmeg, myrrh and frankincense are also used for aches and pains. In addition, some more unexpected ingredients – including lead and turpentine – are also cited. Catchmay includes recipes borrowed from other authors. She cites Mr Smith's 'Electuary for the Cough of the Lungs' which is composed of marshmallow root, honey, liquorice powder, cinnamon and saffron. She also refers to Dr Owen's 'Cure for the Plague'. He is called a doctor of 'physick'. As well as citing the remedies of others, Catchmay's book is in several hands, at least seven, and some recipes are written in Latin, presumably indicating that she was not the sole author. In addition to the recipes designed to cure common ailments, Catchmay, in common with many other women authors, includes recipes related to female conditions, such as childbearing. She wrote that a 'woman's breast curdled with milk, cause a woman to be delivered with child'. The odd cosmetic recipe is also present: for the whitening of hands use blanched almonds, and to whiten teeth, dried sage, pepper and bay leaf. Lastly, again in common with many other similar works, Catchmay provides remedies for depression or 'melancholy'. For melancholy, she recommends cinnamon and rosemary.

Jane Jackson's book intended to aid those tending for the sick dates from 1642 (MS 373). It is entitled, 'A very shorte and compendious Methode of Phisicke and Chirurgery'. This book demonstrates its author's knowledge of both Galenic medicine and the properties of common herbs. The most common ailments for which remedies are provided are cholera, constipation and colic. One remedy for the cholera is to take the 'syrup of rose, opezaccharum, compound of each, water of endive and chicory. Meddle them well together and give the sick to drink in mornings in the spring of day whether it be winter or summer a little warm on the fire.' For constipation, she recommended taking 'caspia, rose, diaprum's laxative, dissolve in endive water and parsley and give to the sick an hour before springs and a little on the first and let the sick keep his bed'. There were pills for purges, several types of laxative remedies, and cures for the stone, arm and back problems. In addition she provides receipts to relieve melancholy. The ingredients in this book are common to other recipe books at this time: rose syrup, endive, chicory, wormwood, eggs, thyme, mint, English saffron.

Other books are those of Jane Parker and Elizabeth Okeover. Jane Parker's collection, simply entitled, 'Mrs Jane Parker her Boock' (1651; MS 3769) includes remedies for a disease as serious as scurvy, but the majority of ailments are minor in nature. These include worms, green sickness, coughs, boils, nosebleeds, toothaches, vomiting, various aches and pains. Elizabeth Okeover's book, 'Collection of medical receipts' (MS 3712), is a collective enterprise dating from between approximately 1625–1725. Once again, there are common disorders listed: from plague and smallpox (found in almost every book from the 1600s to mid-1700s) to colds, sore throats, gas (wind in the spleen), fever, cramps, swellings and piles. Remedies for disorders of the nervous and cardiovascular systems such as palsy and strokes are also discussed. Birthing methods and child afflictions such as rickets are also covered. There are remedies for ailments that one would not find today, for example, quicksilver to relieve the king's evil. Finally, herbal concoctions to cure the jaundice, the bloody flux, the flux, the falling sickness and green sickness are suggested.

Sarah Palmer's work, Sarah Palmer and others, 'Collection of medical receipts' (MS 3740), consists of contributions by various individuals. Once again, the commonest illnesses and complaints are listed with a few additions, some cosmetic in nature such as 'salve for face break outs' and 'salve to take away freckles and sunburn'. Warts and corns are also mentioned. The same may be said about Frances Springatt and others, 'Collection of cookery and medical receipts, 1686–1823' (MS 4683) (although the book actually dates from 1686 to 1824) and many similar collections.[97] Springatt's book contains receipts for plasters, salves, various drinks for the stone and colic.

She borrowed receipts from other women, among them Mrs Mathais's 'medicine for the stone'.

Anne Neville's book, 'Collection of medical receipts' (MS 3585), from the mid-eighteenth century, contains recipes for many recognizable ailments, including plague sore, consumption, scurvy, burns and scalds, gangrene, boils, swelling of the throat, joint pains, cough and phlegm, canker sores, toothache, stone in the bladder, convulsions, shingles, sciatica, dog bites, bile, ringing in the ears, ordinary ague and nosebleeds. Once again, there are many children's ailments included: colic, problems with children's teeth, 'child bounded in the body' and worms. Detailed instructions are provided for making 'oil of St. John', which is extracted from St John's Wort and used for relieving pain from sunburn and other burns as well as for nerve pain relating to repetitive motion injuries, strains and shingles.

The 'Receipt book' (MS 3087) by Charlotte van Lore Johnstone, Dowager Marchioness of Annandale (1700–62) is entirely medicinal in nature.[98] It resembles other books of this time in terms of ailments and ingredients used; however, its receipts are more varied in nature and demonstrate evidence of shared information from physicians and others. It contains a prescription for an infusion for fever from a Dr Lower. The book proposes 'Lucatella's Balsam' as a cure-all. This potion will relieve burns, aches in bones, the wind, colic, plague and pox, and will expel poison. It is made from fat, turpentine, rose water and red saunders (also red sandalwood). Other prescriptions cited are Dr Butler's 'Cordial water for healing melancholy' which is 'much approved', and '(RX) for Yellow Jaundice Recommends Dr. Hobb's Receit for Rickets' which is made from oil of chamomile and powder of orris. The child should be 'anointed' with this salve. There is also Dr Burgess's medicine against the plague and smallpox. The Honourable Mrs Catherine Shawell's receipt for rickets apparently cured several children in Hampshire. She gave them two spoonfuls of juice of white horehound, three mornings together, anointing their joints and back with oil of chamomile. Like many other books, Johnstone's collection includes an extensive alphabetical index arranged by ailment and disease and in some cases, cures, particularly drinks. The index begins with aches and end with wounds.

An unusual book is the anonymous 'Book of Medical Receipts in English and French', dating from the latter part of the seventeenth century (MS 4052). Its authorship is unknown. It could have been compiled by a French woman who had married an Englishman or by an educated upper-class Englishwoman who had some knowledge of French and threw in some French receipts. In most respects it is similar to other receipt books, but it specializes in aches, purges, back pain, canker and throat sores, 'green sickness', consumption, and various kidney and stomach problems. From drinks to pills, purging appears to be the remedy of choice for all ailments.

Although it was primarily upper-class Englishwomen who compiled these recipe books they do not have the monopoly on their creation. French language receipt books appear in the collection as early as the sixteenth century. One is Anne de Croy's 'Recueil d'aulcunes confections et medicines' (1533; MS 222). Another example is a 'Collection of medical receipts' (c. 1750–75; MS 2777), written in French with the name of a Sister of Charity, Magdelaine Hanuche, on the frontispiece. The book has two compilers. One hand ends on page forty. The afflictions and remedies listed closely resemble those named by the women of England: childhood diseases, colic, the plague, haemorrhoids, dysentery, fever, wind, various coughs, problems with teeth – primarily toothache and discolouring, epilepsy and difficult childbirth. The ailments are treated with the application of various salves, topical creams and potions in addition to drinks made from herbs and other natural substances.

The majority of these manuscript recipe books from all sources date from the first half of the seventeenth century. Reasons for their decline in the second half of the century underscore the argument in this book that the professionalization of medicine meant that women's medical care was no longer considered to be legitimate and acceptable. During the mid-seventeenth century with the Restoration monarchs, published medical recipes collected primarily by men overtook the earlier unpublished women's collections.[99] Reform of the medical profession was a major reason for this phenomenon. Physicians were suspicious of elite women who practised empirical and charitable medicine. They were also keen to gain new patients and the professionals renewed their attacks on the kitchen physic. In the frontispiece to Robert Wittie's translation of James Primrose's *Popular Errours*, Wittie critiqued the popular remedies used by elite women, which he claimed did more harm than good, while recommending the Hippocratic and Galenic methods of taking the pulse, examining urine and the colour of the face before giving the patient purging plants.[100] The popularization of ladies' recipes made them less respectable. Since their 'secrets' were now public, they carried less credibility.

In France, Madame de Sévigné (1626–96),[101] the famous letter-writer, provides an excellent case-study of a seventeenth-century lady for whom self-medication and family health were obsessions. Madame de Sévigné wrote more than 1500 letters between 1646 and 1696, most of them addressed to her daughter. Many were on the subject of health and domestic medicine and they are a rich source of information concerning her medical views, her practice of family medicine, which was primarily composed of a discussion of her own health problems and suggested cures, her advice to her daughter, other family members and friends. They provide specific details concerning ailments and cures that she prescribed herself and cures recommended by other amateurs. Unlike her contemporary, Marie de Maupeou Fouquet, Madame de Sévigné did not publish a book of medical receipts. Nor did she practice charitable medicine.[102] Apparently, she developed an intense interest in all things medical in 1676 when she fell ill with rheumatic fever and was nursed by her son.[103] De Sévigné acknowledged that: 'I think of nothing but my health...'[104] The rheumatism from which she continued to suffer[105] was excruciatingly painful. At times, she was unable to use her hand to write to her daughter and friends. Others such as her son, Charles, would finish her letters: 'Some other hand must finish, for mine will proceed no further.' She complained of swollen hands, arms and feet.[106]

In addition to her own health concerns, she was also preoccupied with the health of her daughter, Françoise-Marguerite, Madame de Grignan, and to a lesser extent, with that of other relatives and friends. Madame de Grignan suffered from a number of health problems including smallpox, from which she died in 1696. Sévigné's preoccupation with her daughter's health increased over time. In 1677, she wrote. 'I cannot manage wholly to conceal from you the fact that your health gives me some concern. I pity you for harboring similar concern for mine.'[107] A few years later, in 1684, the concern was more pronounced: 'Your health often occasions me many uneasy moments.'[108] Writing to a friend, she confessed that her daughter's health caused her 'a thousand and one pangs of sorrow, daily'.[109] And to her cousin she revealed her concerns: 'I must confess that the ill health of that Provençale [Madame de Sévigné referred to her daughter as la Provençale because she lived in the countryside rather than in Paris] fills me with sadness. I tremble at the delicacy of her chest...'[110]

De Sévigné's daughter went through five pregnancies in as many years.[111] In 1671, when her daughter was pregnant again, Madame de Sévigné wrote to her of her sadness about this 'misfortune' and her disapproval of her son-in-law, criticizing him for being 'the cause of this evil'.[112] De Sévigné was prolific on the subject of obstetrics mainly because of her daughter's many pregnancies, miscarriages and births, which were the source of great consternation to her. For her daughter's first birth, Sévigné had her come to Paris. She counselled her daughter to take special care of herself to avoid premature delivery, which so often resulted in a stillborn baby. She warned her against dancing and falling, and she recommended rest.[113] Sévigné advised her not to travel to Marseilles: 'Think of your delicate health, and remember that it was only by being careful that you carried to term, last time.'[114] She chided Madame de Grignan for not taking better care of herself during pregnancy. She was not drinking enough broth so Sévigné recommended chicken broth and cow's milk. After the birth of her seventh child, Madame de Grignan lost a great deal of weight, so her mother again recommended cow's milk.[115] She advised her daughter to stay away from blood-letting and drugs, to take a good diet and plenty of rest.[116]

Madame de Sévigné also freely offered advice on contraception, which in the seventeenth century meant sexual abstinence or coitus interruptus. She advised her daughter to sleep in a separate room from her husband to avoid temptation.[117] When Madame de Grignan was not pregnant, her mother was elated, writing, 'I am thrilled, my darling, that you are not pregnant!'[118]

Madame de Sévigné made her own diagnoses and took or advised others to take medications devised from her home remedies or those prepared by other amateurs. She diagnosed herself with 'a slight colic, composed of bile and other human miseries...'[119] In another diagnosis, she described the symptoms of a disorder in her leg: 'About four days ago this wicked leg took the fancy to swell, burn and break out in little watery pimples...' Her remedy was to retire to bed and the 'leg discharged plentifully, and I am convinced this will be my cure, for nothing was able to dissolve the hard lumps in the calf of my leg but such a discharge'. She wrote again in vivid detail on her leg and a remedy recommended by the Capuchin monks:

> The skin indeed is discolored and neither the lotion nor the arquebusade water will restore it to its natural hue; there are also marks, *fructus belli*, but these are only the unusual consequences of such complaints. I know not whether my cure is performed by sympathy, but the wound grows better by degrees, as the herbs with which it is steeped, and which are afterwards buried, rot in the ground. I was inclined to laugh at this conceit, but the Capuchins tell me, that they have daily experience of the proof of such effects.[120]

Rather than sending for a doctor, she called in the Capuchins from Rennes.[121]

Another description of an ailment and cure related to her foot: 'It is the funniest thing about my foot. One day, it is painful, the next day, fine. I shall postpone curing myself of all my ailments until I get back to Grignan.'[122] A few years later, she claimed to have an 'attack of bilious and nephritic colic'.[123]

On the subject of remedies, she wrote that she 'carried with me an infinite number of remedies, good or bad, they are all well recommended and prescribed to me by neighbors and friends. I hope, however, this magazine of medicines will be of little use to me, for I am extremely well in health.'[124] She followed Madame de Lavardin's regimen, which involved purging, and taking special waters including linseed tea, at the end of the month.[125] She praised Madame de Nemond's recommendation of 'asses milk' as a salutary remedy for lung problems.[126] Other remedies she covered were those for the hands: composed of 'deer's marrow, and Hungary water, which according to some, is to perform miracles ... I cannot move my right side. Your Hungary water will have cured me before this letter has reached Paris.'[127] On another occasion de Sévigné informed her daughter that Madame de Rochebonne sent her a case of the Queen of Hungary's water.[128] Although she wrote that she had suffered a negative reaction to the water, and advised her daughter against taking it, Sévigné refused to stop taking it herself, 'for it is still a craze with lots of people, including me sometimes'.[129] She had the same attitude towards products like tea and coffee.

Sévigné's cousin, Roger, Comte de Bussy de Rabutin, wrote to her about the virtues of urine: 'It is said to be good for all fevers.' He provided her with a receipt: 'You take the urine of the patient and cook it in an egg; give it to a dog and the dog dies and the patient lives.'[130]

When writing to her daughter in September 1676 on the illness of Madame de Coulanges, a relation through marriage, de Sévigné described both symptoms and cure in great detail: 'Violent fever, attended with shiverings. She was seized at Versailles ... she has been bled. Her lungs are very much affected.'[131] A few days later: 'I have witnessed the terrible bleedings the physicians prescribe to the poor creatures who happened to be afflicted with it.'[132] She continued: 'It is the fourteenth day of Mme de Coulanges's illness ... she hasn't been purged because of the haemorrhoids that are extremely painful ... This morning they wanted to give her an emetic ... she was forced to swallow five or six miserable sips.'[133] By October, she seemed to have recovered: 'Neither the fever nor the fits have yet entirely left her; but as the crisis is past, and she is no longer subject to delirium, she may consider herself as being on the high road to convalescence.'[134] In another letter, she wrote that Monsieur de Coulanges was 'a candidate for gout'. This was a correct diagnosis, for a few weeks later she exclaimed that he was indeed suffering from this ailment and was in great pain.[135]

While in England, Madame de Sévigné met the Princess de Tarente,[136] who was also an amateur medical practitioner. She designated the princess 'my physician when I am ill'. The princess gave advice and recipes to Madame de Sévigné. One of these was 'an essence completely miraculous which healed these horrible vapours ... Three drops are to be taken in any liquid and you are cured, if by magic.'[137]

In addition to the Princess de Tarente, Madame de Sévigné obtained medical advice from other amateurs: Madame de Marbeuf, the Duchess de Lude, Madame de Lavardin, M de Lorme, the Abbé de Tetu, Friar Ange, a Capuchin doctor and the Capuchin monks.[138] She consulted with Friar Ange whose remedies she characterized as, 'mild, strengthening and refreshing'. They were effective as they had 'cured the Maréchal de Bellefond, the Queen of Poland and a thousand others'.[139]

The Capuchins possessed a whole armoury of drugs for all ailments. For flatulence, the Capuchins advised the powder of crab's eyes every morning.[140] They recommended a 'tranquil balsam' mixed with ten to twelve drops of urine for nephritic complaints and chest pains.[141] De Sévigné described the monks' various medicinal drinks as 'pleasant as a glass of lemonade'. She praised the Capuchins' treatment of her legs with herb tea and herb bathing. They were 'enemies of purgative salts'.[142] Her daughter was taking herbal tea as recommended by them and her daughter-in-law was 'immersed in dosing herself with the remedies of our Capuchin brethren, which consist of potions and herb baths'.[143] She claimed that the Capuchins had saved the lives of two women, one of whom had 'been weakened by twelve bleedings'.[144] Even when the Capuchins were unsuccessful and a patient in their care died, she continued to sing their praises and absolve them from blame: 'One of the women [of] whom our Capuchins had the care died lately; but do you know how it happened? Because they could not find out a method to make her a new pair of lungs; it seems half her own were wasted when she first applied to them; indeed, they insisted they would never promise more than to preserve her life for a short time, and enable her to make a comfortable end; and they have kept their word.'[145] She praised Capuchin water as a miracle cure to her daughter. It was a 'marvel for all pains of the body, blows on the head, contusions and even cuts...'[146] She recommended chicken broth to her unwell adult daughter on the basis that it had aided the recovery from her own health problems of Mlle de Frenoi. M Delorme gave her 'opening powders' which she insisted were a 'never failing remedy'.[147] She used the powder for purging as a cure-all remedy. It was a 'true remedy for all sorts of ailments'.[148] From Friar Ange, she took a 'purgative infusion' which had a positive effect.[149]

Madame de Sévigné's son Charles was also in poor health, suffering from gonorrhea, which he had contracted from one of his mistresses. His symptoms included terrible headaches, fever and boils.[150] Madame de Sévigné was much more positive about the medicine provided by the Capuchins than she was of that provided by doctors, as she wrote: 'My son has a little disorder flying about him for which he takes the Capuchins tisanes that did me so much good.' Whereas 'a rascally surgeon at Paris, after having made him swallow medicine after medicine, assured him that he was cured and had nothing more to do with it, than to follow a milk diet for a short time, to cool and purify his blood. Your brother followed his advice but soon found himself in a state that made him curse both the surgeon and the regimen.'[151]

She was also a proselytizer for a new medicine – cinchona bark – which she referred to as the English remedy (it was introduced into England in 1665 from Peru under the names of Jesuits' powder, fever bark and Peruvian bark). Thomas Sydenham is credited with developing the remedy as a cure for malaria around 1676.[152] The medicine came to France with Dr Robert Talbor who had been recommended to Louis XIV by Charles I to treat the dauphin.[153] Madame de Sévigné praised the medicine as a cure for the cold, flux of the chest (inflammation of the lungs) and fever.[154] She described it in the following manner: 'The Englishman has been to visit the good Abbé on account of the cold which gave us all so much uneasiness: he put something sweet into his bark, of such sovereign virtue, that the good Abbé is cured...'[155]

She had great confidence in herbal medicine and very little in licensed physicians even though she was often under their care. In many instances, she refused to take medication prescribed by physicians, yet she still consulted them.

> My little powder of antimony is the prettiest thing in the world; it is the staff of life as old de Lorme tells me; but by the bye, I must tell you that I disobey good M. de Lorme a little, for he wishes me to go to Bourbon, but the experience of a thousand people, the fine air and less company, determine me to go to Vichy ... My fingers will not close yet, and I have a pain in my knees and shoulders; in short, I am so full of serosities, as they are called, that I absolutely must have these marshes drained, which can only be done by drinking warm chalybeate waters, and then I think I shall do pretty well.[156]

On physicians and their remedies, she commented that 'Extraordinary remedies are necessary for persons of extraordinary character; physicians would never have dreamed of such a one as I have mentioned.' She does not indicate her superior remedy here.[157] At times she displayed contempt for physicians: 'Your philosophical physician shoots from far too great a distance to hit; he thought me ill, when I am perfectly recovered ...'[158] On educated physicians as opposed to amateur lady healers, she insisted that: 'Mlle de Méri has acquired more skill by her experience in sickness, than a physician in health ever did by his learning and practice...'[159] When writing about French doctors in particular, Madame de Sévigné could be very sarcastic: 'I shall speak with Du Chêne relative to your little physician, whom we employ in killing a few patients in our quarter, that we may have an opportunity of seeing how he succeeds; it would be a thousand pities that he should be deprived of the privilege of killing with impunity.'[160] Although she would use their medicines: 'I use a wash for my hands, which old Delorme has recommended me...' She did not have great faith in them: '...it [the medicine] has given me hopes and that is all'. In another letter on the same subject, she wrote, 'I continue to use Delorme's wash, but the cure goes on so slowly that I have much more hope from the weather than from all the herbs in creation.'[161] She had greater faith in herself as a physician. 'Ask the Chevalier de Grignan if I have not taken great care of him, if I did not procure him to a good physician, and if I am not an excellent one myself. I treat the Chevalier's health very seriously; I see how his medicines operate and leave him in a good way before I quit him.'[162]

And for the physicians at Vichy, she had nothing but contempt – she called them 'unbearable' except for one young doctor, 'genteel, neither a quack nor a bigot ... he amuses me'.[163] Another exception was a physician named Amiot recommended to her by friends. She approved of his medicine because he did not subscribe to conventional academic medicine. He did not bleed his patients and he 'approved the method of our Capuchins...' He was also 'a great advocate of the waters of Vichy'.[164]

In addition to writing about her own health, and that of family and friends, the most common medical subjects on which de Sévigné wrote were the practice of blood-letting, obstetrics and general medicines. She often went against the grain in terms of the treatment of phlebotomy. Bleeding or blood-letting was a common practice in medicine at this time,[165] but Madame de Sévigné believed it to be a harmful as well as a painful practice. She claimed to have 'witnessed the terrible bleeding the physicians prescribe to the poor creatures who happen to be afflicted with it'.[166] When her sickly daughter was bled for a leg ailment, she wrote that she would be at ease if her blood was not flowing uselessly: 'You have been ill, have been bled twice, have had reason to fear a return of your quinsy, and have been spitting blood. They say it proceeded only from the throat, but pray this is the blood that was in so good a state?'[167] At times, she did give in to being bled, as she did when she was suffering from a bad cold.[168] She related the contradictory advice of two doctors, one French, the other English. Gusioni, the French physician, advised her to be bled to cure her rheumatism, while the English physician 'says it is death to be bled for the rheumatism, and that if I take away the blood which destroys the watery humours, I shall be as ill as I was four years ago. Which of the two am I to believe? I will take the middle course...' This meant drinking linseed tea and taking medicines once a month.[169] Soon after, she wrote that the Englishman's medicine, 'which will soon be made public, renders all your physicians, with their purgings and bleedings perfectly useless'.[170] Later, she was of the opinion that her three-year-old granddaughter should not be bled. Oddly, she believed that to bleed one person from a family sufficed for all family members due to the principle that they were all of the same blood.[171]

On the other hand, Madame de Sévigné approved heartily of blood transfusions for those suffering from anaemia. When her daughter had been weakened by a successive series of miscarriages and births, Madame de Sévigné wrote to her cousin, M de Coulanges,

> Three months ago, she was afflicted by some kind of illness which was not supposed to be dangerous, but I found that it was the most horrific that one could suffer from ... The latest was so violent that she was bled in the arm: a strange remedy, which makes the blood flow, when there is none left to flow! That is burning the candle at both ends. What would be preferable, my dear cousin, would be to send her ... blood, strength, and health through a transfusion.[172]

She took water cures for her rheumatism at the popular aristocratic watering resorts of Vichy and Bourbon-L'Archambault. Sévigné found the waters of Bourbon to be superior to those of Vichy, particularly in curing the gout.[173] Her friend Madame de Lavardan had recommended the waters of Vichy to her, which she took and praised: 'I am now taking medicine, and am drinking the waters which Madame de Lavardan relates such wonders; I shall observe her regimen under every aspect of the moon and planets, in short, I find myself much better after it, without offence to the linseed tea.'[174]

She wrote that she 'drank dozens of glasses of Vichy water which caused a purge'.[175]

She claimed that the hot showers, the pump treatments which brought 'profuse perspiration', cured her knees. She described the pump operation which she denoted as 'no bad rehearsal for purgatory' as follows. 'The patient is naked in a little subterraneous apartment where there is a tube of hot water, which a woman directs wherever you choose.' She was convinced that the 'waters and pumping have evacuated a great quantity of humors'.[176]

Diet and nutrition were also of great concern to Madame de Sévigné. Several of her letters are dedicated to the medicinal uses of tea, coffee and chocolate. These products were new to France in the seventeenth century. Chocolate, she believed, cured sleeping problems, as she wrote to her daughter: 'But you are not well; you have not slept lately. Chocolate will also do you good.'[177] A few months later, she urged her daughter not to consume chocolate; much to her chagrin, her daughter did not follow this piece of advice.[178] In addition to causing heart palpitations, kidney pain, and 'vapors', Sévigné thought it would 'burn the blood...'[179] She was determined to understand the impact chocolate had on her daughter's bowels.[180] However, she herself decided to consume chocolate as an aid to digestion and as a between meals snack, 'by way of nourishment, to enable me to fast till supper time' and 'it had the desired effect'. Some years later, however, she recognized its 'special virtues'.[181]

Coffee was still a rare commodity in seventeenth-century France. It was first brought into France by a Marseilles merchant, P. de la Roque in 1644. His son Jean de la Roque accompanied the French ambassador to Turkey, and introduced Turkish coffee to French aristocrats when he returned from Constantinople some twenty-five years later. Soliman Aga, Turkish Ambassador to France, brought coffee with him to the court of Louis XIV and it soon became something of a fad amongst the upper classes.[182] Although the doctors advised taking coffee, Madame de Sévigné had mixed feelings: 'I entreat to deliver you from this pang; I still have but too many left. Madame de Schomberg advises, if you must at all events drink coffee, to sweeten it with Narbonne honey instead of sugar; this is good for the lungs...'[183] Madame was convinced that 'coffee does not do any good...' She was against coffee because it had differing results with different people She thought it made 'some fat, makes others lose weight'.[184] She advised her daughter not to drink coffee about which she was anxious. She believed that 'coffee increases the circulation of the blood too much and heats it'. Barley waters and chicken broth were better.[185]

Madame de Sévigné's views on coffee may well have been influenced by other than primary medical interests. As an aristocratic women who was often at court, Sévigné expressed the fashion of the day as she wrote, 'Coffee is entirely out of style at court.'[186] Tea, on the other hand, was very much de rigueur as a remedy and a fashionable beverage. It was used to relieve complaints of the spleen and highly recommended by the Princess de Tarente who took as many as fourteen or fifteen cups a day. It was 'the panacea of all her disorders'.[187] De Sévigné claimed that the princess was the 'best doctor in the world', and that it was the princess's nurse who was 'good and skilfull' who came to dress her leg daily and in fact 'was the first to diagnose the ailment' and 'to give it a name'. This name was 'erysipelas' which today would be called phlebitis. Apparently the nurse, Charlotte, 'cures everyone in Vitré'.[188]

It is clear that Madame de Sévigné had much to say about domestic remedies and fashionable cures, both those that she used herself and those that she recommended to family members and friends. Her obsession with self-medicating and her rather contradictory views on physicians were probably not uncommon for people at this time. She and many others exemplify the fact that domestic medicine was situated in the realm of the family and that women were those who had and who passed on the theoretical and practical knowledge of healing. Contemporaries seem largely to agree that women were both well-qualified and skilled in inventing, collecting and compiling medical receipts.

9

The Wise-Woman as Healer: Popular Medicine, Witchcraft and Magic

This chapter concentrates on wise-women, who were healers and, to a lesser extent, midwives,[1] and who were often designated as 'witches'. In the Early Modern era, these women could find themselves accused of practising witchcraft even though healing was their chief objective. The witch-hunt[2] as applied to wise-women can be interpreted as another step in the removal of women from healing. Wise-men and wise-women were important healers in Early Modern Europe and women retained a pivotal role in village medicine in the pre-industrial era.[3] In rural areas of Europe, amateur healers, many of whom were women, were ubiquitous. They cured all descriptions of illnesses with herbs, poultices, prayers and ointments. This traditional healing role was threatened during the Renaissance because at this time, 'the first concerted efforts were made to remove medicine from the realm of popular culture and establish it as the preserve of a restricted profession'.[4] Furthermore, this was the period when 'medicine and science lost their spiritual dimensions; as healers, magicians, and witches lost their claim to manipulate the spiritual forces of the world, the ground was prepared for a mechanization of the world picture'.[5] It was during this period that a number of strategies were taken to eliminate women and other 'popular' healers from the medical 'profession'. One of these was the licensing of various practitioners. A second method was the prescription of university training – denied to women – for physicians.[6] Another involved the accusation of witchcraft against irregular practitioners, such as 'old wives'. Women's work as village healers and midwives and their methods of healing through spells and potions made them vulnerable to attacks from the emerging medical profession, the state and the Church. Magical healing had existed since the Stone Age, but it was only around the late fifteenth century and under the Inquisition that it seems to have been considered as a form of witchcraft.[7] As the era of the witch-hunts coincided with a tightening of the regulations as to who could and who could not practise medicine, *The Act for the Appointing of Physicians and Surgeons*, drafted by the Royal College of Physicians and Surgeons of

London, condemned unlicensed practitioners of medicine as those 'who try to cure with the use of sorcery and Witchcraft ... to the high displeasure of God, great infamy to the Faculty ... most especially of them that cannot discern the uncunning from the cunning'.[8]

A tradition going back to ancient times existed in European society of people practising various forms of magic,[9] and during the Middle Ages, accusations of witchcraft would be made against men and women from all sectors of society, from the peasantry to monks and priests, who practised various healing methods. Male clergy often learned about herbs from wise-women and other 'quacks', while the men of the cloth taught lay people about healing charms. Monasteries had their infirmaries for sick and elderly brothers and sisters and often took in and cared for sick travellers.[10] The clergy had been involved in healing since Christianity began and were engaged in a form of magical healing of their own: the transubstantiation of the Mass, magical cures through holy water and the power of relics of saints. Although women could not be priests because of their sex, some had practised a form of spiritual healing through visions with the help of the supernatural. During the Middle Ages, women such as the Virgin Mary and living female saints were credited with important works of healing; however, times had changed and female healers of any description were no longer welcome. The Church viewed these women with suspicion, construing traditional practice as forms of superstition and even of making a mockery of the rituals of the Church.

In contrast to developments in the Early Modern period, throughout the Middle Ages, women had been praised for healing through the supernatural. Women saints were lauded and appealed to for intercession and the tradition was continued into the Early Modern period. Catherine of Siena was renowned for her healing powers in times of plague.[11] In the city of Bologna, men and women appealed to the Virgin Mary, and to Caterina Vigri, a fifteenth-century nun. During Vigri's canonization proceeding a witness proclaimed that, 'there isn't one sick person in this city who does not resort to her'.[12] Touching the body of this saint was reputed to have cured many. Other women who were renowned for their healing powers were Caterina Fieschi, a married aristocrat from Genoa who had a vision of Christ who endowed her with his healing powers.[13] However, the sixteenth century Church was ambitious to reclaim any spiritual power it had lost to lay people, women in particular, and it aimed to do this through whatever means necessary, including the Inquisition.[14] The influence and power of these lay healers was strong when the cure worked, and their magical cures often rested on the power of words.[15] According to Mary O'Neil, in sixteenth-century Modena, the Church was keen to eliminate what it interpreted as 'ignorance and superstition' (superstition meaning belief in magic) amongst the ordinary people. The Church wished to reinforce its own spiritual power and claimed complete monopoly over access to the supernatural.[16]

People turned to local healers for various reasons, one of which was the dubious reputation of university educated doctors. They feared surgery and disliked the painful remedies associated with Galenic medicine. Francis Bacon, when writing about the merits of physicians versus non-professionals, commented that: 'Empirics and old women were more happy many times in their cures than learned physicians.'[17] Another contemporary writer and founder of the Muggletonian Puritan sect, Lodowick Muggleton (1609–98), noted that: 'Doctors of physic ... were the greatest cheats ... in the world. If there were never a doctor of physic in the world, people would live longer and live in better health.'[18]

Popular women healers performed tasks from blood-letting, bone-setting and diagnosis to prescribing curative herbal concoctions. In essence, they duplicated the roles of barbers, surgeons and physicians while also being faith healers or magic workers. Professional practitioners resented the incursion of ill-educated women into their territory. The power and respect they commanded on a local level increased the perception of women healers as a threat.[19]

Many of the substances developed by wise-women were effective in healing illnesses. The testimony by Andres Hernandez de Laguan, a Spanish physician who was employed by the city of Metz, demonstrates the importance of the medicinal efficacy of the substances developed by wise-women. An older couple, accused of witchcraft, had been arrested on suspicion of bewitching the Duke of Lorraine. Dr Laguan was sent to their cabin where he found various remedies, including an ointment which he thought the couple had been using to anoint themselves. Laguna was asked to examine this; he thought that it looked like *unguentum populeum*, a narcotic salve made from the buds of black poplar (which gave it the green colour) plus leaves of poppy, henbane and deadly nightshade. He sniffed the little pot, and recognized the heavy odour of nightshade and henbane.[20] The doctor tested its efficacy by applying it to one of his patients, who was the wife of the city's executioner. She had been experiencing sleeping problems. Apparently, she slept for three days and woke up with a grin and a story of having cuckolded her husband.[21] The unguent thus proved to be effective.

The Italian physician Girolamo Cardano (1501–76) also wrote about vegetable-based ointments prepared by 'witches' which had positive medicinal effects in inducing sleep. In a section entitled 'On Marvels' in Book Eighteen of his *De Subtilitate* (1550) he discussed the impact of a plant called Melissa[22] on sleep and dreams. He described the ointment's composition and its medicinal effects: 'We speak now of the witches' ointment, which makes one see wonderful things, which are not real but appear to be so.'[23]

Witchcraft has been defined in many different ways from the practice of black magic to the worship of Satan, but historically speaking it may be defined as 'a composite phenomenon drawing from folklore, sorcery, demonology, heresy and Christian theology'.[24] Anthropologists such as

E.E. Evans-Pritchard have suggested a difference between 'sorcery', as comprised of rituals and chants, and witchcraft, which implies a special power inherent in the witch herself.[25] Another definition, provided by historian Richard Kieckhefer, is more inclusive. He defined witchcraft as sorcery, diabolism, invocation or any combination of the three.[26] Contemporary sources indicate that witchcraft was perceived as comprising two types of activities. These were the practice of harmful, black or maleficent magic, which entailed the performance of malicious acts by means of extraordinary, mysterious, occult and supernatural power, and the practice of white witchcraft or white magic, sometimes known as helpful rather than harmful magic. Black magic involved acts such as inducing a person's death by piercing a doll made in his/her image, inflicting sickness on a child by reciting a spell and so on. In Latin, these acts are called *maleficia* or witchcrafts. They were characterized as magical rather than religious, as harmful rather than beneficial. They concerned the relationship between the witch and the devil, between the woman or man and the supernatural foe of the Christian God, the very personification of evil. Such a witch performed harmful magic, had made a pact with the devil and made some sort of homage to him. Witchcraft thus equalled diabolism or worship of the devil and it was the devil from whom the witch received her/his powers. A witch was not merely a magician, but was also believed to be a devil worshipper. As one who had rejected Christianity the witch was a threat to society.[27] This sort of witchcraft was identified in the sixteenth and seventeenth centuries by 'Christian witch theorists', from both the clerical and legal professions. It was particularly pursued on the European continent in German and French-speaking regions, and in Scotland.[28] Although we have used both male and female pronouns above, by far the majority of people identified as witches were women: 80 per cent of those accused of witchcraft and 85 per cent of those executed, were women. Between 1400 and 1700, about 500,000 people were burned at the stake as witches.[29]

Common people, usually rural and poor, received their medical care from 'cunning folk' often identified by contemporaries as witches. As novelist Daniel Defoe wrote in his *Journal of the Plague Year 1665*: 'The common people who [are] ignorant and stupid in their Reflections ... ran to Conjurers and Witches and all Sorts of Deceivers to know what should become of them; who fed their Fears and kept them always alarm'd and awake, on purpose to delude them and pick their Pockets. So they were as mad upon running after Quacks and Mountebanks and every practicing Old Woman for Medicines and Remedies.'[30] And according to scholar and Anglican cleric Robert Burton (1577–1640), 'Cunning men, Wizards, and white-witches' were 'in every village. Cunning women had curative powers...'[31]

Historians maintain that the average age of a witch was fifty although some were as old as sixty.[32] George Gifford (d. 1620), an Essex clergyman, defined a witch as 'one that worketh by the Devil, or by some curious art either hurting or healing, revealing things secret or fortelling things to come, which the devil hath devised to entangle and snare men's souls ... The conjurer, the enchanter, the sorcerer, the diviner, and whatsoever odd sort there is, are indeed compassed within this circle.'[33] He also described them as 'old bags' and 'poor' as well as simply 'old', as in the following extract from his *Dialogue concerning Witches and Witchcraft*: 'Daniel: "You had no hurt done yet, had you, by any witch?" Sam: "Trust me I cannot tell, but I feare me I have, for there be two or three in our town which I like not, but especially an old woman. I have been as careful to please her."'[34] Commonly considered to be eccentric, these women would often exhibit some kind of physical deformity or pock-marked faces. One contemporary described witches as having 'long teeth and cloven feet'.[35]

According to Heinrich Kramer, also known as Institoris, and James Sprenger, both German Dominican Inquisitors and the authors of a highly influential witch-hunter's manual, the *Malleus Maleficarium* or *The Hammer of Witches* (1486), women were more likely to be witches than men because of their inherent inferiority, which manifested itself in several ways.[36] They were 'more superstitious, more credulous, and more impressionable'. They were 'weaker, they have slippery tongues, and they wish to vindicate themselves through witchcraft. All wickedness is but little to the wickedness of a woman.' Women were also 'more carnal than men and since all witchcraft comes from carnal lust, which is in women insatiable'.[37] For the first time, the link between heresy, witchcraft and women was established. To justify their views, Kramer and Sprenger drew upon Greco-Roman, Old Testament and medieval misogynist texts about women.[38]

This chapter is primarily concerned with 'white witchcraft', the practice of various types of traditional healing from folk medicine to positive magic using the recitation of prayers or chants and sometimes the use of objects such as magnets to bring about health and well-being.[39] Magic is traditionally characterized as having three components: natural magic, demonology and symbology. The Italian natural philosopher Giambattista della Porta (1531–1615), who wrote *Magia naturalis* (four books, 1558; 'Natural Magic', 2nd edn, 20 books, 1589), characterized magic as a 'practical part of natural philosophy. It involved natural magic, the generation of plants and animals, the use of alchemy, strange cures involving cookery and cosmetics.'[40] Loosely defined, magic was a 'practical art which used the natural powers of things to achieve certain desired effects'. This includes physiological changes which could heal the body from disease. These changes could be brought about through the use of herbs or charms. Even in the context of healing magic charms were commonly considered to have originated from some kind of contact with Satan and were thus condemned by the Church and other authorities.[41] Contemporaries such as Agrippa and Paracelsus divided magic into two categories: angelic and demonic. They endeavoured to make magic a positive force to help rather than hinder human beings.

Magicians and witches were not the same things. Unfortunately, their efforts were not successful. The alchemists Agrippa and Paracelsus, both of whom had associations with wise-women, themselves came under attack from the Church.[42]

White witches were common throughout the countryside in England and on the continent. As one expert on witchcraft has maintained, 'Few settlements could have lain more than five miles from the residence of one of these good witches.'[43] The English country gentleman, Reginald Scot (1538?–99), supported the stereotype of the old woman as witch, writing that, 'Witches are women which be commonly old: lame, bleary-eyed, pale, foul and full of wrinkles; poor, sullen, superstitious, and papists; or such as know no religion: in whose drowsy minds the devil hath gotten a fine seat ... they are easily persuaded ... It is indifferent to say in the English tongue, she is a witch or she is a wise-woman.'[44] However, while he believed in the devil, Scot was possibly one of a minority of men of the age who did not believe that witches were 'flying nightwalkers, infant boilers, child eaters, sabbat attendees'.[45] He did not believe that Satan endowed humans with magical powers, but that people believed in satanic witchcraft because of ignorance. He did consider that the effect of witchcraft could be 'good, as whereby sick folk are healed',[46] and that diseases which were blamed on witches were brought on by natural causes.

Scot's book, *Discoverie of Witchcraft* (1584), challenged many of the contemporary views about witches. Scot provided examples of the recipes used not only by old women to heal those in their villages, but also by 'bad physicians and lewd surgeons' to prove that 'they know not how to cure, and in truth are good stuff to shadow their ignorance...'[47] Book 9 in Chapter 14 provides examples of people who were healed by charms. 'For the falling evil', Scot recommended that one 'take the sick man by the hand and whisper these words softly in his ear, I conjure thee by the sun and moon'. Sections of his book dealt with charms, such as 'A charm for the headache', and 'A Charm to heal the King's or Queen's Evil or any soreness in the throat'. In his discussion of 'Charms used while collecting medicinal herbs', he wrote that: 'An old woman's charm wherewith she did much good in the country and grew famous thereby, healed diseases of cattle.'[48]

Scot's book proved highly unpopular; particularly disliked was his denial of the existence of black magic. He was attacked by the British authorities and copies of his book were burned. Several intellectuals wrote tracts in response to *Discoverie of Witchcraft* including James I and VI, king of Scotland and England. James's own treatise on witchcraft, *Daemonologie*, was published in Edinburgh in 1597.[49] James himself believed that witchcraft was a sin prohibited by God. He cited the Old Testament as his authority for this opinion.[50]

A good number of women accused of witchcraft were traditional healers who did not engage in the practices associated with magic. They were healers and cooks in the household and midwives in their local community, which alone made them more likely to be accused of witchcraft than men.[51] These were often women who, although lacking formal education, were very knowledgeable healers. The French historian Jules Michelet wrote in his nineteenth-century study of witches that 'witch' at one point meant a 'woman of superior knowledge'. He argued that witches were healers who 'were able to perceive the hidden principles of all vegetable or mineral substances'.[52]

In Spain during the Middle Ages the custom was to associate witchcraft with *sanadoras* or *curativas* (healers), and thus many were accused of practising witchcraft. Witchcraft – white magic – and healing were both rural and urban phenomena. In the cities, witches 'were accused of being able to distill the essence of the plague, depositing it in products and unguents with which to contaminate diverse points of the city'. This created panic among the masses. For the most part, these healers were women past middle age, who fitted the typical profile of a witch. They worked as cooks, preparing their foods with herbs combined with 'magical' products. In reality, these healers frequently used medicinal plants in their remedies which seemed to add a magical formula. As in other European countries, they helped those who were unable to receive any other type of cure or assistance. When a sick person died, the healers were open to accusations of witchcraft.[53]

Traditional healers treated diseases in humans and animals, including ailments that people thought were caused by witchcraft. They also foretold the future and made love potions. Wise-women treated the sick with organic medicines made from herbs – remedies not unlike those employed by licensed physicians.[54] However, wise-women also engaged in magical practices, such as 'girdle measuring' and the transferral of illnesses from the patient to themselves.[55] A number of wise-women and men were faith healers, and used the power of touch that was supposed to emanate from God.[56] However, healers also employed many of the same substances and methods as those involved in sorcery or black magic, which made them easy targets for witch-hunters. Such techniques involved a combination of potions, charms and amulets, which were utilized specifically as preventative medicine. Typical amulets would be a hare's foot, worn to avoid danger, or a sprig of rosemary placed over a doorway to prevent snakes from entering the home.[57]

Wise-women, 'white witches' or traditional female healers, gathered herbs that they made into a variety of folk remedies, waters and ointments, using what were often considered to be magical formulas. Healers were vulnerable if something went wrong, if their remedy did not cure, or worse, if the patient died. Belief in magic was widespread amongst the ordinary people. Although 'white magic' had been condemned by the medieval Church, it continued to be practised and was not widely considered to be evil. Rather, people considered it to be a 'shield against misfortune...'[58] Accusations of witchcraft against those practising folk medicine 'were encouraged both by the appearance of certain disease ... and by those distrusted by the authorities or their clients'.[59]

In such a climate, wise-women and wise-men who were capable of recognizing the work of witches and illnesses that they believed had been induced by witchcraft were themselves wide open to accusations of witchcraft. At the time, people believed that 'magic was identified by magic'.[60] George Gifford believed that seeking a cure from wise-women and wise-men, those making use of charms and sorcery, was harmful to the soul.[61] White witches were also attacked by physicians for their ignorance of medical matters and of practising magic rather than medicine: 'They know not the cause of Disease, refer it unto charms, witchcraft, magnifical incantations, and sorcery, vainly and with a brazen forehead, affirming that there is no way to help them but by characters, circles, figure-castings, exorcisms, conjurations, and other impious and godless means.'[62] Sprenger and Kramer referred to a woman from Modena who would heal as well as harm.[63] Many women who were prosecuted as witches throughout Europe and England were wise-women, in other words those involved in magical healing. Almost half of the cases which were heard as appeal cases before the Paris Parlement, were cases which dealt with healing.[64]

Although a European-wide phenomenon, there were a number of significant regional variations to the witch-hunt. It was most severe in German-speaking lands and in those countries which bordered German lands, such as Poland. It was also vigorous in France, a country which was torn apart by religious wars and where the Catholic Church attempted to enforce its control over female sexuality.[65] Less severe in the witch-craze were countries like England, where there was no Inquisition and where common rather than Roman Law was practised. The law in England forbade torture and there was no belief in the Sabbat. The Mediterranean countries of Italy and Spain brought many women to trial, many of whom were folk healers, but few of them were actually executed.[66]

Church and secular courts united in their prosecution of witches through inquisitional courts in Spain and Italy to Church courts. Secular courts gradually superseded Church courts throughout the sixteenth century. They adopted the inquisitional methods used by Church courts, usually involving torture.[67]

Cases involving superstition were marginal to the Spanish Inquisition's concern in the sixteenth century. The Spanish Inquisition, established by the Catholic monarchs in 1478, had as its goal the eradication of the Jewish and Muslim minorities. Even though the Jewish population had been expelled in 1492, the so-called '*conversos*' were suspected of practising their original religion. Although forced to convert to Christianity, by the sixteenth century, there were still a large number of Muslims in Aragón, Valencia, Murcia and particularly eastern Andalucia.[68] What drew the attention of the inquisitors to the Muslim healers was their use of magical healing. The Jews, on the other hand, were not brought before the Inquisition for their medical practices, but for their religious beliefs.[69] During the sixteenth century, cases of magic, including various types of healing, composed up to one-fifth of the Inquisition's cases. Reforming bishops, the post-Tridentine clergy and the Inquisition treated folk practices harshly,[70] while until the sixteenth century, the Roman Inquisition was mostly concerned with stamping out Protestantism. Where Protestantism was less of an issue, such as in Naples, magic was the most commonly prosecuted crime after 1570.[71]

Historians have proposed many explanations as to why the witch-hunts began at this particular time in history. Their upsurge was intertwined with economic, political and cultural events which resulted in the growth of heresy and the loss of the Church's control in the south of France and other parts of Europe. This was an era of religious uncertainty when the elite of society demanded security.[72] Thus, as we have seen, in France much of the fervour against so-called witches was correlated with the Wars of Religion and the attempt to root out heresy by the Church.[73]

Family structure was changing as couples delayed marriage, while rural poverty and mendicancy were on the rise. In England this was in part an outcome of the Enclosure Acts. Natural disasters such as illnesses, epidemics and plagues were also contributing factors.[74] Inflation rose as did the population. The revival of trade along the Mediterranean made possible the growth of a cosmopolitan society in the south of France. Here migrated a heretical sect from Bulgaria, known as the Cathars. Women, in particular, were associated with this sect.[75] The Cathars were able to convert local people including members of the clergy and nobility.[76] The Pope intervened to root out this heresy by creating the Dominican order and when peaceful tactics, such as preaching, failed to halt the spread of the heresy, Innocent III demanded a military crusade. Although the Church claimed a victory, the heresy was not eliminated and the Inquisition was established. This church court was modelled on Roman treason trial procedures. These included forced confession by torture, no legal representation and confiscation of the victims' property. The inquisitors were primarily Dominican fathers.[77] The Inquisition was originally created to eliminate the Albigensian heresy, in which it was successful, but eventually it received official endorsement for rooting out witches. The Church had previously held the view that witchcraft was an illusion.[78] A witch-hunt was started in Toulouse and Normandy by Pope John XXII in 1326 following demands by his Dominican inquisitors. Most of the victims were peasant women. This hunt lasted until the 1430s.[79] A few years later, in 1451, the Pope appointed Hugh le Noir, who was already prosecuting peasant women in northern France, as Inquisitor General in France.[80]

Although the practice of witchcraft was not new in the Early Modern era, the idea that the witch's powers came from the devil only emerged in the later Middle Ages.[81] Caesar Carena, a consultant of the Roman Inquisition appointed by Urban VIII and the Congregation, wrote in his work on sorcery that among the powers of demons, 'they can induce incurable disease and cure all curable diseases'.[82] A leading witch-hunter held that, 'A Witch was accused of evil deeds from murder to having sexual relations with the Devil to healing.' Witches were not only 'those which kill and torment, but all Diviners, Charmers, Jugglers, all Wizards, commonly wise men and wise-women ... and in the same number we reckon all good Witches, which do no hurt but good, which is not to spoil and destroy, but save and deliver...'[83]

During the later medieval period, the practice of magic became a crime. Specific cases provide illuminating insight into women healers accused of magical healing. One of the earliest cases of a woman who was tried for practising magic took place in 1375 in Florence. Monna Caterina di Agostino had been accused by Vieri di Michele Rondinelli, perhaps a neighbour. He certainly lived in the same parish as Caterina. Apparently, she had been 'motivated by a diabolical spirit' which caused her to commit 'numerous and various acts of sorcery and magic and also invoked demons' to provoke men into committing 'libidinous acts with her'. Her trial was conducted by the municipal court but her sentence was cancelled three years later.[84]

One of the more interesting cases is that of the Italian healer or wise-woman, Matteuccia Francisci of Todi. A specialist in folk medicine, including contraceptives, she was charged with sorcery by the Inquisition in 1428. She was accused of practising magic of all kinds, including 'love magic' which involved providing women with love potions composed of herbs that aroused men's feelings. She cured by burying a bone from an unbaptized baby at a crossroads and chanting prayers and various formulae.[85] Interestingly, her prayers were all Christian in nature, including calling upon the Trinity, the Virgin Mary and other saints. She prescribed all manner of folk remedies composed of herbs, she made unguents from baby fat, and she practised rituals involving wax images placed over the fire. She rooted out curses, destroyed spells and transferred ailments from one person to another. Women, among them the mistress of a priest, came to her for contraceptive drinks made from a mixture of wine and the hoof of a female mule. Matteuccia was renowned for her cures and people travelled to be treated by her.[86] In the first part of her trial, Matteuccia was charged with various forms of sorcery, primarily love magic, incantation, and beneficent magic. In the second part, she was charged with diabolism and killing children. She was sentenced to burning by the municipal court.[87]

Remedies used by these women, the concoctions of herbs and other natural ingredients combined with the recitation of prayers and chants were confusing to the authorities. The cases of Maria la Medica, who was tried at Brescia by Brother Antonio Petsoelli, a Dominican, for diabolism, invocation (love magic) and sorcery, and of Lucia Ghiai illustrate the fine line between religion, magic and medicine. Maria la Medica was accused of showing her patients ways to 'abuse' holy oil by spreading it on their bodies for healing purposes. She combined this abusive application of holy oil with the chanting of the Roman Catholic prayers Pater Noster and the Ave Maria three times 'in the name of the Trinity'.[88] However, the authorities interpreted this as honouring the devil. Likewise, Lucia Ghiai used holy oil, crucifixes, prayers and rosaries to bring about cures. She was called a witch by a Franceschina of Frattuzze, the woman she had attempted to cure, who denounced her to local inquisitors at the monastery of San Francesco in Portogouaro.[89] Further cases in which 'Witches use something of Religion in Healing and Sickness' are cited by Brother Francesco Maria Guazzo in his *Compendium Maleficarum,* published in 1608. This work is concerned with pacts made by witches with Satan, harmful magic and related topics. Brother Guazzo wrote:

> For witches observe various silences, measurings, vigils, mutterings, figures and fires, as if they were some expiatory religious rite; and worse still, they transfer the sickness to certain pious men, alleging that it is a punishment for having dishonored their deity. Most intolerable of all, they often mingle with their prayers all sorts of filth and dung and excrement, than which nothing can be imagined more foreign to the purity which is proper to Divine worship and ceremonies.

One case he cited was that of Theonotte, a witch at Nancy, who, when asked to heal a sick neighbour (for she was supposed to have such power) said that the sickness had been caused by Saint Fiacre, an Irish abbot in Ireland who died in 670. In order to effect the cure, the abbot needed placation which involved taking gifts to his shrine: 'First she measured the sick woman crosswise with a waxed linen cloth, lit the cloth at his shrine and then walked three times around the chapel.'[90]

Accused of witchcraft by a former client for whom her cure of a two-year-old child was unsuccessful, Diamente de Bisa from Modena used a healing procedure which involved ashes and water. This was one of her few failures and Diamente, described as a 'big, old and ugly woman', was well-respected in her village. She cured worms by using the sign of the cross and repeating a refrain that went as follows: 'On Holy Monday, Holy Tuesday, Holy Wednesday, Holy Thursday, Holy Friday, Holy Saturday, Easter Sunday, the worm dies and decays.' Although the Inquisition did not prosecute her as a witch, it classified her as a 'superstitious healer' and she was forced to do penance which was a minor penalty. Her penance involved being placed at the front of the church during Mass, having only bread and water on certain holy days and reciting the rosary.[91] In Venice, the majority of folk healers were older women, usually widows. These women transmitted their 'secrets' to their younger female relatives thus assuring that the remedies were passed from one generation to the next. One practice, which may not have been in the original receipt, involved licking the patient's head.[92]

The case of Elena Draga or Crusichi, a folk healer examined by the Inquisition for witchcraft in Venice in the 1570s, illustrates the extensive knowledge possessed by these healers. Although Draga made two appearances before the tribunal, she was never convicted. While the tribunal did not approve of her methods of healing, for unstated reasons, she was given no 'more than a lecture and spiritual penances'.[93] Evidently, the Venetian tribunal was most concerned with the methodology of healing, which it considered to be heresy, in that it involved summoning the devil and abusing the sacraments.[94] Draga's cures and methods did not appear to do either.[95] They were composed of a great variety of natural remedies: herbs, unguents and the like. The herbs in her collection included rue, laurel, ambrosia to make lotions to treat epilepsy and catarrh. Other ingredients, such as incense, garlic, barley, almond oil and chestnuts, were commonly used for backaches. These natural remedies were accompanied by various chants invoking Christian icons:

> I go and take five sprigs of rue and of ambrosia and five of incense and five star herbs and five cloves of garlic, and while preparing it I say five our fathers and five ave marias in honour of the five wounds of Jesus Christ. And I also took soot from Christmas Eve, and I crush all these things between two pieces of marble, and then I put on that five pennies worth of bay: and the child should be anointed with that poultice in a cross starting with the arm right down the body, saying: 'In the name of Christ and the glorious virgin Mary and of the Most Holy Trinity that the Lord should be the one to heal you from this illness.'[96]

Midwives were at particular risk of accusations of witchcraft. There were several reasons for their vulnerability. Childbirth was a totally female affair, there was a high rate of infant mortality, and infanticide was fairly common. Official documents from the Roman Inquisition, established by Pope Paul III in 1542, specifically connect the midwife or witch to infanticide. As one inquisitor related, midwives employed body parts of the dead infant: 'Del Rio says the ointment used is made of various foolish things, but chiefly of the fat of slain infants; sometimes the staff is anointed, sometimes the thighs or other parts of the body. The transport could be effected without it, but the demon insists on it to stimulate infanticide. This is shown by the fact that the first time the witch can use ointment afterwards she must make it herself.'[97] Some midwives were prosecuted and even put to death shortly after the plague around 1360.[98] Revenge by parents was generally a motive for prosecution.[99]

Witch-hunts frequently started with the local midwife who was accused of bringing various types of evil into the village through her medical practices.

She was suspected of performing abortions and infanticide and making couples sterile. When a fifteenth-century Parisian midwife named Perrette gave a nobleman suffering from leprosy an unguent made from the fat of a stillborn baby, she found herself in prison on suspicion of witchcraft. Although she was later released and pardoned by the king after appeals by friends, this incident demonstrates the fine line between healers and witches.[100] According to Kramer and Sprenger, midwives 'surpassed all other witches in their crimes'. Midwives made use of herbs such as ergot, poppy, henbane and bryony root to bring about labour and to ease the pain of childbirth. This alone was considered suspect by Kramer and Sprenger, as relieving the pain of childbirth was held to be against the natural order of things. Women were supposed to endure childbirth as God's punishment for Eve's original sin.[101] In Chapter XIII of the *Malleus*, 'How Witch Midwives commit most Horrid Crimes when they either Kill Children or Offer them to Devils in most Accursed Wise', they recount the story of a midwife from Zaburn, accused of witchcraft for inflicting a curse on a pregnant woman. The midwife, described as a 'vile woman', apparently extracted the 'entrails' of the pregnant woman.[102] Inevitably midwives were also held responsible when babies died.

Birth control was now included as one of the 'crimes' committed by midwives according to Sprenger and Kramer. Indeed, one of the goals in writing their tract was to communicate the duty to procreate.[103] They described 'the seven methods by which they [the witches] infect with witchcraft the venereal act and the conception of the womb'. These methods were detrimental to reproduction in the following ways: 'First, by inclining the minds of men to inordinate passion; second, by obstructing the generative force; third, by removing the members accommodated to that act; fourth, by changing men into beasts by their magic art; fifth, by destroying the generative force in women; sixth, by procuring abortion; seventh, by offering children to devils.' In addition, they considered birth control as 'injuries towards men' brought about by witches. In a section entitled, 'That Witches who are Midwives in Various Ways Kill the Child Conceived in the Womb, and Procure an Abortion; or if they do not this Offer New-born Children to Devils', they expand on this theme: 'It is witchcraft, not only when anyone is unable to perform the carnal act ... but also when a woman is prevented from conceiving or is made to miscarry after she has conceived ... Without the help of devils, a man can by natural means, such as herbs, savin for example, or other emmenagogues, procure that a woman cannot generate or conceive.'[104]

Midwives in many parts of Europe were forced to swear an oath against sorcery before a local bishop in order to be licensed and to baptize newborns. With infant mortality a common occurrence, immediate baptism was considered a necessity. Frequently, there was not time to get the child to a church official, thus this important ritual was in the hands of the midwife.

The practice of taking oaths began in France in the fifteenth century, but after the Council of Trent, it became universal as the church cracked down on witchcraft.[105]

The Papal Bull issued by Innocent VIII, '*Summis desiderantes affectibus*' also known as the 'Witch-Bull' (5 December 1484) coordinated the battle against midwives throughout Christendom.[106] It also confirmed the Church's belief in witchcraft, stressing the harmful manifestations of witchcraft, such as bringing about inclement weather, inflicting illness in animals and destroying crops. The bull also made clear the Church's responsibility in eradicating heresy – including the practice of contraception:

> many persons of both sexes ... who by their incantations, spells, conjurations, and other accursed charms and crafts, enormities and horrid offences, have slain infants yet in the mother's womb...; they hinder men from performing the sexual act and women from conceiving, whence husbands cannot know their wives nor wives receive their husbands.[107]

Priests regularly accused midwives of sorcery. On 1 October 1587, Don Vincenzo Amorosi, a priest in the town of Cesena, Italy, accused the midwife Caterina Domenatta of sorcery 'when a certain woman gave birth to an infant who came into the world feet first, this guilty sorceress persuaded the mother that if she did not want her child to become a benandante or a witch, she should place him on a spit and then turn him over the fire, I do not know how many times'. The priest recommended imprisonment for the midwife. He described her as 'a woman of low life, full of incantations and sorceries'. Because the midwife admitted to making the recommendation of this custom, with complete approval by the parents, she received a lighter sentence. She was 'condemned to make public penance and an adjuration'.[108]

Between the fifteenth and seventeenth centuries, a number of handbooks were written to aid the inquisitors with their work. One of the most influential was entitled *Flagellum haereticorum Fascinariorum*, written in 1458 but not published until 1581. The author was an inquisitor by the name of Nicolas Jacquier (Jaquerius), who put forth the view that the sect of witches differed significantly from other heresies. Witches attended the Sabat or ceremonies where they copulated with demons, and ate unbaptized infants.[109]

When Kramer and Sprenger published *The Hammer of Witches* the Papal Bull of 1484 was placed at the start of the tract. Kramer and Sprenger used St Augustine as their guide, citing Book 83 where Augustine wrote: 'This evil, which is of the devil, creeps in by all sensual approaches...' The Church denounced female healing as heresy: 'If a woman dare to cure without having studied, she is a witch and must die.' This statement went hand in hand with the medical profession's attempt to eliminate women from practising medicine.[110] It was the most influential of the witchcraft handbooks, and went through fourteen editions between 1487 and 1520. It led to an increase in witch trials.[111] Most of the content in *The Hammer of Witches* was not new. Much of the text merely reiterated what had already been said by men like Jaquerius. However, there was one important addition, a section that asked questions such as, why did the devil possess women? Why did women become witches? Unlike men, why were women so easily possessed? The answer was found in the nature of woman, which was evil, weak, frivolous and malicious and of course, inferior to man. *The Hammer of Witches* not only provided inquisitors with a witch-hunter's handbook, but it justified hunting women down.

Churchmen in particular railed against witches. As we have seen, the witch-hunt began with the Church's fear of heresy, which threatened its control and authority. One expert on the witch-hunts has argued that 'lethal misogyny' flourished in the Church at this time.[112] The Church permitted healing and medical treatment by physicians (for those who could afford to pay), yet healing by peasants, females in particular, was forbidden. Secondly, the Church differentiated between what it defined as medicine and magic. Court physicians practised medicine while witches practised magic. The devil or Satan, whom the Church believed to have real power, worked through women,[113] who employed charms and incantations in addition to a host of herbal remedies. The same remedies were often used by physicians and the witch or wise-woman to relieve the symptoms of minor ailments: aids for digestion and pain killers, especially to relieve the pain of childbirth, for which ingredients such as ergot and belladonna were used.[114] Digitalis, which is used today for heart problems, was another drug that witches used.[115]

Perhaps the most famous lawyer to write a demonology tract is better known in history as the founder of political science rather than as an anti-witch crusader. This was Jean Bodin (1530–96), writer, scholar and lawyer from Angers. His treatise, *On the Demon-Mania of Witches* (1580), influenced later writers such as Pierre de Lancre and Henri de Boguet.

There are a number of shared themes in Bodin's *On the Demon-Mania of Witches* and Kramer and Sprenger's *Hammer of Witches* even though they were written almost a century apart.[116] In many respects, Bodin's treatise was a new and revised edition of Kramer and Sprenger's work. Bodin's *Demon-Mania* became the handbook for the state courts as Kramer and Sprenger's *Hammer* had served that function for the Church courts. However, one difference between the two books was Bodin's critique of a physician by the name of Jean Wier. Wier was a sceptic when it came to the existence of witches and he protested against the unscientific nature of the evidence used at witch trials.[117] Bodin reiterated Sprenger and Kramer's ideas on birth control and midwives. He affirmed that: 'Now the most wicked murder among animals is of man, and among men that of an innocent child. It is the most pleasing to Satan, like the case we described of witches who receive children and offer them to the Devil and immediately put them to death before they have been presented to God…' Next, Bodin cited the trial of one 'witch' by the name of Stadlin ' in the diocese of Lausanne, who, confessed to having killed seven children in their mother's womb…'[118] In addition to abortion and infanticide, Bodin added contraception to his characterization of witchcraft:

> Since whosoever practices the [magical] art, he unequivocally violates the divine laws of God and of nature: this is because he obstructs the purpose of the marriage which was constituted by God. This leads subsequently to either divorce or to *childlessness*, and this undeniably constitutes a sacrilege or a desecration of the sacred act. In addition, he cannot deny becoming a killer. A person, therefore, who obstructs the conception or birth of children must be considered just as much a murderer as the person who cuts another's throat.[119]

Birth control was not only condemned in various tracts, but in 1556, the Parlement of Paris passed an anti-abortion edict requiring all pregnant women to register their pregnancy and have someone witness the birth. If these practices were not followed and the child died, the woman could be prosecuted for murder.[120]

Demonology tracts were written by Protestants and Catholics during an era of religious turmoil but there was little difference between them when it came to witchcraft. Protestant ministers and others were engaged in rooting out witches from their communities as much as were the Roman Catholic priests.[121] In terms of the Reformation and magic, reformers on both sides of the divide spoke out and wrote against popular magic. Witchcraft was superstitious and thus idolatrous, magicians appealed to the devil. Clerics were concerned with spiritual welfare of the people and witchcraft endangered this.[122] Neither was it only Roman Catholics such as Kramer and Sprenger who condemned the use of pain relief in childbirth, Protestants were equally scathing.[123] However, there were some differences between Protestants and Catholics which should be made clear. Protestants wanted to eliminate the whole magical aspect of Christianity – faith healing, healing by saints, relics, shrines – in other words, the use of the supernatural in healing.[124] One example of the attempt to eliminate superstition, magic and conjuration by the Protestants was the case of 'Coxe alias Devon'. A priest named John Devon, who had 'celebrated mass in the house of Sir Thos Wharton of Newhall, Essex' as well as in other homes and places, was punished for his 'magic and for his conjuration'. He was accused of having made use of 'Popish books' and 'superstitious ornaments'.[125]

In addition, Protestants did not believe that the priests had the power to exorcise the devil from the possessed.[126] Luther's views on witchcraft may be found in his *Commentary on the Epistle to the Galatians*. Here he wrote that witches made a pact with the devil.: 'For witchcraft covenanteth with the devil; superstition or idolatry covenanteth with God: albeit, not with the true God, but with a counterfeit god.'[127] Calvin viewed witches as heretics. Both Protestants and Catholics condemned them to death.[128] Both Protestant and Catholic clergy were concerned to enforce their standards on the ordinary man and woman.

Although less harsh than the continent's treatment of witches, England passed legislation against witches in 1542 (repealed in 1547), 1563 (repealed in 1604) and 1604 (repealed in 1736).[129] These laws made practising witchcraft a criminal offence. The 1563 Act 'against Conjurations, Enchanchments, and Witchcrafts', imposed the death penalty for a first conviction, for using 'witchcraft, Enchantment, Charme or Sorcerie, whereby any person shall happen to be killed or destroyed'. The 1604 act was directed against popular healers, those unauthorized people who tried to 'cure' could now be accused of witchcraft. It added necromancy, laming, wasting men's bodies or goods and harbouring familiar spirits as offences.[130]

In France, both Church and state worked against witches. The first secular law passed against witches was by Emperor Charles V in the Codification of Imperial Law, known as the Carolina, 9 October 1490. He decreed that 'enchanters, invokers of evil spirits' were to be arrested, imprisoned and condemned to death. These were considered to be offences pertaining to the Church and they would be handled by the *Ordinaires*. The property of offenders would be sequestered. The Prevost of Paris ordered that 'speedy justice be executed on charmers, diviners, invokers of bad and damned spirits, those persons using prohibited arts and sciences'.[131] The decree passed by the Fifth Lateran Council of 1514 applied to both civil and canon law. It prohibited 'sorceries by the invocation of demons, incantations, and superstitious divinations'. The laity as well as priests were subject to the terms of this law. It did not refer specifically to witchcraft.[132] The Tridentine Reforms were enforced in France. Several councils held during the course of the sixteenth century ruled against practices associated with witchcraft, including magic. These included the Council of Evreux (1576), which passed a decree against magic; Rouen (1581), which decreed against 'maleficos, atheistos et libertinos'; Rheims (1583), which concluded against the use of biblical texts 'for incantations and divinations. Excommunication for soothsayers, for ligature of married folk and for other injury to persons'; Bordeaux (1583), where priests were 'ordered to warn their flocks against use of magic arts, astrology and divination...'; and the Council of Tours (1583), which specifically ordered priests to teach people the wrongs of the practices 'of magicians, enchanters, *malefici* and other superstitious persons'.[133]

Throughout the seventeenth century, the professions, both medical and legal, allied with the Church to take on female healers who they believed to be witches.[134] A 'cunning man', who acted as an intermediary between the accusers and the judiciary, decided if a witch had been at work and if there was a case to be prosecuted. The 'cunning man' in most cases was a physician. He provided the entire proceeding with scientific legitimacy. By law, a physician had to be consulted before a prosecution could occur: it was the physician who often determined 'whether an illness is caused by witchcraft or by some natural physical defect'.[135]

Consequently, in both continental Europe and England, the doctor's evidence at a trial was crucial in determining whether or not sickness or death was attributable to witchcraft.[136] Physicians would also serve as general advisers to the court. The witch would be examined first by a physician and second by a clergyman, especially in cases of poisoning. The process is described by one authority, Johann Weyer, MD, who wrote extensively on the witch-hunt:

> First of all ... recourse should be had, as ordained by God, to a man renowned with respect to his profession, his learning, and his experience, who will thoroughly distinguish diseases and their differences and signs and causes – that is to say, a learned and experienced physician of strong moral sensibilities – because such rare and severe symptoms often arise in diseases that stem from natural causes but are immediately attributed to witchcraft by men of no scientific experience and little faith.[137]

A physician, or if there was none available, a barber-surgeon or barber, examined the witch's mental and physical state. He would determine how fit she was to withstand torture.

Unlike England, with no Inquisition, and where Roman law and Papal authority were weak, in continental Europe, the Inquisition gave the doctor power over life and death. After a doctor had diagnosed an illness as the witch's fault, the Church took over.[138]

Almost certainly, the country to produce the largest body of literature against witches was France. A great number of these works were produced by lawyers, such as Henri Boguet and Pierre de Lancre. Henri Boguet, (1550–1619), a chief prosecutor and chief justice of the district of Saint-Claude in the Franche-Comté was one of the most important instigators of the witch-hunt in France.[139] As a judge, he was notorious for excessive harshness in his sentencing of the twenty-eight men and women he condemned. He believed in burning witches alive rather than having them strangled first. He primarily conceived of witches as female, although he did prosecute a few men.[140]

Boguet's *Discours des Sorciers*, translated as *An Examen of Witches*, was as popular as the *Malleus Maleficarum* and other treatises of the same genre. It went through twelve known editions. Boguet borrowed from the *Malleus Maleficarum* as well as from witch-hunting authorities Jean Bodin and Nicolas Rémy, but at the core of his text are the more than forty cases he tried: 'I have founded the following Examen upon certain trials which I have myself conducted, during the last two years, of several members of this sect, whom I have seen and heard and probed as carefully as I possibly could in order to draw the truth from them.'[141] All the usual suspects appear in his book: the midwives, the wise-women. Borrowing from Bodin and Kramer and Sprenger, he argued that witches 'kill the children they deliver', not only before they have been baptized, but while they are still in their mother's wombs. He seems to have believed that this was a common practice among midwives.[142]

Bouguet also believed that witches could heal as well as harm. First, he discussed the maladies they could bring about in man and beast. Witches could bring about all sorts 'of ills of the stomach and the head and feet, with cholic, paralysis, apoplexy, leprosy, epilepsy, dropsy, and stranguary'.[143] With the help of Satan, they make people drink 'certain poisons and drugs; or perhaps the witches themselves mix them with their food and drink'. They dry up wet-nurses' milk, 'making them swallow a certain powder, which they throw in their broth…' Wise-women (witches) were also blamed for impotence in men and for causing illness among 'cattle, crops and fruits of the earth' by administering powders, ointments or even from a certain glance.[144]

As far as healing was concerned, he provided plenty of examples to prove his point that, yes indeed, witches or 'old women', could heal. From the Emperor Hadrian cured of dropsy by a witch to more contemporary cases which involved healing through prayer – but the witches' prayers are 'full of superstition and impiety'; his witches were healers but any credit for their healing belonged to Satan.[145] He made it clear that healing is the province of the doctor not the witch. To give validity to his argument, he quoted medical authorities such as Galen and Avicenna who healed with 'medicine not chants and superstitions'.[146] Witches were not scientific healers in the manner of physicians as they 'make use of characters and words when they heal, and yet nothing can be more certain than that such words and characters have no healing properties'.[147] Witches did employ substances, but their substances were contrary to nature.[148] It is interesting to note that Boguet acknowledged that so-called witches who worked through Satan employed treatments that were the same as those used by physicians: 'And he does so by making use of second and natural causes and the methods used by physicians. For as the learned Cardinal Bellarmine stated, when a sickness is naturally curable the Devil can bring remedies to the sick man.'[149] However, unlike the physician, whose motives were always good and pure, 'there is always this evil in cures effected by witches, or rather by the Devil'. If a woman is the healer, then 'the cure is only effective for a limited time, or else it is necessary for the sickness to be transferred to someone else; and sometimes we find both these conditions operating at the same time'.[150] He 'proves' his first point with the case of a French gentleman whose battle wounds, which had been, 'charmed away', reappeared some three years later, causing the man to die. As far as transferring illnesses from one patient to another, he cites the case of Mumol, Grand Master of France whose life was saved by witches only by causing the death of King Childebert's grandson. Other examples are taken from Bodin. Finally, he contended that witches routinely cast spells on beasts to heal men.[151]

Lawyers such as Pierre de Lancre (1553–1631) assisted the Church in its quest for greater authority over 'assertive, unruly and devilish females with ominous and destabilizing effects within nature's realm'.[152] De Lancre, a counsellor for the Bordeaux Parlement, was sent in 1609 by Henri IV to investigate witchcraft in the Pays de Labourd, a Basque-speaking region in south-western France. He presided over trials in Gascony and was assisted by a surgeon. In addition, he was the author of a treatise on demonology, *Tableau de l'Inconstance des mauvais anges et demons* (1612). Clearly a misogynistic text, influenced by the *Malleus*, he equates the witches in Labourd with Eve: they eat nothing but apples, they drink only apple juice '....which was prohibited by our first father'. He described them as 'Eves who gladly seduce the children of Adam with their naked heads live among the mountains in complete liberty and naivete as Eve did in Paradise, they listen to the Demons and giving their ears to the serpents who they want to seduce, and while frequenting cemeteries night and day which they cover with their crosses and aromatic herbs...'[153] Like Kramer and Sprenger, he asked why, throughout history, there had always been more women witches than men? His own answer was that women have a natural inclination for sorcery which men lack. It is not the fragility of the female sex that leads them to witchcraft but the strength of the 'bestial cupidity which pushes them to extremes where they voluntarily throw themselves to satisfy their appetites and curiosities'. He quoted from Book III of St Augustine's *City of God* where Augustine stated that women have a terrible inclination to be more opinionated than men. Infidelity, ambition and luxury were also more prominent in women than men. Why were women so evil? De Lancre found his answer in Genesis where Eve is held responsible for the fall of man, for the first evil. Eve is seduced by the devil in the form of a serpent and enters into league with him.[154]

The image of the witch as evil, a direct descendant of Eve, draws on the misogynistic literature prevalent in medieval Europe.[155] As with the witchcraft treatises, the authors were primarily medical, legal and ecclesiastical authorities. Women were regularly depicted as inferior to men in every way, corrupt and inconstant. George Gifford referred to the Genesis story of the fallen woman, placing woman as the origin of all evil: Eve seduced by the devil himself.

The English clergyman John Gaule argued that women were fitter than men for the practice of witchcraft because of their 'infirmity, ignorance, impotence of passions and Affections, melancholy, solitariness, timorousness, credulity, inconstancy, etc.'[156] Richard Bernard, who authored *A Guide to Grand Jurymen with respect to Witches* (London, 1627), echoed other writers in asserting that the evil nature of woman started with Eve. He wrote that, women were 'more credulous, more apt to be misled and deceived ... They are more impatient, more superstitious and thus fitter instruments for the Devil.'[157]

Adhering to the writings of Saint Augustine was not uncommon for demonologists. In Spain, Alonso de Madrigal (1409–44), bishop of Avila, was one such, while Fray Lope de Barrientos, bishop of Cuenca (1382–1469), who wrote a treatise on divination, followed the *Canon episcopi*.[158]

In a similar vein, Nicolas Rémy, privy counsellor to Duke Charles III of Lorraine, who was made attorney general in 1591, wrote a treatise on demonology, published in 1595. The book had tremendous success and was reprinted the following year in Cologne. Rémy dedicated the book, which consists of a compendium of his cases, to Charles of Lorraine. Rémy claimed to have presided over 900 cases in fifteen years although this is probably an exaggeration.[159] He devoted a considerable part of the book to cases dealing with magical healing which were connected to spells and the *maleficia* of black witchcraft. He condemned the practice of the country people or peasants in seeking out the care of a witch.[160]

In Book I, he cited cases where women employed the use of plants and herbs to make efficacious poisons. He was struck by the sheer number and diversity of plants they used. He also referred to 'magical unguents' which were applied to the body.[161] These women distributed their herbs, powders and other items in order to bring about illness and cause death. He cited the cases of several women who caused death or grave illness to men by their herbs. He argued that healing and sickness can result in the same method and object: 'It is almost impossible to cure an illness with this aspersion by a remedy other than wanted by witches and that which constitutes a medicine, which most of the time, is ineffective.' The women he named, Odile, femme de Boncourt, Rose Gérardin, Isabelle, and Marthe Mergelat, all received their herbs from the devil. Rémy refers to a number of cases of women who were witches, although he did not prosecute them. One of these women was a healer named Theonotte. She diagnosed and treated diseases through the use of folk magic and Christianity. In addition, she charged for her services, as Rémy related:

> When the price of her services had been settled, she first measured the sick woman cross-wise with a piece of waxed linen, and then folded the linen a certain number of times and placed it in her bosom as if for safety. For the whole of the following night she kept watch before the door of the sick woman's hourse and at the break of day set out on her way without ever uttering a word. When she came to the shrine of S. Fiacre she entered and set fire to the linen, and with the wax that had dropped from it traced figures in the form of a cross on the steps of the

> High Altar; and then went out and walked three times round the chapel, the linen meanwhile giving out spluttering and violet coloured flames... And having performed all of this, she returned to town.[162]

The most powerful institutions of the Early Modern era were united in their attempt to eradicate the witch or wise-woman. The Roman Catholic Church, various European states, the legal and medical professions, all joined forces in their attacks against the witch. They worked in tandem to eradicate these female healers. They were unsuccessful in eliminating the lower-class female healer, but her reputation was greatly damaged among the middle and upper classes.

Epilogue

This book has considered the role and contributions of late medieval and Early Modern European women to health and healing in a selection of countries. Beginning with the later Middle Ages, we have witnessed the extensive contributions made by women practitioners, famous and not so famous. Anna Comnena and Trotula are two names which come to mind when chronicling important medical women of Byzantium and Salerno, but there were countless women whose names we will never know who treated the sick at this time.

The professionalization of medicine had a detrimental impact on female practitioners. The establishment of the licensing process as well as the male-only system of university trained physicians did not bode well for women and other 'irregular' healers. These medical men, who competed with the traditional healer for patients, did their best to bar all others from taking care of the sick. Notwithstanding the introduction of innumerable licensing regulations and a system designed to keep out women, they continued to heal regardless of whether or not they were legally permitted to do so.

Contemporary societal views and expectations of women buttressed the official legal and institutional framework which officially banned women from medicine. Legal, theological and medical commentators contributed to the debate. Some physicians held that women were incomplete and deformed males, while others held more positive views. Ideas on what was the appropriate role for women varied between countries and cultures with the Spanish recommending a very cloistered life for women, either in the home or the convent, while the French, such as the Cartesian philosopher Poulain de la Barre, wrote a curriculum for women which included medicine. Although most Renaissance men recommended an education for women, it was not an education that prepared them for the public sphere. In spite of receiving an inferior education when compared with their male counterparts, exceptional women, among them Dona Oliva Sabuco de Nantes in Spain and Marie de Maupeou Fouquet in France, were able to publish significant medical treatises. Not all women, however, published their works.

Many kept their receipt books at home or shared them with neighbours. This was particularly true in England where we find hundreds of such 'receipt books', with healing receipts often combined with cooking recipes, in family collections. These collections of traditional medicines provide evidence that women were practising medicine from the home and that they understood the basics of herbal medicines.

Nurses have played a crucial, yet often overlooked and denigrated role within the healing community. The chapter dealing with nurses, who were often nuns, aimed to highlight the medical care that they gave to the sick and poor in earlier times. Similarly, midwives, often accused of being witches, dominated childbirth until the eighteenth century. Midwives' duties frequently extended beyond the immediate help and care with the process of childbirth, caring for mother and baby before, during and after birth. Midwives were not the only group of female health-care workers designated as witches in the past. Wise-women, who were popular, or local village healers, those who used spells and potions to heal and relieve pain, were also called witches during the period of the great witch-hunts. Through tenacity and creative strategies, women were able to overcome these obstacles in the world of medicine. In the nineteenth century, several brave women would lead the battle to gain access to what they had been denied for centuries: access to medical school.

Notes

Introduction

1. 'Medicine', in William Morris, ed., *The American Heritage Dictionary* (Boston: Houghton Mifflin, 1976); 'medicine *n.*', in *The Oxford American Dictionary of Current English, Oxford Reference Online* (Oxford University Press, 1999), University of Toronto Libraries, http://www.oxfordreference.com.myaccess.library.utoronto.ca/views/ENTRY.html?subview=Main&entry=t21.e19038 [accessed 22 August 2008].
2. The term doctor was derived from the Latin *docere*, to teach. See Vern Bullough, 'The Term Doctor', *Journal of the History of Medicine*, 18 (1963): 284–7.
3. Dorothy Porter and Roy Porter, *Patient's Progress: Doctors and Doctoring in Eighteenth-Century England* (Cambridge: Polity, 1989), p. 11.
4. I am indebted to many previous scholars who have worked on popular healers. See particularly work by scholars such as Margaret Pelling, Roy Porter, Monica Green, Andrew Weir, Doreen Nagy, Danielle Jacquart, Nancy Siraisi, Luis García Ballester, Matthew Ramsey, Colin Jones and Lawrence Brockliss. Mary Lindemann, Merry Weisner, Katharine Park, Carole Rawcliffe and Joseph Shatzmiller have brought to light the importance of both the multiplicity of medical practitioners that have existed throughout history, and the fact that most of these were not university trained. This is in no way a complete list of the authors I have consulted in preparation of this book; however, their studies have been ground-breaking in terms of stressing the importance of popular healers.
5. This collection contains excellent specialized articles on different aspects of female health-care and midwifery in medieval Iberia, and Early Modern Germany, England and France. The articles are not comparative in nature.
6. Monica H. Green, 'Midwives and Other Female Practitioners', in Thomas Glick, Steven J. Livesey and Faith Wallis, eds, *Medieval Science, Technology and Medicine: an Encyclopedia* (New York and London: Routledge, 2005), p. 216.
7. Chapter 8 looks at unpublished medical receipts and remedies produced by women who, although not formally trained as medical practitioners, provided medical services to their communities.
8. See Elaine Hobby for a discussion of the authorship of this text, *Virtue of Necessity: English Women's Writing: 1649–88* (Ann Arbor: University of Michigan Press, 1989), p. 175.
9. Hannah Woolley, *The Gentlewoman's Companion, or, A Guide to the Female Sex* (London: A. Maxwell, 1673), p. 10.
10. Sabuco de Nantes preceded British physicians, Thomas Willis (1621–75) and Francis Glisson (1597–1677) in their work on the nervous system by about thirty years. The editors and translators of the *Nueva Filosofia* note that these scientists did not credit Sabuco de Nantes even though their works are very similar in content. See *New Philosophy of Human Nature*, trans. and ed. Mary Ellen Waithe, Maria Colomer Vintro and C. Angel Zorita (Champaign, IL: University of Illinois Press, 2007).
11. Chapter 5 relies heavily on the work of others in this field of medicine. The literature on the history of midwifery is enormous. Subsequent notes should provide readers with a guide to the literature.

12. For some negative stereotypes which historians of medicine had traditionally held concerning female medical practitioners in general and nurses in particular, see Margaret Connor Versluysen, 'Old Wives' Tales? Women Healers in English History', in *Rewriting Nursing History* (London: Croom Helm, 1980), pp. 175–99. She writes, 'Organised medicine, especially its most prestigious branches, has formally barred women from its ranks for most of its known past. History has reflected this sexual exclusivity and has been primarily the story of a socially privileged group of male healers' (p. 177).
13. William L. Minkowski, 'Women Healers of the Middle Ages: Selected Aspects of their History', *American Journal of Public Health*, 82(2) (February 1992): 289; Thetis M. Group and Joan I. Roberts, *Nursing, Physician Control, and the Medical Monopoly: Historical Perspectives on Gendered Inequality in Roles, Rights, and Range of Practice* (Bloomington: Indiana University Press, 2001), p. 24.
14. Midwives come up frequently in the demonology literature, but cases where women were actually prosecuted for practising their craft are much fewer in number than those where women were accused of healing. See the provocative article by David Harley, who poignantly makes this point, arguing that 'historians have been led astray by a tradition that derives from the discredited work of Margaret Murray'. 'Historians as Demonologists: the Myth of the Mid-Wife-Witch', *Social History of Medicine* (1990): 99–124.
15. Primary source material for witch persecutions consist of trial records, demonology handbooks and witch-hunters' textbooks, contemporary pamphlets of eyewitness accounts, theoretical works by believers and sceptics. For an excellent guide to sources, see Jean-Pierre Coumont, *Demonology and Witchcraft: an Annotated Bibliography* (Utrecht: Hes and DeGraaf, 2004).
16. This role was not unique to European society, but can also be found in the Middle East and Latin America where women's healing practices were widespread. Anne Llewellyn Barstow, *Witchcraze: A New History of European Witch Hunts* (San Francisco: Pandora, 1994), p. 207, n. 1.
17. John Henry, 'Doctors and Healers: Popular Culture and the Medical Profession', in Stephen Pumfrey, Paolo L. Rossi and Maurice Slawinski, eds, *Science, Culture and Popular Belief in Renaissance Europe* (Manchester and New York: Manchester University Press, 1991), p. 191.
18. Guido Ruggiero, *Binding Passions: Tales of Magic, Marriage, and Power at the End of the Renaissance* (Oxford: Oxford University Press, 1993), p. 17.

1. The Medieval Contribution

1. Christine de Pizan, *The Book of the City of the Ladies*, trans. Earl Jeffrey Richards, foreword, Marina Warner (New York: Persea Books, 1972), p. 26.
2. Monica H. Green, 'Midwives and Other Female Practitioners', in Thomas Glick, Steven J. Livesey and Faith Wallis, eds, *Medieval Science, Technology and Medicine: an Encyclopedia* (New York and London: Routledge, 2005), p. 216.
3. Nursing and midwifery are considered in Chapters 5 and 6. These were areas of health-care which were open to women in the Early Modern period. Midwifery was women's speciality.
4. Jennifer Lawler, *Encyclopedia of the Middle Ages* (London and Jefferson, WI: McFarland, 2001), p. 122.
5. See Monica Green's chapter, 'Documenting Medieval Women's Medical Practice', in Luis García Ballester, ed., *Practical Medicine from Salerno to the Black Death* (New York: Cambridge University Press, 1994), pp. 322–52.

6. See Thomas G. Benedek, 'The Roles of Medieval Women in the Healing Arts', in Douglas Radcliff Umstead, ed., *The Roles and Images of Women in the Middle Ages and Renaissance* (Pittsburgh: University of Pittsburgh Publications on the Middle Ages and Renaissance, 1975), III, pp. 145–59. Geneviève Dumas adds that the study of medieval medical practitioners is a relatively recent one and that women are very under-represented in the sources. Geneviève Dumas, 'Les Femmes et les pratiques de la santé, dans le "Registre des plaidoiries du Parlement de Paris", 1364–1427', *Canadian Bulletin of Medical History/Bulletin canadien d'histoire de la medicine*, 13 (1996): 3–27.
7. Cited in Eileen Edna Power, *Medieval Women*, ed. M.M. Postan (New York: Cambridge University Press, 1975), p. 86, n. 17.
8. Anna Comnena, *The Alexiad of the Princess Anna Comnena*, ed. and trans. Elizabeth A.S. Dawes (New York: Barnes & Noble, 1967), Preface, I, p. 1.
9. Muriel Joy Hughes, *Women Healers in Medieval Life and Literature* (Freeport, NY: Books for Libraries Press, 1968), p. 37.
10. Rae Dalven, *Anna Comnena* (New York: Twayne Publishers, 1972), p. 78.
11. Comnena, *Alexiad,* IV, pp. 1, 99–100; XIV, pp. 4, 370–1; VI, pp. 6, 147.
12. Comnena, *Alexiad*, I, X, p. 26.
13. Alain Touwaide, 'Galen', in Thomas Glick, Steven J. Livesey and Faith Wallis (eds), *Medieval Science, Technology and Medicine: An Encyclopedia* (New York and London: Routledge, 2005), p. 179.
14. Comnena, XIV, pp. 4, 434; XIV, pp. 7, 449, cited in Georgina Grenfell Buckler, *Anna Comnena: A Study* (London: Oxford University Press, 1929), p. 216, n. 8.
15. Comnena, XV, pp. 11, 419– 20.
16. Comnena, XV, pp. 11, 422.
17. Comnena, XV, Sec. 11, p. 422; XV, Sec. 11, pp. 424, 426.
18. Comnena, Preface, Sec. 3, p. 3.
19. Comnena, VI, Sec. 6, p. 147.
20. Demetrios Constantelos, *Byzantine Philanthropy and Social Welfare*, 2nd revised edition (New Rochelle, NY: Aristide D. Cartazas, 1991), p. 129; G.C. Pournaropoulos, 'The Real Value of Greek Medicine (Byzantium)' in *XVIIe Congrès International d'histoire de la medicine*, I (Athens, 1960), p. 357.
21. G.C. Pournaropoulos, 'Hospital and Social Welfare Institutions in the Medieval Greek Empire (Byzantium)', *XVIIe Congrès International d'histoire de la medicine*, I (Athens: The Congress, 1961), p. 378.
22. Comnena, *Alexiad*, XV, pp. 7, 409–10; Marilyn French, *Beyond Power: on Women, Men and Morals* (New York: Ballatine Books, 1986), p. 159.
23. Excerpts from the *Typikon* are cited in Demetrios J. Constantelos, *Byzantine Philanthropy and Social Welfare* (New Brunswick, NJ: Rutgers University Press, 1968), pp. 172–5.
24. Constantelos, *Byzantine Philanthropy*, p. 129.
25. Timothy S. Millar, 'Byzantine Hospitals', *Dumbarton Oak Papers*, 38, *Symposium on Byzantine Medicine* (1984): 61.
26. Ferdinand Chalandon, *Jean II Comnène 1118–1143 et Manuel I Comnène 1143–1180* (New York: B. Franklin, 1960), I, 84–7; Comnena, *Alexiad*, Book XV, p. 7.
27. Vern Bullough and Bonnie Bullough, *The Emergence of Modern Nursing* (New York: Macmillan, 1969), p. 44; Millar, 'Byzantine Hospitals', p. 61.
28. Constantelos, *Byzantine Philanthropy*, p. 175.
29. See especially the writings of the Byzantium monastic reformer, Theodore of Studium (d. 826) in Constantelos, *Byzantine Philanthropy*, p. 184.

30. Robert de Sorbonne founded the first college in 1275 in Paris. Mortimer Chambers et al., *The Western Experience, Vol. 1: To the Eighteenth Century*, 9th edn (Boston: McGraw–Hill, 2006), p. 251.
31. John Walton, Paul B. Beeson and Ronald Bodley Scott, eds, *The Oxford Companion to Medicine* (Oxford: Oxford University Press, 1986), II, p. 1457.
32. J.A. Lekstrom, 'Medical Literature of Medieval Salerno: Evolution of the Modern Medical Professional', *Pharos*, 53(1) (1990): 24.
33. Orderic Vitalis, *The Ecclesiastical History of Orderic Vitalis*, ed. and trans. with introduction and notes by Marjorie Chibnall (Oxford: Clarendon Press, 1968), Book III, Vol. II, pp. 76–7. For a detailed study of the School of Salerno, see Paul Oskar Kristeller, 'The School of Salerno: Its Development and Contribution to the History of Learning', *Bulletin of the History of Medicine*, 17 (1945): 138–94.
34. H.J. Mozans, *Women in Science: with an Introductory Chapter on Woman's Long Struggle for Things of the Mind*, preface Cynthia Russett, introduction Thomas P. Gariepy (Notre Dame, IN: University of Indiana Press, 1991), pp. 283–4.
35. Fragments of manuscripts signed by her are in Breslau in addition to those in Leipzig, Florence and the Bibliothèque Nationale in Paris where there is the oldest manuscript dating from the thirteenth century, Fonds Latin, no. 7056. Mélina Lipinska, *Les Femmes et le progrès des sciences médicales* (Paris: C. Jacques, 1930), pp. 28–30.
36. H.P. Bayon, 'The Masters of Salerno and the Origins of Medical Practice', in E.A. Underwood (ed.), *Science, Medicine and History* (London: Oxford University Press, 1953), I, pp. 203–19.
37. From Josette Dall'ava-Santucci, *Des Sorcières aux Mandarines Histoire des femmes Médecins* (Paris: Calmann-Lévy, 1989), p. 43.
38. Benjamin F. Shearer and Barbara S. Shearer, eds, *Notable Women in the Life Sciences: a Biographical Dictionary* (Westport CT: Greenwood Press, 1996), pp. 382–5.
39. Wolff cited in John F. Benton, 'Trotula, Women's Problems, and the Professionalization of Medicine in the Middle Ages', *Bulletin of the History of Medicine*, 59(1) (Spring 1985): 36, and Margaret Alic, *Hypatia's Heritage: a History of Women in Science from Antiquity through the Nineteenth Century* (Boston: Beacon Press, 1986), p. 54.
40. Dall'ava-Santucci, *Des Sorcières aux Mandarines*, p. 45.
41. Benton, 'Trotula', pp. 30–53.
42. Walton et al., *Oxford Companion to Medicine*, II, p. 1458.
43. Lekstrom, 'Medical Literature', p. 23.
44. Trotula, *The Trotula: a Medieval compendium of Women's Medicine*, ed. and trans. Monica H. Green (Philadelphia: University of Pennsylvania Press, 2001), pp. xi–xii, 17, 48–51.
45. Green, *The Trotula*, p. 135.
46. Ibid., p. 37.
47. Cited in Edward Grant, ed., *A Sourcebook in Medieval Science* (Cambridge, MA: Harvard University Press, 1974), p. 763.
48. Grant, *Sourcebook*, p. 765.
49. Ibid., p. 766.
50. Green, *The Trotula*, pp. 129, 131.
51. Cited in C.H. Talbot, 'Dame Trot and her Progeny', *Essays and Studies in Honour of Beatrice White* (London: J. Murray, 1972), p. 1.
52. Anne Echols and Marty Williams, *An Annotated Index of Medieval Women* (Princeton, NJ: Princeton University Press, 1993), p. 375.

53. The titles of Guarna and Abella's works are cited in Marcello Segré's 'Dottoresse Ebree Nel Medioevo', *Pagina di Storia della Medicina*, 14(5) (1970): 100 and in James J. Walsh, *Medieval Medicine* (London: A & C Black, 1920), pp. 157–8.
54. Published in 1943 reprinted in 1968 and 1987, Muriel Joy Hughes's *Women Healers in Medieval Life and Literature* (Freeport, NY: Books for Libraries Press, 1968) remains the only monograph dedicated to medieval European women healers. Particularly useful is Appendix I: Women Practitioners of the Later Middle Ages, 138–47, More recently, Monica Green has published several scholarly articles on this subject.
55. Echols and Williams, *An Annotated Index*, p. 310.
56. The primary documents concerning her were destroyed during the Second World War. They were in the Archivo Angiono, Reg. 1422, fol. 20. A reference to them may be found in Salvatore De Renzi, *Storia documentata della Scuolo Medica di Salerno* (Naples, 1857; reprinted Milan, 1967), cxxx, no. 338, 569 and in Paul Oskar Kristeller, 'Learned Women of Early Modern Italy: Humanists and University Scholars', in Patricia H. Labalme, ed., *Beyond their Sex: Learned Women of the European Past* (New York and London: New York University Press, 1980), p. 115, n. 52; Bonnie S. Anderson and Judith P. Zinsser, *A History of their Own*, Vol. 1, *Women in Europe from Prehistory to the Present* (New York and Oxford: Oxford University Press, 2000), pp. 416–17; Hughes, *Women Healers*, pp. 148–9; Talbot, 'Dame Trot', p. 13.
57. M.P. Huppert, 'Italian Women Doctors in the Middle Ages', *History of Medicine Quarterly*, 5(3) (Autumn 1973): 26.
58. David C. Lindberg, ed., *Science in the Middle Ages* (Chicago: University of Chicago Press, 1998), p. 408.
59. See Helen Lemay, 'Women and the Literature of Obstetrics and Gynecology', in Joel T. Rosenthal, ed., *Medieval Women and the Sources of Medieval History* (Athens and London: University of Georgia Press, 1990), p. 193.
60. *Collectio Salernitana*, cited in Julia O'Faolain and Laura Martines, eds, *Not in God's Image: Women in History from the Greeks to the Victorians* (London: Temple Smith, 1973), p. 165.
61. Hughes, *Women Healers*, p. 142; Echols and Williams, *An Annotated Index*, p. 247.
62. This licence to practise 'the art of surgery...' is dated from September 1309 to April 1310, and found in Raffaele Calvanico, ed., *Fonti per Storia della Medicina e della Chirurgia per il Regno di Napoli nel periodo Angioinio*, doc. 1165 (Naples: L'Arte tip., 1962), p. 141. Cited in Ronald J. Doviak, 'The University of Naples and the Study and Practice of Medicine in the Thirteenth and Fourteenth Centuries', unpublished PhD dissertation, City University of New York (1974), p. 37.
63. Her licence was renewed from September 1330 to August 1331. Calvanico, *Fonti*, doc. 3195, p. 229.
64. Raymunda's licence is dated September 1334. Calvanico, *Fonti*, doc. 3643, p. 277.
65. Calvanico, *Fonti*, docs 3226 and 3598, pp. 232, 236. Judging by the dates of the licence, September 1331 to August 1333, Polisena practised for a minimum of eleven years.
66. Doviak, 'The University of Naples', p. 44.
67. C.H. Talbot and E.A. Hammond, *The Medical Practitioners in Medieval England: A Biographical Register* (London: Wellcome Historical Medical Library, 1965), pp. 13–14.
68. Echols and Williams, *Annotated Index*, p. 315.
69. Talbot and Hammond, *Medical Practitioners*, p. 13.

70. Doviak, 'The University of Naples', p. 43.
71. Hughes, *Women Healers*, p. 142.
72. Monica H. Green, 'Documenting Medieval Women's Medical Practice', in Ballester, *Practical Medicine from Salerno*, p. 322, n. 3; Echols and Williams, *Annotated Index*, p. 410.
73. Echols and Williams, *Annotated Index*, p. 28.
74. See R. Olry, 'Medieval Neuroanatomy: The Text of Mondino dei Luzzi and the Plates of Guido da Vigevano', *Journal of the History of Neurosciences*, 6(2) (August 1997): 113–23.
75. Thomas N. Haviland and Lawrence Charles Parish, 'A Brief Account of the Use of Wax Models in the Study of Medicine', *Journal of the History of Medicine and Allied Sciences*, XXV (1970): 52.
76. This tablet was written by Otto Agenius Lustrulanus, her fiancé and another assistant to Luzzi. Cited in Michele Medici, *Compendio storico della Scuola Anatomica di Bologna dal rinascimento dell scienze e delle lettere a tutto il secolo XVIII: con un paragone fra la sua antichità a quella delle scuole di Salerno e di Padova* (Bologna: Tipografia governativa Della Volpe e del Sassi, 1857), p. 30.
77. Similar information about Bucca is found in Elisabetta Caminer Turra, *Selected Writings of an Eighteenth-Century Venetian Woman of Letters*, ed. and trans. Catherine M. Sama (Chicago: University of Chicago Press, 2003), p. 177; Marilyn Bailey Ogilvie, *Women in Science: Antiquity through the Nineteenth Century, a Biographical Dictionary with Annotated Bibliography* (Cambridge, MA: MIT Press, 1986), pp. 11, 42; Richard H. Popkin, ed., *The Columbia History of Western Philosophy* (New York: Columbia University Press 1999), p. 767; Ethel M. Kersey, *Women Philosophers: A Bio-Critical Source Book* (Westport, CT: Greenwood, 1989), p. 8.
78. Monica Green, 'Women's Medical Practice and Health Care in Medieval Europe', *Signs*, 14 (1989): 443.
79. Jean Dangler, *Mediating Fictions: Literature, Women Healers and the Go-between in Medieval and Early Modern Iberia* (Lewisburg: Bucknell University Press, 2001), p. 21; Luis García-Ballester, Michael McVaugh and Augustin Rubio Vela, *Medical Licensing and Learning in Fourteenth Century Valencia* (Philadelphia: American Philosophical Society, 1989), p. 30.
80. A copy of this licence found in Document LXVIII of *Frorilegio documental del reinado de Pedro IV de Aragón* is published in Amada López de Menses, 'Cinco Catalanas Licenciadas en Medicina por Pedro el Ceremonioso (1374–1382)', *Correro Erudito*, V(37) (1957): 252.
81. Archivo de la Corona de Aragón. Registro I.891, f. 90v–91r. in Document II, Documentos culturales de Pedro el Ceremonioso (Zaragosa, 1953) cited in López de Menses, 'Cinco Catalanas', p. 252, n. 3.
82. Archivo de la Corona de Aragón. Cancilleria real, Registro 943, in López de Menses, 'Cinco Catalanas', p. 253, n. 5.
83. Jean Dangler, *Mediating Fictions*, pp. 20–4.
84. Michael R. McVaugh, *Medicine before the Plague: Practitioners and their Patients in the Crown of Aragon, 1285–1345* (Cambridge: Cambridge University Press, 1993), p. 105.
85. McVaugh, *Medicine before the Plague*, p. 162.
86. 30 July 1496 (C.R. Leg 100, fol. 62, Archivo General de Simancas) cited in Juan M. Jiménez Munoz, 'Salario de medicos, cirujanos, boticarios y enfermeras', *Asclepio: Archivo iberomaeircano de historia de la medicina y antropología médica*, Vols 26–7 (1974–1975): 548.

87. Archives C1296/8 and C 1297/215r–v, cited in McVaugh, *Medicine before the Plague*, p. 104.
88. McVaugh, *Medicine before the Plague*, p. 106.
89. Margaret Wade Labarge, *Women in Medieval Life* (London: Hamish Hamilton, 1986), p. 174.
90. Ernest Wickersheimer, *Dictionnaire biographique des Médecins en France au Môyen Age*, 2 vols (Paris: E. Droz, 1936) and Danielle Jacquart, *Le milieu médical en France du XIIe au XVe siècle* (Geneva : Droz, 1981), 47 and annexes.
91. Wickersheimer, *Dictionnaire biographique*, I, pp. 21, 39; II, pp. 750, 505.
92. Hercule Géraud, *Paris sous Philippe-le Bel, d'après des documents originaux, et notamment d'après un manuscrit contenant le rôle de la taille imposée sur les habitants de Paris en 1292* (Paris: Crapelet, 1837).
93. Géraud, *Paris sous Philippe-le Bel*, p. 57.
94. Paris tax roll of 1292, cited in Echols and Williams, *Annotated Index*, p.133.
95. Géraud, *Paris sous Philippe-le Bel*, p. 47; Hughes, *Women Healers*, p. 140; Jacquart, *Le milieu médical*, p. 443.
96. Wickersheimer, *Dictionnaire*, I, p. 39.
97. Wickersheimer, *Dictionnaire*, II, pp. 506, 537, 538.
98. Ibid., p. 505.
99. Wickersheimer, *Dictionnaire*, III, p. 222.
100. Wickersheimer, *Dictionnaire*, I, p. 31; II, p. 750.
101. Wickersheimer, *Dictionnaire*, II, p. 747.
102. Echols and Williams, *Annotated Index*, p. 199; Marilyn Bailey Ogilvie and Joy Dorothy Harvey, *The Biographical Dictionary of Women in Science: Pioneering Lives from Ancient Times to the Mid-20th Century* (London: Routledge, 2000), I, p. 502.
103. Hersend's name as 'magistra Hersend physica' can be found with those of nineteen other doctors who worked for royalty and nobility from the thirteenth to the fifteenth centuries. See 'Catalogue des archives de M. de Joursanvault', *Bulletin de la société de l'histoire de France* (Paris, 1855–56), p. 144, n. 2. For information about Hersend, see Hughes, *Women Healers*, pp. 88–9; Echols and Williams, *Annotated Index*, p. 218; Labarge, *Women in Medieval Life*, p. 174, Wickersheimer, *Dictionnaire*, vols. I–II, pp. 294–5.
104. L. Douët-a'Arcq, ed., *Compte de l'Hôtel des Rois de France au XIVe et XVe siècles* (Paris: Société de l'Historie de France, 1865), p. 377; Hughes, *Women Healers*, p. 89; Labarge, *Women in Medieval Life*, p. 174.
105. Jacquart, *Le milieu médical*, p. 52.
106. Wickersheimer, *Dictionnaire*, II, p. 538.
107. The Châtelet was one of the two great law courts of *ancien régime* Paris. The other was the Parlement, a higher court.
108. Dumas, 'Les Femmes', p. 11, n. 50.
109. Wickersheimer, *Dictionnaire*, II, p. 537.
110. E. Coornaert, *Les corporations en France avant 1789* (Paris: Les Editions ouvrières, 1968), pp. 184, 190.
111. Faye Marie Getz, *Medicine in the English Middle Ages* (Princeton, NJ: Princeton University Press, 1998), p. 5.
112. Getz, *Medicine*, p. 9.
113. Ibid., p. 94, n. 7.
114. Talbot and Hammond, *Medical Practitioners*, pp. 10, 28, 100.
115. Echols and Williams, *Annotated Index*, pp. 39–40.

116. Eileen Power, 'Some Women Practitioners of Medicine in the Middle Ages', *Proceedings Royal Soc Med*, 15(3): 23. Citing and translating, PRO Ancient Petitions, file 231, no 11510. A.L. Wyman, 'The Surgeoness, the Female Practitioner of Surgery 1400–1800', *Medical History*, 28 (1984): 22–41.
117. Getz, *Medicine*, pp. 263, 256, 269. Her information for Lady Beauchamp is based on a Wellcome Manuscript, MS 542, fols. 17v–18, Balliol College, MS 89 fol 398.
118. 'Man and women are able to heal.' Cited in Edmée Charrier, *L'évolution intellectuelle feminine* (Paris, A. Mechelinck, 1931), p. 447.
119. Dorothy Whitelock, *The Beginnings of English Society* (Harmondsworth: Penguin, 1979), pp. 94–5.
120. Edward J. Kealey, 'England's Earliest Women Doctors', *Journal of the History of Medicine and Allied Sciences*, 40 (1985): 473–5.
121. Getz, *Medicine*, p. 95, n. 26.
122. Talbot and Hammond, *Medical Practitioners*, p. 200.
123. Getz, *Medicine*, p. 11 and Sidney Young, *Memorials of the Craft of Surgery in England, from Materials Compiled by John Flint South*, ed. D'Arcy Power (London: Cassells, 1886), p. 19; D'Arcy Power, 'English Medicine and Surgery in the 14th Century', *Lancet*, II (1914): 176–83.
124. Robert Steven Gottfried, *Doctors and Medicine in Medieval England, 1340–1530* (Princeton, NJ: Princeton University Press, 1986), p. 88.
125. Breviary of Practice I, 38, cited in Lynn Thorndike, *A History of Magic and Experimental Science* (New York: Columbia University Press, 1923; reprint 1964), II, pp. 843, 853.
126. Thorndike, *History of Magic*, II, p. 226.
127. Cited in Thorndike, *History of Magic*, II, p. 482.
128. Thorndike, *History of Magic*, II, p. 482.
129. Ibid., p. 483.
130. Guy de Chauliac (c.1300–1368) was the most prominent surgeon in Europe during the fourteenth century. He was Pope Clement VI's doctor in Avignon. His major work, *Chirurgia Magna* (1363) was highly influential and used by doctors for three centuries.
131. Cited in Thorndike, *History of Magic*, IV, p. 383.
132. See Bacon's *Epistola de Secretis operibus* for his views on magic cited in Thorndike, *History of Magic*, II, p. 661. Very little is known about Bacon's life. What is known is that he studied at Oxford and Cambridge and completed his studies in 1240. He was an Aristotelian specialist. See Allison Kavey, *Books of Secrets: Natural Philosophy in England, 1550–1600* (Chicago & Urbana: University of Illinois Press, 2007), pp. 36–7.
133. The first edition was printed in 1478, shortly after the invention of the printing press. Chauliac received the highest medical degree of his time, the Clerk and Master of Medicine. James E. Pilcher, 'Guy de Chauliac and Henri de Mondeville: A Surgical Retrospect', *Annals of Surgery*, 21(1) (January 1885): 87.
134. See the introduction to Chauliac's *Chirurgia magna. English. Selections,* Ann Arbor, Michigan, Early English Books Online Text Creation Partnership (2002) Original publication, *Chirurgia magna* (London: printed by Robert Wyer for Henry Dabbe and Rycharde Banckes, 1542); see also, Guy de Chauliac, *The Cyrugie of Guy de Chauliac*, ed. Margaret S. Ogden (London and New York: Published for the Early English Text Society by the Oxford University Press, 1971), p. 10.
135. John of Arderne (b. 1307), author of *Practica*, written in the 1370s was an English surgeon, famous for his work on fistula-in-ano.

136. John Arderne, *Treatises of Fistula in Ano, Haemorrhoids and Clysters from an early fifteenth century manuscript translation*, ed. and trans. D'Arcy Power (London: Published for the Early English Text Society by Kegan Paul, Trench, Trübner, 1910), pp. 44, 49.
137. John of Mirfield, cited in G.R. Owst, *Literature and the Pulpit in Medieval England* (Oxford: Oxford University Press, 1933), pp. 349–50.
138. Regulations against clergy practising medicine were passed at councils in Rheims in 1131 and the Lateran Council of 1139. See Pearl Kibre, 'The Faculty of Medicine at Paris, Charlatanism, and Unlicensed Medical Practices in the Later Middle Ages', *Bulletin of the History of Medicine*, 28 (January–February 1953): 4.
139. See Monica Green, 'Books as a Source of Medical Education for Women in the Middle Ages', *Dynamis*, 20 (2000): 341–60, for a discussion of medical books found in European convents during the Middle Ages and the general literacy level in these female institutions.
140. For excerpts from Hildegard's medical writings on diseases and their treatments, see Margret Berger, *Hildegard of Bingen: on Natural Philosophy and Medicine: Selections from 'Cause et cure'*, translated from Latin with introduction, notes and interpretive essay (Cambridge and Rochester, NY: D.S. Brewer, 1999).
141. Marilyn Bailey Ogilvie, *Women in Science*, p. 9.
142. Cited in Monica Green, 'Books as a Source of Medical Education', p. 342, n. 33; Labarge, *Women in Medieval Life*, p. 171,
143. P.H. Cullum, 'Cremetts and Corrodies: Care of the Poor and Sick at St Leonard's Hospital, York in the Middle Ages', *Borthwick Papers*, 79 (1991): 13.
144. John Henderson, 'The Hospitals of Late Medieval and Renaissance Florence: a Preliminary Survey', in Lindsay Granshaw and Roy Porter, eds, *The Hospital in History* (London and New York: Routledge, 1989), p. 82.
145. George James Aungier, *The History and Antiquities of Syon Monastery* (London: J. B. Nichols & Son, 1840), p. 395.
146. See the testimony of Rabbi Asher of Toledo who had been treated by a female Jewish oculist in the mid-1300s. Reprinted in Joseph Shatzmiller, *Jews, Medicine and Medieval Society* (Berkeley: University of California Press, 1994), p. 111.
147. Paracelsus, cited in David B. Ruderman, *Science, Medicine and Jewish Culture in Early Modern Europe* (Tel-Aviv: Tel-Aviv University, 1987), p. 6.
148. David M. Feldman, *Health and Medicine in the Jewish Traditions* (New York: Crossroad, 1976), p. 41.
149. Norman Roth, ed., *Medieval Jewish Civilization: an Encyclopedia* (London and New York: Routledge, 2003), p. 437.
150. Shatzmiller, *Jews, Medicine*, pp. 23, 109.
151. Roth, *Medieval Jewish Civilization*, p. 438.
152. Archivo de la Corona de Aragón ACA, R. 863 f. 163, cited in A. Cardoner Planas, 'Mujeres Hebreas Practicando la Medecina', *Sefarad*, 9 (1949): 442.
153. C 873/160v, 1 July 1342 in McVaugh, *Medicine before the Plague*, p. 107.
154. Evelyn Rose Benson, *As We See Ourselves: Jewish Women in Nursing* (Indianapolis: Center Nursing Publishing, 2001), p. 13.
155. Woodcut from Liber Chronicarum, H. Schedel, Nuremberg, 1493, the Wellcome Library, London, cited in Natalia Berger, ed., *Jews and Medicine, Religion, Culture, Science* (Tel-Aviv: Beth Hatefutsoth 1995), p. 76; Madeleine Pelner Cosman, *Women at Work in Medieval Europe* (New York: Facts on File, 2000), p. 39. See also Cecil Roth, 'Qualifications of Jewish Physicians in the Middle Ages', *Speculum*, 28 (1953): 834–43.

156. The date of the manuscript is 28 August 1326. The manuscript is cited in Latin by Shatzmiller, *Jews, Medicine*, p. 197, n. 36, and she is also mentioned by Talbot and Hammond, *Medical Practitioners*, p. 3.
157. Feldman, *Health and Medicine*, p. 43; Michael Nevins, *The Jewish Doctor* (London: Jason Aronson, 1996), p. 99.
158. Joseph Shatzmiller, *Médecine et Justice en Provence Médiévale Documents de Manosque* (Aix-en-Provence: Publications de l'Université de Provence, 1989), pp. 6, 8–9.
159. ADBR Doc No 47, cited in Shatzmiller, *Médecine et Justice*, p. 25.
160. Echols and Williams, *Annotated Index*, p. 241.
161. Géraud, *Paris sous Philippe-le Bel*, p. 149.
162. Shatzmiller, *Jews, Medicine*, pp. 20–2, 111. Her case will be examined in detail in Chapter 2.
163. Shirley Guthrie, *Arab Women in the Middle Ages* (London: Saqi Books, 2001), p. 53.
164. '...Aalimatin fi sinaat al tibb wa al mudawah' ['two lady scholars in medicine and therapeutics with good experience in the treatment of ladies'] as stated by Ibn Abi Usaibia the famous thirteenth-century medical historian, cited in Rabie E. Abel-Halim, 'Ibn Zuhr (Avenzoar) and the progress of surgery', *Saudi Medical Journal*, 26(9) (2005): 1334.
165. See Charles Singer, *From Magic to Science: Essays on the Scientific Twilight* (New York: Boni & Liveright, 1928), p. 80.
166. Cited in Edouard Nicaise, *La Grande Chirurgie de Guy de Chauliac* (Paris: Alcan, 1890), pp. lxiii, lxiv.
167. Cited in James William Brodman, *Charity and Welfare Hospitals and the Poor in Medieval Catalonia* (Philadelphia: University of Pennsylvania Press, 1998), p. 91.
168. Agustín Rubio Vela, 'La asistencia hospitalaria infantile en la Valencia del siglo XIV: Pobres, huérfanos y expósitos', *Dynamis*, 2 (1982): 180.

2. New Medical Regulations and their Impact on Female Healers

1. Ian Mortimer, 'Diocesan Licensing and Medical Practitioners in South-West England, 1660–1780', *Medical History*, 48(1) (January 2004): 62.
2. Harold John Cook, 'The Regulation of Medical Practice in London under the Stuarts, 1607–1704', unpublished PhD dissertation, University of Michigan, 1981, p. 8.
3. Geneviève Dumas, 'Les Femmes et les pratiques de la santé, dans le "Registre des plaidoiries du Parlement de Paris", 1364–1427', *Canadian Bulletin of Medical History/Bulletin canadien d'histoire de la medicine*, 13 (1996): 19.
4. Vern L. Bullough, 'Training of the Nonuniversity-Educated Medical Practitioners in the Later Middle Ages', *Journal of the History of Medicine*, XIV (October 1959): 446–9.
5. *Ordonnances des rois de France de la troisième race: recueillies par ordre chronologique: avec des renvoys des unes aux autres, des sommaires, des observations sur le texte, & cinq tables*, Eusèbe Jacob de Laurière, Denis François Secourses et al (Paris: Imprimerie nationale, 1723–1849) V, pp. 530–1; VI, pp. 197–8.
6. *Ordonnances des rois de France*, XIV, pp. 427–33.

7. David Harley, '"Bred up in the study of that faculty": Licensed Physicians in North-West England, 1660–1760', *Medical History*, 38 (1994): 398.
8. Doreen A. Evenden, 'Gender Differences in the Licensing and Practice of Female and Male Surgeons in Early Modern England', *Medical History*, 42 (1998): 194. Evenden's article focuses on practitioners in London.
9. Evenden, 'Gender Differences', p. 205.
10. Mortimer, 'Diocesan Licensing and Medical Practitioners', p. 63.
11. Nancy G. Siraisi, *Medieval and Early Renaissance Medicine: An Introduction to Knowledge* (Chicago and London: University of Chicago Press, 1990), p. 19.
12. Darrel W. Amundsen, *Medicine, Society and Faith in the Ancient and Medieval Worlds* (Baltimore: Johns Hopkins University Press, 1996), p. 197.
13. Heinrich Denifle and Emile Chatelain, *Chartularium Universitatis parisiensis* (Paris: ex typis fratrum Delalain, 1889), Part I, pp. 77–8. Subsequently cited as *Chart. Univer. Paris.*
14. See Amundsen, *Medicine, Society and Faith*, particularly chapter 8, 'Medieval Canon Law on Medical and Surgical Practice by the Clergy', for a detailed study of church edicts on the prohibition of the practice of medicine by the clergy.
15. Hastings Rashdall, *The Universities of Europe in the Middle Ages: A New Edition in Three Volumes*, eds F.M. Powicke and A.B. Emden, vol. 2, *Italy–Spain–France–Germany–Scotland* (Oxford: Oxford University Press, 1967), pp. 294–5.
16. R.R. James, 'Licences to Practise Medicine and Surgery issued by the Archbishops of Canterbury, 1580–1775', *Janus*, 41 (1937): 41; John R. Guy, 'The Episcopal Licensing of Physicians, Surgeons and Midwives', *Bulletin of the History of Medicine*, 56 (1982): 529.
17. Guy, 'The Episcopal Licensing', p. 529.
18. Ibid., p. 531.
19. Mortimer, 'Diocesan Licensing and Medical Practitioners', p. 50.
20. Jessie Dobson and R. Milnes Walker, *Barbers and Barbers-Surgeons London: A History of the Barbers' and Barber-Surgeons' Companies* (London: Blackwell Scientific Publications for the Worshipful Co. of Barbers, 1979), pp. 6–7, 46–7.
21. Bullough, 'Training', p. 449.
22. Monica Green, 'Women's Medical Practice and Health Care in Medieval Europe', *Signs*, 14 (1989): 456.
23. Jean Dangler, *Mediating Fictions: Literature, Women Healers and the Go-between in Medieval and Early Modern Iberia* (Lewisburg: Bucknell University Press, 2001), p. 35.
24. Roger II cited in H.E. Sigerist, 'The History of Medical Licensure', *JAMA*, CIV (1935): 1057–60.
25. Muriel Joy Hughes, *Women Healers in Medieval Life and Literature* (Freeport, NY: Books for Libraries Press, 1968), p. 64.
26. Siraisi, *Medieval and Early Renaissance Medicine*, p. 7.
27. Ibid.
28. Thomas G. Benedek, 'The Roles of Medieval Women in the Healing Arts', in Douglas Radcliff Umstead, ed., *The Roles and Images of Women in the Middle Ages and Renaissance* (Pittsburgh: University of Pittsburgh Publications on the Middle Ages and Renaissance, 1975), III, p. 149.
29. Katharine Park, 'Medicine and Magic: The Healing Arts', in Judith C. Brown and Robert C. Davis, eds, *Gender and Society in Renaissance Italy* (London and New York: Longman, 1998), pp. 136–8.

30. These boards or tribunals were staffed by university educated physicians, such as the *Protomedicato* of the University of Bologna which was composed of the medical college's physicians. Gabriella Berti Logan, 'Women and the Practice and Teaching of Medicine in Bologna in the Eighteenth and Early Nineteenth Centuries', *Bulletin of the History of Medicine*, 77 (2003): 506–7.
31. Richard Palmer, 'Physicians and the State in Post-Medieval Italy', in Andrew W. Russell, ed., *The Town and State Physician in Europe from the Middle Ages to the Enlightenment* (Wolfenboutel: Herzog August Bibliothek, 1981), pp. 57–61.
32. David Gentilcore, '"All that pertains to Medicine": Protomedici and Protomedicati in Early Modern Italy', *Medical History*, 38 (1994): 123–4.
33. Siraisi, *Medieval and Early Renaissance Medicine*, p. 18.
34. Katharine Park, *Doctors and Medicine in Early Renaissance Florence* (Princeton, NJ: Princeton University Press, 1985), p. 47.
35. Gentilcore, '"All that pertains to Medicine"', pp. 127–30.
36. Ibid., p. 130.
37. Palmer, 'Physicians and the State', p. 58.
38. Cited in James Joseph Walsh, *Medieval Medicine* (London: A.C. Black, 1920), p. 154.
39. Ronald J. Doviak, 'The University of Naples and the Study and Practice of Medicine in the Thirteenth and Fourteenth Centuries', unpublished PhD dissertation, City University of New York, 1974, p. 44. See Chapter 1 for details about their medical practice.
40. Archivo di Stato Rome cited in Gentilcore, '"All that pertains to Medicine"', p. 131, n. 60.
41. Gentilcore, '"All that pertains to Medicine"', p. 123.
42. Gianna Pomata, *Contracting a Cure: Patients, Healers and the Law in Early Modern Bologna* (Baltimore and London: Johns Hopkins University Press), p. 80.
43. Ibid., p. 77.
44. Ibid., pp. 61–3.
45. Gentilcore, '"All that pertains to Medicine"', p. 130, n 70; p. 132.
46. Case cited in ibid., p. 130.
47. Vern L. Bullough, 'The Development of Medical Guilds at Paris', *Medievalia et Humanistica*, XII (1958): 36.
48. *Ordonnances des rois de France*, I, p. 491.
49. Dumas, 'Les Femmes et les pratiques de la santé', p. 19.
50. René de Lespinasse, *Les métiers et corporations de la ville de Paris, 14e–18e siècle* (Paris Impr. nationale 1886–97), III, p. 628.
51. *Ordonnances des rois de France*, V, p. 530.
52. Bullough, 'The Development of Medical Guilds', p. 38.
53. *Ordonnances des rois de France*, XIII, pp. 60–4.
54. Pierre Jacques Brillon, *Dictionnaire de jurisprudence et des arrêts, ou Nouvelle édition du dictionnaire de Brillon, connu sous le titre de Dictionnaire des arrêts et jurisprudence universelle des parlemens de France et autres tribunaux augmentée* (Paris: Chez, Guillaume Cavelier, Pere, Michel Brunet, Nicolas Gosselin, 1727), II, p. 173.
55. G.B. Depping, ed., *Réglemens sur les arts et métiers de Paris, rédigés au 13 siècle, et connus sous le nom du Livre des métiers d'Étienne Boileau. Publiés, pour la première fois en entier, d'après les manuscrits de la Bibliothèque du roi et des Archives du royaume, avec des notes et une introd., par G.B. Depping* (Paris: Imp. Nationale, 1837), p. 603.
56. Henri de Mondeville, *La Chirurgie de Maitre Henri de Mondeville*, ed. A. Bos (Paris: Firmin, Didot et cie, 1897), I, pp. 5–6.

57. Cited in Achille Chéreau, 'Procès intenté à Paris, en 1322, par la Faculté de Médecine, contre une femme exerçant illégalement la médicine', *L'Union Médicale* (7 août 1866): 16.
58. Guy de Chauliac, *La Grande Chirurgie*, ed. E. Niçaise (Paris, 1910), pp. 15–16.
59. Brillon, *Dictionnaire de jurisprudence et des arrêts*, II, p. 172.
60. Ibid., pp. 172–3.
61. Ibid., p. 173; Jean Verdier, *La Jurisprudence de la Médecine en France ou Traité historique et juridique* (Alençon: Malassis le jeune, 1762–63), I, pp. 624–5.
62. R.S. Roberts, 'The Personnel and Practice of Medicine in Tudor and Stuart England: Part I, The Provinces', *Medical History*, 6(4) (October; 1962): 365.
63. Guy, 'The Episcopal Licensing', p. 532.
64. Faye Marie Getz, *Medicine in the English Middle Ages* (Princeton, NJ: Princeton University Press, 1998), p. 65.
65. Getz, *Medicine in the English Middle Ages*, p. 65.
66. Dobson and Milnes Walker, *Barbers and Barbers-Surgeons*, p. 9.
67. Sidney Young, *The Annals of the Barber-Surgeons of London Compiled from their Records and other Sources* (London: Blades, East & Blades, 1890), p. 24.
68. Ibid., p. 260; Carole Rawcliffe, *Medicine and Society in Later Medieval England* (Phoenix Mill: Sutton, 1997), p. 188.
69. D'Arcy Power, 'English Medicine and Surgery in the Fourteenth Century', *Lancet*, II (1914): 176–83; Dobson and Milnes Walker, *Barbers and Barbers-Surgeons*, p. 24.
70. Dobson and Milnes Walker, *Barbers and Barbers-Surgeons*, p. 25.
71. Ibid., p. 31.
72. Ibid., p. 46.
73. Corporation House Book, Egerton MS 2572, in G.A. Auden, 'The Gild of Barber-Surgeons of the City of York', *Proceedings of the Royal Society of Medicine*, 21 (II) (May–October 1928): 1402.
74. *Calendar of State Papers: Domestic Series, Commonwealth, 1649–1660*, M.A.E. Green (London: Longman, 1875–1886), IX (1656), p. 23.
75. See Evenden, 'Gender Differences', p. 197.
76. Rawcliffe, *Medicine and Society*, p. 188, n 54. Her source is Sidney Young, *Annals*, p. 576; see also Toulin Smth, ed. with notes, *English gilds. The original ordinances of more than one hundred early English gilds: Together with the old usages of the cite of Wynchester; the Ordinances of Worcester; the Office of the mayor of Bristol; and the Costomary of the manor of Tettenhall-Regis. From original mss. of the fourteenth and fifteenth centuries.* With an introduction and glossary, &c., by his daughter, Lucy Toulmin Smith. *And a preliminary essay ... On the history and development of gilds*, by Lujo Brentano (Oxford: Early English Text Society, Oxford University Press, 1924), 27; Auden, 'The Gild of Barber Surgeons of the City of York', pp. 1400–6.
77. See Chapter 1 for details on female medieval practice. Robert S. Gottfried, *Doctors and Medicine in Medieval England 1340–1530* (Princeton, NJ: Princeton University Press, 1986), p. 87.
78. *Herbalists' Charter of Henry the VIII: Annis Tircesimo Quarto and Tricesimo Quinto. Henry VIII Regis. Cap. VIII. An Act That Persons, Being No Common Surgeons, May Administer Outward Medicines*, 1543. Posted on the internet by Ralph Fucetola, J.D., http://home.earthlink.net/~lifespirit23/herbcharter.htm.
79. George Clark, *A History of the Royal College of Physicians of London* (Oxford: Clarendon Press, 1964), I, p. 87. R.R. James, 'Licences to Practise', pp. 98–9.

80. John Tate Lanning, *The Royal Protomedicato* (Durham, NC: Duke University Press, 1985), p. 24.
81. Michael Solomon, 'Women Healers and the Power to Disease in Late Medieval Spain', in Lilian R. Furst, ed., *Women Healers and Physicians: Climbing a Long Hill*, (Lexington: University Press of Kentucky 1997), p. 79.
82. Dangler, *Mediating Fictions*, n. 73, 36.
83. Antonio Ballesteros y Beretta, *Las Cortes de 1252* (Madrid: Establecimiento Tip. de Fortanet, Impresor de la Real Academia de la Historia 1911), p. 141.
84. Luis García-Ballester, Michael R. McVaugh and Agustín Rubio-Vela, *Medical Licensing and Learning in Fourteenth Century Valencia* (Philadelphia: Transactions of the American Philosophical Society, 1989), p. 3.
85. Articles 17 and 18 cited in García-Ballester et al., *Medical Licensing*, p. 2.
86. García-Ballester et al., *Medical Licensing*, pp. 3–4.
87. Dangler, *Mediating Fictions*, p. 34.
88. Gentilcore, '"All that pertains to Medicine"', p. 125.
89. García-Ballester et al., *Medical Licensing*, p. 29.
90. Michael R. McVaugh, *Medicine before the Plague: Practitioners and their Patients in the Crown of Aragon, 1285–1345* (Cambridge: Cambridge University Press, 1993), p. 105; and García-Ballester et al., *Medical Licensing*, p. 60.
91. James M. Powell, ed., *Muslims under Latin Rule 400–1300* (Princeton, NJ: Princeton University Press, 1990), pp. 87–8.
92. Dangler, *Mediating Fictions*, p. 45; Powell, *Muslims*, p. 92.
93. See Green, 'Women's Medical Practice', pp. 446–52 and García-Ballester et al., *Medical Licensing*, pp. 30–2.
94. Dangler, *Mediating Fictions*, pp. 47–8.
95. Ibid., p. 87.
96. Aníbal Ruíz Moreno, *La Medicina en la legislación medieval española* (Buenos Aires: El Ateneo: 1946), pp. 24, 25.
97. Lanning, *The Royal Protomedicato*, pp. 15–17.
98. Ibid., p. 17.
99. List of female physicians and surgeons licensed by the Archbishop of Canterbury, 1535–1775, Archbishops' Archives (Vicar General), Lambeth Palace Library, London. This list was sent to me compliments of Jessamy Sykes, Assistant Archivist, Lambeth Palace Library.
100. Doreen A. Evenden has looked at the records left behind by these women in her article, 'Gender Differences'. Evenden's paper argues that gender played a major role in determining whether or not one was issued a medical licence and that male practitioners did not undergo the same rigorous scrutiny as females in the sense that they were not required to present testimonials of their medical expertise before the licensing board. She uses the records to prove this argument. While I do not disagree with her argument, this narrative is focused on the nature of the medical care provided by the women rather than the licensing procedures.
101. Archbishops' Archives, Moore (Elizabeth) VX 1A–10–259–3.
102. Archbishops' Archives, VX 1A-10-259-1, 28 December 1689.
103. Archbishops' Archives, VX 1A-10-259-2.
104. Ibid.
105. Ibid.
106. Archbishops' Archives, VX 1A-10-297-2.
107. Ibid.
108. Archbishops' Archives, VX 1A-10-297-6.

109. Archbishops' Archives, VX 1A-10-223-1.
110. Ibid.
111. Archbishops' Archives, VX 1A-10-223-2.
112. Archbishops' Archives, VX 1A-10-223-3.
113. Archbishops' Archives, VX 1A-10-223-4.
114. Ibid.
115. Ibid.
116. Ibid.
117. Evenden, 'Gender Differences', p. 212.
118. William Minkowski, 'Physician Motives in Banning Traditional Healers', *Women and Health*, 21(1)(1994): 86; Hughes, *Women Healers*, p. 64.
119. See Chapter 7: 'Bachelors: The Scholastic Cloister', in David F. Noble, *A World without Women: The Christian Clerical Culture of Western Science* (Oxford: Oxford University Press, 1992), for a discussion of the clerical nature of the university in northern Europe.
120. Kathleen, F. Lander, 'The Study of Anatomy by Women before the Nineteenth Century', *Proceedings of the Third International Congress of the History of Medicine* (1922), p. 126; see Nancy G. Siraisi, *Medicine and the Italian Universities, 1250–1600* (Leiden, Boston and Köln: Brill 2001).
121. As Lanning claims, 'In no nation of Europe was the requirement of a university degree more persistent than in Spain' (*Royal Protomedicato*, p. 18).
122. Pearl Kilbre and Nancy G. Siraisi, 'The Institutional Setting: The Universities', in David C. Lindberg, ed., *Science in the Middle Ages* (Chicago: University of Chicago Press, 1998), p. 120.
123. See Kilbre and Siraisi, 'Institutional Setting', p. 120.
124. Christine de Pizan recounted this story in her *City of the Ladies*, Book 2, Chapter 36.
125. See Paul Oskar Kristeller, 'Learned Women of Early Modern Italy: Humanists and University Scholars', in Patricia H. Lablame, ed., *Beyond their Sex: Learned Women of the European Past* (New York and London: New York University Press, 1980), p. 114, n. 49.
126. Noble, *A World without Women*, p. 167.
127. There is a copy of the document in the Archivio Antico dell'Università di Padova, MS 365, fols. 24v–26v; Lablame, *Beyond their Sex*, p. 115, n. 53.
128. Alan B. Cobban, *English University Life in the Middle Ages* (London: University College London Press, 1999), pp. 1–3.
129. Getz, *Medicine in the English Middle Ages*, pp. 169, 171.
130. Marilyn French, *Beyond Power: On Women, Men and Morals* (New York: Summit Books, 1985), p. 160.
131. Achille Luchaire, *Social France at the Time of Philip Augustus*, intro. John W. Baldwin, authorized translation from the 2nd edn of the French by Edward Benjamin Krehbiel (New York: Harper & Row, 1967), pp. 72–3.
132. Minkowski, 'Physician Motives', pp. 83, 96.
133. *Chart. Univer. Paris*, I, p. 517.
134. *Chart. Univer. Paris*, I, pp. 488–90. The English translation is found in Lynn Thorndike, *University Records and Life in the Middle Ages* (New York: Octagon Books, 1971), pp. 83–5.
135. *Chart. Univer. Paris*, I, pp. 488–90; Thorndike, *University Records*, p. 84.
136. Benedeck, 'The Roles of Medieval Women', p. 150.
137. *Chart. Univer. Paris*, III, pp. 16–17; Thorndike, *University Records*, pp. 235–6.
138. Archival Records: Archives Nationales: M 70, no. 11 bis, Histoire de la faculté de Médecine, 1395–1434, no 12, Chirurgiens, fols 1r–3r, copied in 17th century;

AN MM 266, 17th Century pp. 3–13. *Chart. Univer. Paris* II, pp. 149–53, nos. 693–693a–c. See Pearl Kilbre, 'The Faculty of Medicine at Paris: Charlatanism and Unlicensed Medical Practices in the Later Middle Ages', *Bulletin of the History of Medicine*, 27 (1953): 1–20.

139. Kilbre, 'The Faculty of Medicine', pp. 7–8.
140. Her story has been told by historians for we have the actual trial records. See Kilbre as cited above and more recently, Montserrat Cabré I. Pairet and Fernando Salmón Muñiz, 'Poder académico *versus* autoridad femenina: la Facultad de Medicina de París contra Jacoba Félicié (1322)', *Dynamis*, 19 (1999): 55–78; Adrian Gamelin, 'Jacoba Félicié: Power and Privilege in Fourteenth Century Medicine', in Peter Cruse, ed., *The Proceedings of the 7th Annual History of Medicine Days* (Calgary: University of Calgary Press, 1998), pp. 69–73. There is an English excerpt from the trial in Lisa DiCaprio and Merry E. Wiesner, eds, *Lives and Voices, Sources in European History* (Boston: Houghton Mifflin, 2001), pp. 129–31 The trial records are in the National Archives of France and were reproduced by Denifle and Chatelain in the *Chartularium Universitatis parisiensis*, 4 vols (Paris: 1889–97).
141. *Chart. Univer. Paris*, II, p. 263, n. 1; p. 255, n. 1.
142. Ibid., p. 257.
143. Ibid., p. 266.
144. Ibid., pp. 255–66.
145. Ibid., pp. 258–9.
146. Ibid., pp. 263–5.
147. Ibid., pp. 257–8.
148. Ibid., p. 260.
149. Ibid., p. 267.
150. Ibid.
151. Brillon, *Dictionnaire de jurisprudence*, IV, p. 337.
152. *Chart. Univers. Paris*, II, pp. 336–7, n. 900.
153. Ibid., pp. 336–7.
154. Brillon, *Dictionnaire de jurisprudence*, II, p. 337.
155. *Chart. Univ. Paris*, I, pp. 489–90; Thorndike, *University Records*, pp. 84–5.
156. *Chart. Univ. Paris*, II, p. 462; Thorndike, *University Records*, pp. 235–6.
157. *Chart. Univ. Paris*, III, pp. 534–5.
158. Benedek, 'The Roles of Medieval Women', p. 152.
159. Ernest Wickersheimer, *Commentaires de la Faculté de médecine de l'Université de Paris (1395–1516)*, collection de documents inédits sur l'historie de France (Paris: Imprimerie nationale, 1915), lxxxvi, p. 60; *Chart. Univ. Paris*, IV, pp. 198–9.
160. Hughes, *Women Healers*, pp. 110, 146; Brillon, *Dictionnaire de jurisprudence*, III, p. 222.
161. Wickersheimer, *Commentaires*, pp. 331–2, 353.
162. See Pedro Lopez Elum and Mateu Rodrigo Lizondo, 'Las mujeres medievales y su ámbito jurídico', in *Actas de las II Jornadas de Investigacion Interdisciplinaria*, Cristina Segura Graiño, introd. (Madrid: Universidad Autónoma de Madrid, 1983), p. 128.

3. Early Modern Notions of Women: Contradictory Views on Women as Healers

1. Space does not permit a detailed analysis of the debate about women which took place in western civilization from Classical times. For an in-depth treatment of

this debate, see Leigh Whaley, *Women's History as Scientists: A Guide to the Debates* (Santa Barbara: ABC-CLIO, 2003).
2. Ian Maclean, 'The Notion of Woman in Medicine, Anatomy, and Physiology', in Lorna Hutson, ed., *Feminism and Renaissance Studies* (Oxford: Oxford University Press, 1999), p. 130.
3. The major Hippocratic writings concerning women were *On Generation, The Nature of the Child* and *The Diseases of Women.*
4. Cited in Bonnie S. Anderson and Judith P. Zinsser, eds, *A History of their Own: Women in Europe from Prehistory to the Present,* 2 vols (New York and Oxford: Oxford University Press, 2000), I, p. 28.
5. Hippocrates and many other medical thinkers, including Galen, held that the womb required to be nourished through regular sexual activity. If the womb did not receive this nourishment, then it would wander throughout the body. If the wandering womb reached the brain, hysteria would result. Kate Phillips, 'Capturing the Wandering Womb', *Haverford Journal,* 3(1) (April 2007): 41.
6. Anderson and Zinsser, *A History of their Own,* I, p. 29; Helen King, *Hippocrates' Women: Reading the Female Body in Ancient Greece* (London and New York: Routledge, 1998), p. 7.
7. Joseph Needham, *A History of Embryology,* 2nd edn (New York: Abelard-Schuman, 1959), pp. 69–74.
8. Joan Cadden, *Meanings of Sex Differences in the Middle Ages* (Cambridge: Cambridge University Press, 1992), p. 11.
9. P. Manuli cited in Helen King, 'Self-help, Self-knowledge: In Search of the Patient in Hippocratic Gynecology', in Richard Hawley and Barbara Levick, eds, *Women in Antiquity: New Assessments* (London and New York: Routledge, 1995), p. 136.
10. Sister Prudence Allen, *The Concept of Woman* (Montreal: Eden Press, 1985), p. 1.
11. Aristotle, *Generation of Animals* 767b 7–9 in *The Complete Works of Aristotle,* ed. Jonathan Barnes (Princeton, NJ: Princeton University Press, 1984), I, p. 1187. Henceforth cited as *GA.*
12. *GA,* 737a 26–31, p. 1144.
13. *GA,* 775a 14–20, p. 1199; 765b 15–20, pp. 1184–5.
14. Maryanne Cline Horowitz, 'Aristotle and Woman', *Journal of the History of Biology,* 9(2) (Fall 1976): 205.
15. *GA,* 716a 5–23, pp. 1112–13.
16. *GA,* 727b 31–33, p. 1130.
17. *GA,* 729a 25–34, p. 1133.
18. Aristotle, *Politics,* 1260a 14, in *The Complete Works,* II, p. 1999. Hereafter cited as *Pol.*
19. *Pol.,* 1260a 20–24, p. 1999.
20. *Pol.,* 1335b 17–19, p. 2119.
21. *Pol.,* 1259b 33, p. 1999; 1252a 15, p. 1987.
22. *Pol.,* 1259b 33, p. 1999; 1252a 15, p. 1987; Aristotle, *Nicomachean Ethics,* 1162a, in *The Complete* Works, II, p. 1836.
23. Aristotle, *Economics,* 1343b30–1344a8, in *The Complete Works,* II, p. 2131.
24. *Pol.,* 1259b 32, 1260a 10, p. 1999.
25. Galen argued that disease resulted from an imbalance in the four humours (blood, phlegm, yellow and black bile) which were associated with the elements. Andrew Wear, *Knowledge and Practice in English Medicine, 1550–1680* (Cambridge: Cambrindge University Press, 2000), p. 87.

26. Michael T. Walton, Robert M. Fineman and Phyllis J. Walton, 'Why Can't a Woman Be More Like a Man? A Renaissance Perspective on the Biological Basis for Female Inferiority', *Women and Health*, 24(4) (1996): 89.
27. Maclean, 'The Notion of Woman in Medicine', p. 132.
28. Avicenna, *A treatise on the Canon of medicine of Avicenna, incorporating a translation of the first book*, trans. O'Cameron Gruner (London: Luzca, 1930), I, pp. 96, 230.
29. Averroes, *Commentary on Plato's Republic*, trans. E.I.J. Rosenthal (Cambridge: Cambridge University Press, 1956), pp. 164–5.
30. Helen Rodnite Lemay, 'Anthonius Guainerius and Medieval Gynecology', in *Women of the Medieval World: Essays in Honour of John H. Mundy* (Oxford: Blackwell, 1985), pp. 320, 333.
31. Ian Maclean, *The Renaissance Notion of Woman* (Cambridge: Cambridge University Press, 1990), p. 30.
32. Maclean, 'The Notion of Woman in Medicine', p. 145. Merry E. Wiesner, *Women and Gender in Early Modern Europe* (Cambridge: Cambridge University Press, 1993), pp. 25–9.
33. Londa Schiebinger argues that even the female skeleton was held to be inferior to that of the male. Schiebinger, 'Skeletons in the Closet: The First Illustrations of the Female Skeleton in Eighteenth Century Anatomy', *Representations*, 14 (Spring 1986): 43.
34. This section will provide a brief summary of the views put forth by the major Christian thinkers For a full discussion of the nature and role of women in Christian thought, see Leigh Whaley, 'The Medieval Woman in Science: Contradictions within the Church', *Women's History as Scientists*, ch. 2.
35. Eugène Portalié, 'Saint Augustine', *New Advent Catholic Encyclopedia on-line*, vol. ii, (New York, Robert Appleton Company, 1907, 1999), http://www.newadvent.org/cathen/02089a.htm.
36. Augustine, *City of God*, Book XIV, 24.1, cited in Kari Elisabeth Borresen, *Subordination and Equivalence* (Washington: University Press of America, 1981), p. 42.
37. Augustine, *City of God*, ed. David Knowles (Harmondsworth: Penguin, 1972), Book IX, pp. 14, 22.
38. Translated as *The Literal Meaning of Genesis* and *Genesis against the Manichees*.
39. Augustine, *City of God*, Book XXII, Chapter 17, p. 1057.
40. Saint Augustine, *The Literal Meaning of Genesis*, trans. John Hammond Taylor SJ (New York: Newman Press, 1982), Vol. II, Book 2, Chapter 34:45, p. 167.
41. Kim Power, *Veiled Desire: Augustine's Writing on Women* (New York: Continuum, 1996), p. 131.
42. Augustine, *Literal Meaning*, Book 11, Chapter 37, p. 171.
43. Ibid., p. 99.
44. Esther Cohen, *The Crossroads of Justice: Law and Culture in Late Medieval France* (Leiden: E.J. Brill, 1993), p. 85.
45. Summarized from ibid., pp. 86–7.
46. Vern L. Bullough, 'Medieval Medical and Scientific Views of Women', *Viator*, 4 (1973): 485–501.
47. Roland Antonioli, *Rabelais et la Médecine*, Etudes Rabelaisiennes, Vol. 12 (Geneva: Droz 1976), p. 121.
48. Antonioli, *Rabelais et la Médecine*, p. 19.
49. François Rabelais, *Gargantua and Pantagruel*, ed. Donald Douglas (New York: The Modern Library, 1928), in 'Women in World History, Primary Sources, Europe', George Mason University, http://chnm.gmu.edu/wwh/p/83.html.

50. Alison Klairmont-Lingo argues that du Breil and du Courval were the only French doctors to write treatises against 'illicit healers in the late sixteenth and early seventeenth centuries'. See her article, 'Empirics and Charlatans in Early Modern France: The Genesis of the Classification of the "Other" in Medical Practice', *Journal of Social History*, 19(4) (Summer 1986): 583.
51. André du Breil, *La police de l'art et science de medecine, contenant la refutation des erreurs, & insignes abus, qui s'y commettent pour le jourdhuy ... Où sont vivement confutez tous sectaires, sorciers, enchanteurs, magiciens* (Paris: Leon Cavellat. 1580), cited in Alison Klairmont-Lingo, 'The Rise of Medical Practitioners in Sixteenth Century France: The Case of Lyon and Montpellier', unpublished PhD dissertation, University of California at Berkeley (1980), pp. 205, 210–11.
52. Thomas Sonnet de Courval, *Satyre contre les charlatans et les pseudo médecins empyriques* (Paris: Jean Milot, 1610), Preface, and pp. 119–20.
53. De Courval, *Satrye contre les charlatans*, p. 120.
54. Ibid., pp. 123–4.
55. Letter to André Falconet, 3 June 1661, in *Lettres de Gui Patin*, ed. J.H. Reveillé-Parise (Paris: J.B. Baillière, 1846), III, p. 372.
56. Letter to Belin, 18 January 1633, cited in Francis R. Packard, *Guy Patin and the Medical Profession in Paris in the XVIth century* (New York: Paul B. Hoeber, 1925), p. 249.
57. Juan Huarte, *Examen de Ingenios or the Trial of the Wits*, trans. Mr Edward Bellamy (London: Richard Sare, 1698), pp. 408–10.
58. Cited in Michael Solomon, *The Literature of Misogyny in Medieval Spain: The Arcipreste de Talavera and the Spill* (Cambridge: Cambridge University Press, 1997), p. 155.
59. Roig, *Spill*, 4614-44, cited in Solomon, *The Literature of Misogyny*, p. 156.
60. Solomon, *The Literature of Misogyny*, pp. 160–1.
61. Ibid., pp. 3–7.
62. James Hart, *[Klinike], or the diet of the diseased* (London: J. Beale for R. Allot, 1633), p. 2.
63. Ibid., p. 2.
64. Ibid., p. 8.
65. James Primrose, *Popular Errours or the People in matter of Physick First written in Lataine by the Learned Physician James Primrose, Doctor of Physick* (London: Printed by W. Willson for Nicholas Bourne, 1651), p. 19.
66. Ibid.
67. John Cotta, *A Short Discoverie of the Unobserved Dangers of several sorts of ignorant and unconsiderate Practitioners of Physicke in England* (London: William Jones and Richard Boyle 1612), p. 1.
68. Ibid., p. 8.
69. Ibid., pp. 24, 28.
70. Richard Whitlock, *Zwotomia, Or Observations on the Present Manners of the English* (London, 1654).
71. Richard Whitlock, *Observations on the Present Manners of the English Briefly Anatomizing the Living by the Dead. With an Usefull Detection of the Mountebanks of Both Sexes* (London, Thomas Roycroft, 1654), p. 56.
72. Whitlock, *Zwotomia*, p. 50.
73. Ibid., pp. 57–9.
74. Cited in Hughes, *Women Healers in Medieval Life and Literature* (Freeport, NY: Books for Libraries, 1968), p. 85.

75. Burton, the pioneering author of *The Anatomy of Melancholy* (1621), is arguably the first major writer in the history of western cognitive science, see http://www.rc.umd.edu/cstahmer/cogsci/burton.html.
76. Jean Verdier, *La Jurisprudence de la Médecine en France ou Traite historique et juridique* (Alençon: Malassis le jeune, 1762–63), I, p. 615.
77. Ibid., p. 618.
78. Ibid., pp. 623–4.
79. See Chapter 5 below for a discussion of Hecquet's views on midwifery and the attempts of male surgeons to replace female midwives.
80. Cited in Lemay, 'Medieval Gynecology', pp. 323, 327.
81. Phillipus Aureolus Theophrastus Bombastus von Hohenheim, known as Paracelsus, was born in Zurich in 1493.
82. Cited in Marie-Christine Pouchelle, *The Body and Surgery in the Middle Ages* (New Brunswick, NJ: Rugters University Press, 1990), p. 64, n. 16, and Allen G. Debus, *The Chemical Philosophy: Paracelsian Science and Medicine in the Sixteenth and Seventeenth Centuries* (New York: New York Science History Publications, 1977), I, p. 54. See Andrew Wear, *Knowledge and Practice*, p. 87, for details on the differences between Galenists and the Paracelsians.
83. Ambroise Paré, *Collected Works Translated out of the Latin by Thomas Johnson from the first English edition, 1634* (New York: Milford House, 1968), p. 27.
84. Paré, *Collected Works*, p. 902.
85. Paré, *The Apologie and Treatise of Ambroise Paré: Containing the voyages made into divers places, with many of his writings upon surgery*, ed. and intro. Geoffrey Keynes (London: Falcon Educational Books, 1951), p. 140.
86. Thomas Sydenham, *Observationes medicae* (London, 1676). Some experts consider that this statement may have been made by John Locke, friend and colleague of Sydenham. See Robert L. Martensen, 'Habit of Reason: Anatomy of Anglicanism in Restoration England', *Bulletin of the History of Medicine*, 66 (1992): 533, n. 99.
87. Jean Liébault, *L'Agriculture, et maison rustique de M.M. Charles Estienne, & Jean Liébault, docteurs en médecine* (1564), cited in Susan Broomhall, *Women's Medical Work in Early Modern France* (Manchester and New York: Manchester University Press, 2004), p. 145.
88. Liébault, cited in Broomhall, *Women's Medical Work*, pp. 145–6.
89. Olivier de Serres, *Le théâtre d'agriculture*, f. 885V-887R in Alison Klairmont-Lingo, 'Empirics and Charlatans in Early Modern France: The Genesis of the Classification of the "Other" in Medical Practice', *Journal of Social History*, 19 (4) (1986): 593.
90. Lula McDowell Richardson, *The Forerunners of Feminism in French Literature of the Renaissance from Christine of Pisa to Marie de Gournay* (Baltimore: Johns Hopkins University Press, 1929), p. 91.
91. 'Catalog of the Scientific Community', Agrippa, Heinrich Cornelius [Agrippa von Nettesheim], in *The Scientific Revolution, Westfall Catalogue*, Robert A. Hatch, University of Florida, 1998, http://web.clas.ufl.edu/users/rhatch/pages/03-Sci-Rev/SCI-REV-Home/resource-ref-read/major-minor-ind/westfall-dsb/SAM-A.htm.
92. M. Aug. Prost, *Corneille Agrippa sa vie et ses oeuvres* (Paris: Champion, 1881), I, p. 166.
93. Cornelius Agrippa, *Sur la noblesse* (Leiden: T. Haak, 1726), pp. 37, 75, 118.
94. Maité Albistur and Daniel Armogathe, *Histoire du féminisme français* (Paris: Des Femmes, 1977), p. 53.
95. Enid McLeod *The Order of the Rose: The Life and Ideas of Christine de Pizan* (Totowa, NJ: Rowman and Littlefield, 1976), pp. xvii–xxv; Antoine Campaux, *La Question des Femmes au Quinzième Siècle* (Paris: Berger-Levrault, 1865), pp. 8–9.

96. Arthur Piaget, *Martin Le Franc. Prévôt de Lausanne* (Lausanne: Payot, 1858), p. 73.
97. McLeod, *Order of the Rose,* p. 68.
98. Rose Rigaud, *Les Idées Féministes de Christine de Pisan* (Geneva: Slatine Reprints, 1973), p. 64.
99. Ernest Langlois, 'Le traité de Gerson contre le *Roman de la Rose*', *Romania* (1919): 29–48.
100. Christine de Pizan, *The Book of the City of the Ladies*, trans. Earl Jeffrey Richard, Foreword Marina Warner (New York : Persea Books, 1972), pp. 62–3.
101. Ibid., p. 64.
102. Pierre Dubois, *De Recuperatione Terre Sancte: traité de politique générale* (Paris: A. Picard, 1891), p. 118.
103. François Poulain de la Barre, *De L'Education des Dames pour la conduite de l'esprit dans les sciences et dans les mœurs. Entretiens* (Paris: Jean du Puis, 1674), p. 120.
104. François Poulain de la Barre, *De L'Egalité des deux sexes* (Paris: Jean du Puis 1673), pp. 4–5.
105. Ibid., p. 1.
106. Ibid.
107. Ibid., pp. 6–7.
108. Michael A. Seidel, 'Poulain de la Barre's The Woman as Good as the Man', *Journal of the History of Ideas*, 35 (1974): 499–508; Poulain de la Barre, *De L'Egalité*, pp. 6–8.
109. Poulain de la Barre, *De L'Egalité*, 117.
110. Ibid., p. 109.
111. Ibid., p. 194.
112. Ibid., p. 162.
113. Sally-Ann Kitts, *The Debate on the Nature, Role and Influence of Woman in Eighteenth-Century Spain* (Lewiston: Edwin Mellen Press, 1995), p. 249, n. 1. For a more recent summary of the Early Modern debate about women which raged in Spain, see Theresa Ann Smith, *The Emerging Female Citizen, Gender and Enlightenment in Spain* (Berkeley: University of California Press, 2006), pp. 18–28.
114. Kitts, *Debate on the Nature*, p. 1.
115. Milagros Ortega Costa, 'Spanish Women in the Reformation', in Sherrin Marshall, ed., *Women in Reformation and Counter Reformation Europe: Private and Public Worlds* (Bloomington and Indianapolis: Indiana University Press, 1989), pp. 88, n. 3, 110. The *Liber Judicoram* (Book of Judges) was a Visigoth law code, promulgated in 694, consisting of a common law. It was incorporated into the Fuero Juzgo of Ferdinand III in the thirteenth century. Linda Lewin, *Surprise Heirs*, Vol. 1, *Illegitimacy, Patrimonial Rights and Legal Nationalism in Luso-Brazilian Inheritance 1750–1821* (Stanford: Stanford University Press, 2003), p. 4.
116. Malcolm R. Read, *Juan Huarte de San Juan* (Boston: Twayne, 1981), pp. 18–19.
117. Cited in Mary E. Giles, ed., *Women in the Inquisition: Spain and the New World*, (Baltimore and London: Johns Hopkins University Press, 1999), p. 10.
118. Vives, cited in Ortega Costa, 'Spanish Women in the Reformation', p. 90.
119. Virginia Walcott Beauchamp, Elizabeth H. Hageman and Margaret Mikesell; contributing editors, Sheila ffolliott and Betty S. Travitsky; other contributors, Denise Albanese, Introduction to Juan Luis Vives, *The Instruction of a Christen Woman* (Urbana: University of Illinois Press, 2002), p. xvi.
120. Ibid.

121. Emilie Bergmann, 'The Exclusion of the Feminine in the Cultural Discourse of the Golden Ages: Juan Luis Vives and Luis de Léon', in Alain Saint-Saëns, ed., *Religion, Body and Gender in Early Modern Spain* (San Francisco: Mellen Research University Press, 1991), p. 127.
122. Vives, *Instruction*, p. xlviii.
123. Cited in Kitts, *Debate on the Nature*, p. 249, n. 6.
124. Ibid., p. 1.
125. Juan Luis Vives, *Education*, cited in Paul Rousselot, *La Pédagogie Féminine* (Paris, Delgrave, 1881), p. 37; Catherine R. Eskin, 'The Rei(g)ning of Tongues in English Books of Instruction and Rhetorics', in Barbara J. Whitehead, ed., *Women's Education in Early Modern Europe: A History, 1500–1800* (New York: Garland, 1999), p. 116. See also Margaret L. King, *Women of the Renaissance* (Chicago: University of Chicago Press, 1991), p. 165.
126. Vives, *Instruction*, p. 23.
127. Ibid., p. 24.
128. Bergmann, 'The Exclusion of the Feminine', p. 133.
129. John A. Jones and Javier San José Lera, eds, *A Bilingual Edition of Fray Luis de Léon's La Perfecta Casada The Role of Married Women in Sixteenth-Century Spain*, trans. and intro. Jones and San José Lera, Spanish Studies, Vol. 2 (Lewiston: Edwin Mellen, 1999), p. xxv.
130. Jones and Lera, *La Perfecta Casada*, p. 81; Kitts, *Debate on the Nature*, p. 21.
131. Cited in Kitts, *Debate on the Nature*, pp. 2, 104.
132. Bergmann, 'The Exclusion of the Feminine', p. 135.
133. Julian Weiss, 'Qué demandos de los mugeres? Forming the Debate about Women in Late Medieval Spain with a Baroque Response', in Thelma S. Fenster and Claire A. Lees, eds, *Gender and Debate from the Early Middle Ages to the Renaissance* (New York: Palgrave, 2002), pp. 243–4.
134. Ibid., pp. 243–5.
135. Ibid., p. 249, n. 35.
136. Ibid., pp. 249–50.
137. Ibid., 250–2.
138. Smith, *The Emerging Female Citizen*, p. 19.
139. Smith, *The Emerging Female Citizen*, p. 17.
140. Benito Jerónimo Feijoo, *Defensa de la Mujer*, ed. Victoria Sau (Barcelona: Icaria, 1997), p. 15.
141. Ibid., pp. 18–19.
142. Cited in Ivy Lilian McClelland, *Benito Jerónimo Feijóo* (New York: Twayne, 1969), p. 6.
143. Feijoo, *Defensa*, p. 24.
144. Ibid., p. 25.
145. Ibid., p. 30.

4. Medical Treatises and Texts Written by Women and for Women

1. Chapter 8 will consider unpublished medical receipts and remedies produced by women who, although not formally trained as medical practitioners, provided medical services to their communities.
2. Elaine Hobby, *Virtue of Necessity: English Women's Writing: 1649–88* (Ann Arbor: University of Michigan Press, 1989), p. 175.

3. Hannah Woolley, *The Gentlewoman's Companion, or, a Guide to the Female Sex* (London: A. Maxwell, 1673), p. 10.
4. Eva Martin Sartori, ed., *The Feminist Encyclopedia of French Literature* (Westport, CT: Greenwood Press, 1999), p. 529.
5. Mélina Lipinksa, *Les Femmes et le progrès des sciences médicales* (Paris: Masson et Cie, 1930), p. 49.
6. Given that in his will her father claimed to be the true author, there has been some doubt as to Sabuco de Nantes's authorship of the *Nueva Filosofia*. However, in the only English version of the text, it is convincingly argued by the editors that it was indeed the daughter, rather than the father, who was the author. This information was drawn from a site publishing information by the authors/translators of the new edition that is no longer available. For information about the text, see Women-philosophers.com by Kate Lindemann, http://www.women-philosophers.com/Oliva-Sabuco.html.
7. Mary Ellen Waithe, 'Oliva Sabuco de Nantes Barrera', in Mary Ellen Waithe, ed., *A History of Women Philosophers*, Vol. 2, *Medieval, Renaissance and Enlightenment Women Philosophers A.D. 500–1600* (Dordrecht: Kluwer Academic, 1989), p. 265.
8. Mary Ellen Waithe, Maria Colomer Vintro and C. Angel Zorita have translated and edited the first English edition of the *Nueva Filosofía* (Chicago and London: University of Illinois Press, 2007). They base their translation upon two copies: the first edition of the text found at the Biblioteca de la Universitat de Barcelona and the version held at the Universitat de Valencia Facultad de Medicina. See their 'Introduction' (p. 14) for details.
9. Ernesto Beya Alonso, 'Una precursora farmacéutica del Renacimiento', *Boletin de la Sociedad Espanola de Historia de la Farmacía* (December 1984): 246.
10. Waithe et al., 'Introduction', *New Philosophy*, pp. 14, 30, 32–3.
11. 'Oliva Sabuco de Nantes y Barrera and Octavio Cuartero Cifuentes', *Obras de Dona Oliva Sabuco de Nantes, escritora del siglo XVI* (Madrid: Establecimento Tipográfico de Ricardo Fé, 1888), pp. xxiii–xxiv.
12. Waithe, 'Oliva Sabuco de Nantes Barrera', p. 263.
13. See Waithe et al., 'Introduction'.
14. Waithe, 'Oliva Sabuco de Nantes Barrera', p. 278.
15. See section on d'Arconville below.
16. Waithe et al., 'Introduction', pp. 13–14.
17. Sabuco de Nantes, 'Colloquy of the Knowledge of Thyself', in *Nueva Filosofía de la naturaleza del hombre* (Madrid: Editora Nacional, 1981), p. 9.
18. Sabuco de Nantes, cited in Waithe et al., *New Philosophy*, p. 112.
19. Ibid., pp. 31, 71.
20. Ibid., pp. 51, 83–4, 119–20.
21. Ibid., 70, 74–6, 84–5.
22. Waithe et al., *New Philosophy*, p. 35, n. 5.
23. Ibid.
24. Cited in Waithe et al., 'Introduction', pp. 2–3.
25. Miguel Marcelino Boix y Moliner, *Hippocrates aclarado* (Madrid: En la Imprenta de Blàs de Villabueva, 1716), p. 71.
26. Waithe, 'Oliva Sabuco de Nantes Barrera', p. 265.
27. A. Martin-Araguz, C. Bustamante-Martinez and V. Fernandez-Armayor, 'Sabuco's Suco Nerveo and the Origins of Neurochemistry in the Spanish Renaissance', *Revista de Neurologia*, 36 (12) (2003): 1190–8.
28. Mary Ellen Waithe, 'Oliva Sabuco de Nantes Barrera', p. 264.

29. Rudolph M. Bell, *How To Do It: Guides to Good Living for Renaissance Italians* (Chicago: University of Chicago Press, 1999), pp. 8–9.
30. William Eamon, 'From the Secrets of Nature to Public Knowledge: The Origins of the Concept of Openness in Science', *Minerva*, 23(3) (September 1985): 329.
31. Men who wrote 'Books of Secrets' were often physicians, such as Gabriele Fallopio, but often they were not university educated. See William Eamon, 'Science and Popular Culture in Sixteenth Century Italy: The "Professors of Secrets" and their Books', *Sixteenth Century Journal*, 16(4) (Winter 1985): 472–5.
32. Bruce T. Morin, *Distilling Knowledge: Alchemy, Chemistry, and the Scientific Revolution* (Cambridge, MA: Harvard University Press, 2005), p. 61.
33. Cortese to Mario Chaboga, no date, in *I Secreti*, pp. 19–21, cited in William Eamon, *Science and the Secrets of Nature: Books of Secrets in Medieval and Early Modern Culture* (Princeton, NJ: Princeton University Press, 1994), p. 164.
34. Isabella Cortese, *I Secreti* (Venice: Giacomo Fornett, 1584), Book I, pp. 15–19.
35. Cited in Bell, *How To Do It*, p. 44.
36. Cortese, *I Secreti*, Book I, pp. 30–1.
37. The War of the Fronde was composed of a group of uprisings between 1648 and 1653. See John Lough, *An Introduction to Seventeenth Century France* (London: Longmans, Green & Co., 1995), pp. 20, 127–32; Colin Jones, 'Perspectives on Poor Relief, Healthcare and the Counter-Reformation in France', in Ole Peter Grell, Andrew Cunningham and Jon Arrizabalga, eds, *Health Care and Poor Relief in Counter-Reformation Europe* (New York: Routledge, 1999), pp. 227–8.
38. Louis de Rouvroy, Duc de Saint-Simon, *Mémoires de Saint-Simon* (Paris: Gallimard, 1958), V, p. 265.
39. Jacques de Maupeou, 'La mere de Foucquet', *Hommes et mondes: revue mensuelle* (May 1949): 75; A. Chéruel, *Mémoires sur la vie publique et privée de Fouquet surintendant des finances* (Paris: Charpentier, 1862), I, p. 3.
40. The manuscript copy of the original rule is conserved at the Arsenal Library, MS. 2565. Its title is 'Mémoire de ce qui est observé par la Compagnie de dames de la charité de l'Hôtel-Dieu de Paris pour en former d'autres semblables ès autres villes du royame'.
41. Vincent de Paul to Coudray, 25 July 1634, in *Correspondance, entretiens et documents de Saint Vincent de Paul*, ed. Pierre Coste (Paris: Librairie Lecoffre J. Gabalda, 1920–24), I, no. 177.
42. Xavier Azema, *Un Prelat Janseniste: Louis Fouquet: Evêque et Comte d'Agde (1656–1702)*, (Paris: J. Vrin, 1963), p. 7; Susan Dinan, *Women and Poor Relief in Seventeenth-Century France: The Early History of the Daughters of Charity* (Aldershot, Hampshire and Burlington VT: Ashgate, 2006), p. 68. Dinan's book is the most recent study of the Daughters of Charity.
43. De Paul, *Correspondance, entretiens*, XIV, no. 126.
44. Pierre Coste, *Le Grand Saint du Grand Siècle: Monsieur Vincent* (Paris: Desclée de Brouwer et Cie, 1931), p. 325; English translation, Pierre Coste, *The Life and Works of Saint Vincent de Paul*, trans. Joseph Leonard (Westminster, MD: The Newman Press, 1952), I, pp. 238–41.
45. Marie de Maupeou Fouquet, 'Preface', *Recueil de remedes faciles et domestiques, choisis, experimentez, & trés-aprouvez pour toutes sortes de maladies internes, & externes, & difficiles à guerir* (Dijon: Jean Ressayre, 1701).
46. Laurence Brockliss and Colin Jones, *The Medical World of Early Modern France* (Oxford: Clarendon Press, 1987), p. 271.

47. Madame de Fouquet, *Le medecin desinteressé. Ou, l'on trouvera l'élite de plusieurs, remedes infaillibles trés-expérimentés, & à peu de frais. Le tout recueilli par les soins d'un docteur en médecine* (Limoges: Chez J. Farne, 1695)
48. Matthew Ramsey, 'The Popularization of Medicine in France 1650–1900', in Roy Porter, ed., *The Popularization of Medicine, 1650–1850* (London and New York: Routledge, 1992), p. 103.
49. Brockliss and Jones, *The Medical World*, pp. 268, 271.
50. Ramsey, 'The Popularization of Medicine', p. 103.
51. Ibid.
52. Ibid.
53. Dr Delescure, 'Preface', in Marie de Maupeou Fouquet, *Recueil de receptes, où est expliquée la manière de guerir à peu de frais toute sorte de maux tant internes, qu'externes inveterez, & qui ont passé jusqu'à present pour incurables* (Lyon: Certe, 1676), p. 6.
54. The recipes are arranged alphabetically according to the name of the ailment, beginning with abscess. Ailments mentioned here are from Marie de Maupeou Fouquet, *Les remedes charitable de Madame Fouquet, pour guerir a peu de frais toute sorte de maux externs, invéterez, & qui ont passé jusques à present pour incurables* (Lyon: Jean Certe, 1696). See pp. 28, 72–3, 86–93 for the various balms.
55. Stomach cures are listed from pp. 44–6 and 53.
56. Fouquet, 'Dedicatory Epistle', in *Recueil* (1676).
57. Fouquet, 'Dedicatory Epistle' (1675, 1696 editions).
58. Ibid.
59. Ibid.
60. The note in the margin indicates Grégoire 13 – presumably this is Gregory XIII (1502–1585), pope from 1572–85.
61. Préface, *Recueil de Remèdes*, 1701 edition.
62. Jean-Christian Petitfils, *Fouquet* (Paris: Perrin, 1998) p. 171.
63. Pierre Huard and Marie-José Imbault-Huart, 'Jean Pecquet', in Charles Coulston Gillispie, ed., *Dictionary of Scientific Biography* (New York: Scribner, 1970–80), X, 476–7.
64. Letters from Madame de Sévigné to Madame Pomponne, 20 and 24 November 1604, in *Madame de Sévigné, Selected Letters*, ed. Leonard Tancock (Harmondsworth: Penguin, 1982), pp. 13–14, 16.
65. Marie-Laure Girou-Swiderski, 'Vivre la Révolution, L'incidence de la Révolution sur la carrière et la vie de trios femmes de lettres', in Marie-France Brive, ed., *Les Femmes de la Révolution Française 2* (Toulouse-le-Mirail: Presses Universitaires du Mirail, 1990), pp. 239–40.
66. The Jardin du Roi, founded in 1635, later called the Jardin des Plantes, was a centre of scientific teaching, particularly in medicine and pharmacy. At the Jardin, the king's physicians taught courses to future doctors and apothecaries.
67. Yves Laissus and Jean Torlais, *Le Jardin du Roi et le Collège royal dans l'enseignement des sciences au XVIIIe siècle* (Paris: Hermann, 1986), pp. 288, 299.
68. 'Arconville, Geneviève Charlotte d' (1720–1805)' in Marilyn Bailey Ogilvie and Joy Harvey, eds, *Biographical Dictionary of Women in Science: Pioneering Lives from Ancient Times to the Mid-20th Century* (London: Routledge, 2000), I, p. 49.
69. Peter Shaw (1694–1763), physician, writer, lecturer in chemistry and translator of chemical and medical texts, was first doctor to King George II of England. See Jan V. Golinski, 'Peter Shaw: Chemistry and Communication in Augustan England', *Ambix: Journal for the Society for the History of Alchemy and Chemistry*, 30(1) (March

1983): 19. According to Golinski, Shaw pioneered public lectures in chemistry in England. Many followed him throughout the later eighteenth century. Jan Golinski, 'Chemistry', in Roy Porter, ed., *The Cambridge History of Science*, Vol. 4, *Eighteenth-Century Science* (Cambridge: Cambridge University Press, 2003), p. 379.

70. Alexander Monro (Primus) (1697–1767), was a Scottish Professor of Anatomy at Edinburgh University.
71. Golinski, 'Peter Shaw', p. 21.
72. D'Arconville, *Préface, Leçons de chymie, propres à perfectionner la physique, le commerce et les arts* (Paris, 1759), p. xciij.
73. Ibid., p. vi.
74. d'Arconville, *Leçons,* p. 349.
75. Marie-Geneviève-Charlotte Darlus d'Arconville, *Essai pour servir à l'histoire de la putréfaction* (1766), p. xxi
76. Ibid., p. ix.
77. Ibid., p. 1.
78. Ibid., pp. xxvii–xxxviii.
79. Karyna Szmurlo, 'Thiroux d'Arconville, Marie-Geneviève-Charlotte Darlus (1720–1805)', in Eva Martin Sartori, ed., *The Feminist Encyclopedia of French Literature* (Westport, CT: Greenwood Press, 1999), pp. 529–30.
80. D'Arconville, *Essai*, pp. ii–iii.
81. Pringle's primary contribution to medicine was his research dealing with putrefaction processes in the cause of disease. He applied the results of his research to army hospitals in advocating proper hygiene, latrines and ventilation. Because of his revolutionary discoveries and their application to the military, he has been called 'the father of modern military medicine'. He published his results in *Observations on the Diseases of the Army* (1752).
82. This would have been his *Observations on the Diseases of the Army, in camp and garrison: in three parts: with an appendix, containing some papers of experiments, read at several meetings of the Royal Society* (London: A. Millar, 1752, 1753, 1755).
83. D'Arconville, *Essai*, pp. v–vi.
84. Ibid., vi–vii.
85. Table, in ibid., pp. xxxvii–xlvii.
86. D'Arconville, *Essai*, p. xviii.
87. Du Châtelet described herself as Voltaire's secretary. Letters to Pierre Robert le Cornier de Cideville, March 1739 and 27 February 1736, cited in *Lettres de la Marquise du Châtelet*, ed. Theodore Besterman (Geneva: Institut et Musée Voltaire, 1958), I, pp. 346, 100. She aired many of her views in her unpublished 'Feminist Manifesto', written in 1735. Preface to her translation of Mandeville, 'The Fable of the Bees, a Rendering and a Feminist Manifesto', in Ira O. Wade, *Studies on Voltaire with Some Unpublished Papers by Madame du Châtelet* (Princeton, NJ: Princeton University Press, 1947), p. 135.
88. Charles Coulston Gillespie, ed., *Dictionary of Scientific Biography*, 18 vols (New York: Scribner, 1980–90), IX, pp. 479–80.
89. Londa Schiebinger, 'Skeletons in the Closet: The First Illustrations of the Female Skeleton in Eighteenth-Century Anatomy', in Catherine Gallagher and Thomas Laqueur, eds, *The Making of the Modern Body: Sexuality and Society in the Nineteenth Century* (Berkeley and Los Angeles: University of California Press, 1987), p. 77, n. 53. See also Londa Schiebinger, *The Mind has no Sex? Women in the Origins of Modern Science* (Cambridge, MA: Harvard University Press, 1991), pp. 195–200 for a discussion of this issue.

90. Londa Schiebinger, 'Skelettestreit', *Isis*, 94 (2003): 309.
91. Pierre-Henri-Hippolyte Bodard, 'Cours de botanique médicale compare' (Paris, 1810), I, pp. xxvi–xx, cited in Schiebinger, 'Skeletons', 77, n. 53.
92. Wolley, A *Supplement to the Queen-Like Closet, or a Little of Everything* (London: Richard Lowndes, 1674), pp. 10–11 cited in Elaine Hobby, 'A Woman's Best Setting Out is Silence: The Writings of Hannah Wolley', in Gerald Maclean, ed., *Culture and Society in the Stuart Restoration: Literature, Drama, History* (Cambridge: Cambridge University Press, 1995), p. 182.
93. Elaine Hobby, *Virtue of Necessity: English Women's Writing: 1649–88* (Ann Arbor: University of Michigan Press, 1989), pp. 166–7; Hobby, 'A Woman's Best Setting Out', p. 182.
94. English scholar Elaine Hobby claims that three texts have been wrongly attributed to Wolley: *The Gentlewoman's Companion*, which she argues is an anthology based on Wolley's other works, as well as *The Compleat Servant-Maid* (1677) and *The Accomplish'd Ladies Delight* (1677). However, other scholars such as Patricia Crawford and Hilda Smith attribute *The Gentlewoman's Companion* to Wolley as do the British Library and the University of Glasgow Library.
95. *Dictionary of National Biography*, ed. Sidney Lee (London: Smith, Elder, & Co. 1909), XXI, pp. 902–3; Hilda Smith, *Reason's Disciples*: *Seventeenth-Century English Feminists* (Urbana: University of Illinois Press, 1982), p. 106.
96. Hannah Wolley, 'Epistle Dedicatory', to *The Gentlewoman's Companion, or, A Guide to the Female Sex* (London: A. Maxwell, 1673), n.p.
97. Ibid.
98. Wolley, *The Gentlewoman's Companion*, p. 11.
99. Wolley, *The Queen-like Closet or Rich Cabinet. Stored with all manner of rare receipts for preserving, candying and cookery. Very pleasant and beneficial to all ingenious persons of the female sex* (London: R. Lowndes, 1670), p. 2, http://www.gutenberg.org/etext/14377.
100. Ibid., p. 2.
101. Ibid., p. 6.
102. Harold J. Cook, 'The Society of Chemical Physicians, the New Philosophy, and the Restoration Court', *Bulletin of the History of Medicine* (1987): 61.
103. The only account of O'Dowde's life is contained in his daughter's pamphlet, Mary Trye, *Medicatrix, or the Woman Physician* (London, 1675), pp. 25–32.
104. Trye, *Medicatrix*, pp. 44–69; Doreen Evenden Nagy, *Popular Medicine in Seventeenth-Century England* (Bowling Green, OH: Bowling Green State University Popular Press, 1988), p. 30.
105. Trye, *Medicatrix*, p. 120.
106. For a detailed discussion of the conflicts in English medicine during the seventeenth century, see Anne Dunan, 'Mélancolie, enthousiasme et folie: pathologie et inspiration dans la littérature dissidente', *Etudes Epistémè*, 7 (Spring 2005): 65–93.
107. For further discussion of the conflicts occurring in the medical profession in England during the mid-1660s, and Stubbe's role in them, see Harold J. Cook, 'Physicians and the New Philosophy: Henry Stubbe and the Virtuosi-Physicians', in Roger French and Andrew Wear, eds, *The Medical Revolution of the Seventeenth Century* (Cambridge: Cambridge University Press, 1989), pp. 246–71. The only modern full-length study of Stubbe is James R. Jacob, *Henry Stubbe, Radical Protestantism and the Early Enlightenment* (Cambridge: Cambridge University Press, 1983).

108. Lisa Forman Cody, Introduction, *Writings on Medicine. Printed Writings 1641–1700*, Vol. 4, The Early Modern Englishwoman: A Facsimile Library of Essential Works (Aldershot: Ashgate, 2000), pp. xv–xvi.
109. Cook, 'The Society of Chemical Physicians', p. 61.
110. *Dictionary of National Biography*, XIX, pp. 116–17.
111. Jacob, *Henry Stubbe*, p. 43.
112. Stubbe, Preface to *An Epistolary Discourse Concerning Phlebotomy* (1671), cited in Jacob, *Henry Stubbe*, p. 46.
113. University educated doctors were still taught physic which was divided between practical and theoretical. Practical physic involved the study of physiology, pathology, semiotics, hygiene and therapeutics, while the theoretical taught naturals and non-naturals. Even the practical involved a detailed study of Latin grammar and logic. University trained physicians only prescribed medicines (drugs) as a last resort. Cook, 'Physicians and the New Philosophy', pp. 247–248.
114. Stubbe, *Campanella revived or, An enquiry into the history of the Royal Society, whether the virtuosi there do not pursue the projects of Campanella for the reducing England unto Popery* (London: Printed for the author, 1670), EEBO, eebo.chawyck.com; 'To the Reader' in Cook, 'Physicians and the New Philosophy: Henry Stubbe and the Virtuosi-Physicians', p. 263.
115. Stubbe, 'To the Reader' in *Campanella revived.*
116. Trye, *Medicatrix*, p. 83.
117. Ibid., pp. 117–18.
118. Ibid., p. 2.
119. Ibid., pp. 116–17.
120. Ibid., p. 2.
121. Ibid., pp. 2–3.
122. Ibid., p. 106.
123. Ibid., pp. 106–8.
124. Ibid., p. 113.
125. Ibid., pp. 114–15.
126. Ibid., p. 115.
127. A.S. Weber, 'Women's Early Modern Medical Almanacs in Historical Context', *English Literary Renaissance*, 33 (3) (2003): 358.
128. Army Captain Henry Herbert referred to her as such in 1673. This information is cited in Weber, 'Women's Early Modern Medical Almanacs', p. 358, who obtained it from a personal interview with Bernard Capp on 7 December 1998. Capp is a leading expert on English almanacs.
129. Bernard Capp, *English Almanacs 1500–1800* (Ithaca: Cornell University Press, 1979), p. 87.
130. Sarah Jinner, *The womans almanack: or, prognostication for ever: shewing the nature of the planets, with the events that shall befall women and children born under them. With several predictions very useful for the female sex* (London: Printed by J.S. for the Company of Stationers, 1659).
131. Sarah Jinner, *An Almanack, or prognostication for the year of our Lord 1660. Being the third after bissextile or leap year. Calculated for the meridian of London, and may without exception serve for England, Scotland, and Ireland* (London: Printed for the Company of Stationers, 1660).
132. Jinner's medicinal recipes are in both the 1659 and 1660 editions under the section entitled, 'Physical Observations'.

133. Jinner, *An Almanack* (1660).
134. Ibid.
135. Mary Holden, 'Advertisements', in *The Womans Almanack for the Year of Our Lord 1688* (London: Printed by J. Millet for the Company of Stationers, 1688).
136. Doreen Evenden Nagy, *Popular Medicine in Seventeenth-Century England* (Bowling Green, OH: Bowling Green State University Popular Press, 1988), p. 63.
137. Holden, 'Advertisements'.
138. Capp, *English Almanacs*, p. 121.
139. Ibid., p. 17.
140. The only recent study devoted to Blackwell is that by Bruce Madge, 'Elizabeth Blackwell – the Forgotten Herbalist?', *Health Information and Libraries Journal*, 18 (September 2001): 144–52.
141. Ibid., pp. 144–5.
142. Ibid., p. 144.
143. Elizabeth Blackwell, *A Curious Herbal* (1739), I.
144. Ibid., II, Plate 255.
145. Ibid., II, Plate 254.
146. Madge, 'Elizabeth Blackwell', p. 147.
147. Lucia T. Tomasi, *An Oak Spring Flora: Flower Illustration from the Fifteenth Century to the Present Time* (Upperville, Virginia: Oak Spring Garden Library, 1997), pp. 323–4.
148. The following names appear on one of the introductory pages to Blackwell's herbal: R. Mean, G.L. Teissier, Alex Stuart, I.A. Douglas, James Sherard, all medical doctors, and W. Cheseleden, Joseph Miller, Isaac Rand, Rob. Nicholls.
149. Margaret Alic, *Hypatia's Heritage: A History of Women in Science from Antiquity through the Nineteenth Century* (Boston: Beacon Press, 1986), p.100.
150. Madge, 'Elizabeth Blackwell', p. 149.
151. Ibid., pp. 144, 147.

5. Female Midwives and the Medical Profession

1. This chapter relies heavily on the work of others in this field of medicine. The literature on the history of midwifery is enormous. For current studies on European midwives in English, see Lianne McTavish, *Childbirth and the Display of Authority in Early Modern France* (Aldershot, UK and Burlington, VT: Ashgate, 2005), Doreen Evenden, *The Midwives of Seventeenth-Century London* (Cambridge and New York: Cambridge University Press, 2000), and Hilary Marland, ed., *The Art of Midwifery, Early Modern Midwives in Europe* (London and New York: Routledge, 1993). Lisa Forman Cody's *Birthing the Nation: Sex, Science, and the Conception of Eighteenth-Century Britons* (Oxford and New York: Oxford University Press, 2005) contributes to the literature attempting to explain the displacement of female by male midwives in Britain, particularly during the eighteenth century. Subsequent notes should provide readers with a guide to the literature.
2. Datha Clapper Brack, 'Displaced – the Midwife by the Male Physician', *Women and Health*, 1 (1976): 19.
3. Damien Carbón, cited in Teresa Ortiz, 'From Hegemony to Subordination: Midwives in Early Modern Spain', in Marland, ed., *The Art of Midwifery*, p. 95.
4. *Le livre de la Taille de 1292*, cited in Gustave Joseph Witkowski, *Histoire des accouchements chez tous les peuples* (Paris: G. Steinheil, 1887), p. 651.
5. Merry Wiesner, *Women and Gender in Early Modern Europe* (London and New York: Cambridge University Press, 1993), p. 66.

6. Edward Shorter, *Women's Bodies: A Social History of Women's Encounters with Health, Ill-Health and Medicine* (New Brunswick, NJ: Transaction, 1981), p. 36.
7. Wiesner, *Women and Gender*, p. 45.
8. See the case of Jeanne Darc (not the famous Jeanne d'Arc) from 1616 in *Le Réveil du chat qui dort, par la cognoissance de la perte du pucelage de la pluspart des Châbrières de Paris. Avec le moyen de la raccontrer, [...] le rapport des plus signalées Matrones, tant Bearnoises, que Françoises appelées à cet effet. Avec les noms des [...] par elles trouvées dans leurs bas guichets. Mis en lumière, en faveur des bons compagnons à marier* (Paris: Iouxte la Coppie Imprimée par Pierre le Roux, 1616), cited in Witkowsky, *Histoire des accouchements*, p. 652.
9. The names of the midwives were Marie Teste, Jane de Meaux de la Guignans and Magdelaine la Lippue, see Witowsky, *Histoire des accouchements*, p. 652.
10. Henri Stoffart, 'Un avortement criminal en 1660', *Histoire des sciences médicales*, 20 (1986): 72, 78.
11. Gui Patin, *Lettres*, ed. J.H. Reveillé-Parise (Paris: J.-B. Baillière, 1846), III, p. 74.
12. In addition to Patin's correspondence, we also have the proceedings of the trial. They are held at the Archives de la Préfecture de police de Paris: Registre d'écrou de la Conciergerie, 1659–1660. AB 47, fol. 189–90.
13. Trial proceedings, cited in Stoffart, 'Un avortement criminal en 1660', p. 77.
14. Ibid., p. 77.
15. Trial proceedings cited in Ibid., p. 78.
16. Marland, 'Introduction', *The Art of Midwifery*, pp. 1–9.
17. Jacques Gélis, *La sage-femme ou le médecin: une nouvelle conception de la vie* (Paris: Fayard: 1988), pp. 115–18.
18. Jacques Gélis, 'Sages-Femmes et Accoucheurs: l'obstétrique populaire aux XVIIe et XVIIIe siècles', *Annales, Economies, Sociétés et Civilisations* (September–October 1977): 941–6. See Nina Rattner Gelbart's excellent biography, *The King's Midwife: A History and Mystery of Madame du Coudray* (Berkeley: University of California Press, 1998).
19. 'Du Coudray, Angelique', in Marilyn Ogilvie and Joy Dorothy Harvey, *The Biographical Dictionary of Women in Science: Pioneering Lives from Ancient Times to the Mid-20th Century* (London and New York: Routledge, 2000), I, p. 381.
20. Preface to Madame duCoudray, *Abrégé de l'art des accouchemens, dans lequel on donne les préceptes nécessaires pour le mettre heureusement en pratique. On y a joint plusieurs observations intéressantes sur des cas singuliers. Ouvrage très-utile aux jeunes Sages-Femmes, & généralement à tous les élèves en cet art, qui desirent de s'y rendre habiles*, pp. v–viii, cited in Gelbart, *The King's Midwife*, pp. 60–1. Hundreds of du Coudray's machines were made but only one is still in existence. It is at the Musée Flaubert in Rouen (Gelbart, *The King's Midwife*, p. 62). According to Gelbart, the *Abrégé* was published five times in France between 1759 and 1785. See Nina Rattner Gelbart, 'Books and the Birthing Business: The Midwife Manuals of Madame du Coudray', in Elizabeth C. Goldsmith and Dena Goodman, eds, *Going Public: Women and Publishing in Early Modern France* (Ithaca: Cornell University Press, 1995), p. 80.
21. Gélis, *La sage-femme*, p. 178.
22. Ibid., pp. 174, 178; V. Busacchi, 'Benedetto XIV, la Medicina, i Medici', *Storia Medicina*, 3 (1957): 599–612.
23. Gélis, *La sage-femme*, pp. 178–9.
24. Ibid., p. 168.

25. Enrique Perdiguero, 'The Popularization of Medicine during the Spanish Enlightenment', in Roy S. Porter, ed., *The Popularization of Medicine, 1650–1850* (London and New York: Routledge, 1992), p. 166.
26. R.A. Erikson, 'The Books of Generation: Some Observations on the Style of the British Midwife Books, 1671–1764', in P.G. Boucé, ed., *Sexuality in Eighteenth Century Britain* (Manchester: Manchester University Press, 1982), p. 74, n. 11.
27. Helen King, 'As if None Understood the Art that Cannot Understand Greek: The Education of Midwives in Seventeenth Century England', in Vivan Nutton and Roy Porter, eds, *The History of Medical Education in England* (Amsterdam: Rodopi, 1995), p. 189.
28. Adrianna E. Bakos, '"A Knowledge Speculative and Practical" The Dilemma of Midwives' Education in Early Modern Europe', in Barbara J. Whitehead, ed., *Women's Education in Early Modern Europe: A History, 1500–1800* (New York: Garland, 1999), p. 235.
29. See Peter M. Dunn, 'Eucharius Roesslin (c.1470–1526) of Germany and the Rebirth of Midwifery', *Archives of Disease in Childhood*, 79 (July 1998): F 77, http://fnbmjjournals.com/cgi/content/full/79/1/F77.
30. Alfred M. Hellman MD, *A Collection of Early Obstetrical Works* (New Haven, CT: Yale University Press, 1952), pp. 5–6.
31. Eucharius Roesslin, *Rosengarten*, ed. Gustav Klein (Munich: C. Kuhn, 1910), p. 8. For a modern English edition, see *When Midwifery became the Male Physician's Province: The Sixteenth Century Handbook: The Rose Garden for Pregnant Women and Midwives*, trans. and intro. Wendy Arons (Jefferson, NC: McFarland & Co, 1994).
32. Roesslin, 'Contents of the Chapters of This Book', cited in Arons, *When Midwifery became the Male Physician's Province*, pp. 40–1.
33. Thomas Raynalde, *The birth of mankinde, otherwise named The womans booke. Set foorth in English by Thomas Raynalde phisition, and by him corrected, and augmented. Whose contents yée may reade in the table following: but most plainely in the prologue*, Imprinted at London: [By George Eld?] for Thomas Adams. Cum priuilegio [1604], 3–4.
34. The work in English is entitled, *Divers Observations on Sterility, Loss of the Ovum After Fecundation, Fecundity and Childbirth, Diseases of Women and of Newborn Infants, amply treated of and practical with success by L. Bourgeois, called Boursier, midwife to the Queen. A work useful and necessary to everyone.*
35. Bourgeois, *Divers Observations*, I, chs. 1 & 2, pp. 1–17. For difficult births and a summary of cases see, II, pp. 17–25.
36. See *Les Six Couches de Marie de Médicis*, cited in Amanda Carson Banks, *Birth Chairs, Midwives and Medicine* (Jackson, MS: University of Mississippi Press, 1995), pp. 20–1.
37. Dunn, 'Louise Bourgeois (1563–1636): Royal Midwife of France', *Archives of Disease in Childhood and Neonatal Edition* (2004): 89: F185, http://fn.bmjjournals.com/cgi/content/full/89/2/F185.
38. Bourgeois, 'Secrets', *Divers Observations*, 6th edn (1634), cited in Hunter Robb, 'Remarks on the Writings of Louyse Bourgeois', *Johns Hopkins Hospital Bulletin*, 38 (September 1893): 3.
39. Bourgeois, 'Secrets', cited in Lawrence D. Longo, 'Classic Pages in Obstetrics and Gynecology', *American Journal of Obstetrics and Gynecology*, 173 (December 1995): 1893–4.
40. On Carbón, see Antonio Hernández Alcántara, *Estudio historico de la obra toco-ginecológica y pediátrica de Damián Carbón* (Salamanca: Seminario de Historia de la

Medicina, Universidad de Salamanca, 1957). The most recent edition of Carbón's work is Damián Carbón, *Libro del Arte de las Comadres o Madrinas, del Regimento de las Preñandas y de los niños*, transcription de Francisco Susarte Molina (Alicante: Universidad de Alicante, 1995). There is no edition in English.

41. Manuel Usandizaga, *Damían Carbón*, XV Congreso Internacional de Historia de la Medicina, Madrid (Acala, 23–29 September 1956): pp. 1–2.
42. Carbón, *Libro*, pp. 33–4.
43. Carbón, *Libro*, p. iv, cited in Mary Elizabeth Perry, *Gender and Disorder in Modern Seville* (Princeton, NJ: Princeton University Press, 1990), p. 27.
44. Nunez's, *Libro del parto humano en el cual se contienen remedies muy utiles y usuales para el parto dificultoso de las mujeres* (Alcalá, 1580) was reprinted several times during the seventeenth and eighteenth centuries It became very popular with medical practitioners during this time. Ruizes's book is entitled, *Diez privilegios para mujeres prenadas* (Alcalá, 1606). See Hilary Marland, ed., *The Art of Midwifery* (1993), p. 110, n. 24.
45. Cited in Luis Granjel, *La medicina Española del siglo XVII* (Salamanca: Ediciones Universidad de Salamanca, 1978), p. 65.
46. Jacques Gélis, *La sage-femme*, p. 173.
47. Ibid.
48. Ibid., pp. 160–1.
49. Municipal regulation of midwives began in France in 1385, Spain in 1523 and in England in 1902. Thomas R. Forbes, 'The Regulation of English Midwives in the Eighteenth and Nineteenth Centuries', *Medical History*, 15 (1971): 352.
50. Shorter, *Women's Bodies*, p. 41.
51. Richard L. Petrelli, 'The Regulation of French Midwifery during the Ancien Régime', *Journal of the History of Medicine*, 26 (1971): 277.
52. Cited in Thomas Benedek, 'The Changing Relationship between Midwives and Physicians during the Renaissance', *Bulletin of the History of Medicine*, 51 (1977): 553.
53. Petrelli, 'Regulation of French Midwifery', p. 281.
54. Auguste Queirel, *Histoire de la Maternité de Marseille* (Marseille: Ballatier et Berthelet 1899), p. 9.
55. Shorter, *Women's Bodies*, p. xii.
56. Brigitte Jordan, *Birth in Four Cultures* (Montreal: Eden Press, 1978), p. 95, n. 3.
57. An embryotomy is the intentional removal of a foetus from the womb. It is a procedure which takes place when a natural delivery is impossible. E. Wickersheimer, *La médecine et les médecins en France à l'Epoque de la Renaissance* (Paris: A. Malaine, 1906), p. 489.
58. Régistre aux mémoire (Lille, 1458–69 and 1469–82), in E. Leclair, *Un chapitre de l'histoire de la chirurgie à Lille* (Lille: H. Morel, 1910), p. 7.
59. André Pecker, 'François Mauriceau', in *Commentaires sur Dix Grands Livres de Médecine Française* (Mayenne: Floch, 1968), p. 59.
60. François Hacquain, *Histoire de l'art d'accouchement en Lorraine de temps anciens aux Xxe siècle* (Saint-Nicolas-de-Port: Star, 1979), p. 37.
61. Hacquain, *Histoire*, p. 16.
62. Shorter, *Women's Bodies*, p. 42.
63. Compared with English language studies of women in general and midwifery in particular in other European countries, Spain has received scant attention. See Marilyn Stone and Carmen Benito-Vessels, eds, *Women at Work in Spain from the Middle Ages to Early Modern Times* (New York: Peter Lang, 1998) for an example of

an attempt to redress this lacuna. Mary Elizabeth Perry argues that the 'invisible invisibility' is 'especially remarkable in early modern Spain, where Jews, Muslims and Christians had made their homes for centuries'. Mary Elizabeth Perry, 'Weaving Clio and the Moriscas of Early Modern Spain', in Susan D. Amusen and Adele Seef, eds, *Attending to Early Modern Women* (Newark: University of Delaware Press, 1998), p. 58.

64. Ortiz, 'Midwives in Early Modern Spain', p. 98.
65. Ibid.
66. Cited in ibid.
67. Cited in Luis Granjel, *La medicina Española del siglo XVII*, p. 136.
68. Perry, *Gender and Disorder in Modern Seville,* 27. The relationship between witchcraft and medicine will be discussed in more detail in Chapter 9.
69. Rosado's story is told in detail in Ortiz, 'Midwives in Early Modern Spain', pp. 103–7.
70. Ortiz, 'Midwives in Early Modern Spain', p. 106.
71. Archivo General de Simancas (AGS) Sección Gracia y Justicia, leg. 989, f. 695, cited in ibid., p. 104.
72. (AGS), Sección Gracia y Justicia, leg. 989, f. 689, cited in ibid., pp. 104–5.
73. Ibid., p. 105.
74. For information about the nature of Islamic medicine in Spain see José María López Pinero, 'The Medical Profession in 16th Century Spain', in Andrew W. Russell, ed., *The Town and State Physician in Europe from the Middle Ages to the Enlightenment* (Wolfenboutel: Herzog August Bibliothek, 1981), pp. 91–2.
75. Carmen Barceló, 'Mujeres, Campesinas, Mudéjares', in María J. Viguera, ed., *La Mujer en Al-Andalus reflejos históricos de su actividad y categorías sociales: actas de las V Jornadas de Investigación Interdisciplinaria* (Madrid: Ediciones de la Universidad Autónoma de Madrid, 1989), p. 213.
76. M.A. Ladero Quesada, 'Los mudéjares de Castilla en la Baja Edad Media', in *I Simposio Internacional del Mudejarismo* (Madrid: Teruel, 1981), p. 372.
77. Moriscas were Spanish Muslims who had pragmatically converted to Catholicism after the Christian re-conquest of Spain between the eleventh and fifteenth centuries.
78. Ana Labarta, 'La Mujer Morisca: Sus Actitivades', in Viguera, *La Mujer en Al-Andalus*, p. 223.
79. Historical Archives of Madrid (AHN), Inq. Auto de 1607 f, 353, cited in Labarta, 226.
80. (AHN) Inq. Auto 1590 f. 232, cited in Labarta, 'La Mujer Morisca', p. 226.
81. (AHN) Inq. Leg. 548/20 and auto de 1579, f. 232, cited in ibid., p. 226.
82. (AHN), Inq. Libro 990, f. 64, cited in Jacqueline Fournel-Guérin, 'La femme morisque en Aragon', in *Les Morisques et Leur Temps*, Table Ronde International 4–7 July 1981, Montpellier (Paris: Editions du Centre National de la Recherche Scientifique, 1983), p. 525.
83. Trial proceedings are in Archivo Histórico Nacional (Madrid), Leg. 177, no 4 (1536–63) This information is found in Stone and Benito-Vessels, *Women at Work in Spain*, pp. 92–3. See also Renée Levine Melammed, 'Castilian *Conversas* at Work', in Marilyn Stone and Carmen Benito-Vessels, eds, *Women at Work in Spain from the Middle Ages to Early Modern Times* (New York: Peter Lang Publishing, 1998), pp. 81–100. For information on Rodríguez's trial, see Renée Levine Melammed, 'A Sixteenth Century Midwife and Her Encounter with the Inquisition', in Raymond B. Waddington and Arthur H. Williamson, eds, *The Expulsion of the Jews: 1492 and After* (New York: Garland, 1994).

84. Luís S. Granjel, *La Medicina Española Del Siglo XVII*, p. 64.
85. James Walsh, *Medieval Medicine* (London: A.C. Black, 1920), p. 154.
86. For a summary of midwifery in Early Modern Italy, see Nadia Maria Filippini, 'The Church, the State and Childbirth: The Midwife in Italy during the Eighteenth Century', in Marland, ed., *The Art of Midwifery*, pp. 152–67.
87. Gélis, *La sage-femme*, p. 159.
88. Ibid., pp. 162–3.
89. An eighteenth century midwife oath cited in J.H. Aveling, MD, *English Midwives, their History and Prospects* (London: Churchill, 1872), pp. 89–93.
90. Doreen Evenden, *The Midwives of Seventeenth Century London*, pp. xiii–iv.
91. Jean Donnison, *Midwives and Medical Men: A History of Inter-Professional Rivalries and Women's Rights* (New York: Schoken, 1977), p. 6.
92. AD D 82 (Archives Départementales de la Meurthe-et-Moselle), cited in Hacquain, *Histoire*, p. 37.
93. Gélis, *La sage-femme*, p. 176.
94. William Smellie, MD, A *Treatise on the Theory and Practice of Midwifery* (London: D. Wilson, 1752), p. v. William Smellie (1697–1763) was the inventor of a type of forceps. He led the movement against midwives in favour of their replacement by male doctors.
95. The only full length study of Louise Bourgeois Boursier in English is Wendy Perkins, *Midwifery and Medicine in Early Modern France: Louise Bourgeois* (Exeter: University of Exeter Press, 1996). She argues that Bourgeois's medical knowledge exceeded that of most physicians and surgeons. See especially, pp. 111–12.
96. Petrelli, 'Regulation of French Midwifery', p. 279.
97. François Le Brun, *Se Soigner d'autrefois: Médecins, saints et sorciers aux 17e et 18e* siècles (Paris: Temps Actuels, 1983), p. 47.
98. This biographical information is derived from Bourgeois's *Observations diverses sur la sterilité, perte de fruict, foecondité, et maladies des femmes, et enfants nouveaux naiz* (Paris: H. Ruffin, 1652), Book I, dedicated, 'A Madame'.
99. Jacques Gélis, *La sage-femme*, pp. 28–31.
100. P.M. Dunn, 'Louise Bourgeois (1563–1636): Royal Midwife of France', *Archives of Disease in Childhood and Neonatal Edition* (2004), 89: F185, http://fn.bmjjournals.com/cgi/content/full/89/2/F185.
101. Louise Bourgeois, *Observations diverses sur la sterilité* (Paris, 1626), p. 48.
102. Louise Bourgeois, *Apologie contre le rapport des médecins* (Paris: M. Mondière, 1627), p. 17, cited in Perkins, *Midwifery and Medicine*, p. 118.
103. Perkins, *Midwifery and Medicine*, pp. 118–20.
104. It was translated into English by Hugh Chamberlen (c. 1630–1720) in London (printed and reprinted in 1673, 1681, 1683, 1716, 1717). German translations were published in Basel (1680), Nürnburg (1681) and Strassburg (1732. It was published in Italian in Genoa (1727), in Dutch by P. Clamper, Amsterdam (1759) and in Latin in Paris (1861).
105. Benedek, 'The Changing Relationship', p. 564.
106. Bakos, 'The Dilemma of Midwives' Education', p. 238.
107. François Rabelais, Chapter 1.VI. 'How Gargantua was born in a strange manner', *Gargantua and Pantagruel, Complete. Five Books Of The Lives, Heroic Deeds And Sayings Of Gargantua And His Son Pantagruel*, trans. Sir Thomas Urquhart of Cromarty and Peter Antony Motteux, 1653 edition, Project Guttenberg, 8 August 2004 [EBook #1200], p. 47, http://www.gutenberg.org/catalog/world/readfile?fk_files=90155&pageno=47.

108. Cited in Perkins, *Midwifery and Medicine*, p. 99.
109. Paul Portal, a master surgeon and man-midwife, contributed to the advancement of obstetrics in his *La pratique des accouchements* (Paris, 1685).
110. Jacques Guillemeau, *De l'heureux accouchement des femmes où il est traicté du gouvernement de leur grossesse, de leur travail naturel et contre nature* (Paris, 1609), Book II, Chapter X.
111. Laurent Joubert, *La Médecine et le régime de santé, ses erreurs populaires et propos vulgaires*, ed. Madeleine Tiollais (Paris and Montreal: L'Harmattan, 1997), II, pp. 167–8.
112. Wickersheimer, *La médecine et les médecins*, pp. 638–9.
113. Colette H. Winn, Introduction to Louise Bourgeois, *Récit véritable de la naissance de messeigneurs et dames les enfans de France; Fidelle relation de l'accouchement, maladie et ouverture du corps de feu Madame, suivie du, Rapport de l'ouverture du corps de feu Madame; Remonstrance a Madame Bourcier, touchant son apologie* (Geneva: Droz, 2000), p. 14.
114. Joubert, *Traités*, cited in Wickersheimer, *La médecine et les médecins*, pp. 668–9.
115. The 1587 regulations are reprinted in Witkowski, *Histoire des accouchements*, pp. 653–6.
116. Philippe Hecquet, *De l'indécence aux hommes d'accoucher les femmes et de l'obligation aux mères de nourrir leurs enfants*, ed. Hélène Rouch (Paris: Côté-femmes editions, 1990), p. 37.
117. Ibid., pp. 37–40.
118. Ibid., p. 66.
119. Ibid. p. 64.
120. Ibid., pp. 67–8.
121. Ibid., pp. 48–51.
122. Midwifery in England in the Early Modern period has been covered extensively elsewhere. This section will provide a summary of the most important changes and the struggle which took place between midwives and medical men. For an excellent recent discussion of English midwives, see Evenden, *The Midwives of Seventeenth Century London*.
123. James MacMath, *The Expert Mid-wife: a treatise of the diseases of women with child and in child-bed* (Edinburgh: G. Mosman, 1694), cited in Alice Clark, *Working Life of Women in the Seventeenth Century* (New York: Dutton, 1919; reprint, 1968), p. 281.
124. Ibid.
125. Hilda Smith, 'Gynecology and Ideology in Seventeenth Century England', in Berenice A. Carroll, ed., *Liberating Women's History: Theoretical and Critical Essays* (Urbana: University of Illinois Press, 1976), pp. 109–10.
126. Donnison, *Midwives and Medical Men*, p. 13.
127. Ibid., p. 15.
128. Nicolas Culpeper, *A Directory for Midwives* (1671), introductory pages, no numbers.
129. Jane Sharp's *The Midwives Book* and Elizabeth Cellier's *To Dr.— An Answer to his Queries, concerning the Colledg of...* are reproduced in *The Early Modern Englishwoman: A Facsimile Library of Essential Works,* Part I: Printed Writings, 1641–1700: Vol. 4: Writings on Medicine, intro. Lisa Forman Cody (Aldershot: Ashgate, 2000).
130. Lisa Forman Cody, 'Introduction', in *The Early Modern Englishwoman*, p. xi.

131. Jane Sharp, *The Midwives Book or the Whole Art of Midwifery Discovered,* ed. Elaine Hoby (Oxford: Oxford University Press, 1999), pp. 11–12.
132. See chapter 3, '"Daughters are but Branches": English Feminists, 1650–80', in Hilda L. Smith, *Reason's Disciples* (Chicago: University of Illinois Press, 1982).
133. Cellier was a convert to Catholicism who lived during the Restoration. In addition to her activities as a midwife, Cellier was involved in the contemporary political feuds between Catholics and Protestants and it is for this reason that she was in trouble with the law. She became notorious during the 'Meal-tub' or Popish plot of 1679 (in which Catholics had tried to manufacture evidence of a 'presbyterian plot' to counter the fears of the 'popish plot' to overthrow the government of Charles II and assassinate Charles to make way for a Catholic heir revealed by Titus Oates the year before) and also wrote a treatise describing her aid to imprisoned Catholics, and the ghastly conditions of Newgate Prison. The plot was dubbed 'Meal-tub' because the contents of its plan were found in Cellier's meal-tub. The pamphlet was suppressed, and she was put on trial for having published libellous material against Charles II. She was fined one thousand pounds and pilloried for several days at different locations. At each location, copies of her supposedly libellous narrative were burned. See *Malice defeated; or a brief relation of the accusation and deliverance of Elizabeth Cellier* (London: For Elizabeth Cellier, 1680) and Elizabeth Cellier, *The tryal and sentence of Eliz. Cellier* (London: T. Collins, 1680). For an account of Cellier's political activities and her writings, see Penny Richards, 'A Life in Writing: Elizabeth Cellier and Print Culture', *Women's Writing,* 7(3) (2000): 411–25.
134. Elizabeth Cellier, A *Scheme for the Foundation of a Royal Hospital, and Raising a Revenue of Five or Six Thousand Pounds a Year, by, and for the Maintenance of a Corporation of Skilful Midwives and such Foundlings, or exposed Children, as shall be admitted therein'* (1687) reprinted in *The Early Modern Englishwoman: A Facsimile of Essential Works,* Series II Printed Writings, 1641–1700: Part 3, Vol. 5, Elizabeth Cellier, selected and intro. Mihoko Suzuki (Burlington, VT: Ashgate, 2006), pp. 244–5. This pamphlet was alleged to be found in James II's papers in France. Suzuki, 'Introduction', in *The Early Modern Englishwoman,* xi.
135. Cellier, *A Scheme* in *The Early Modern Englishwoman,* p. 247.
136. Ibid., p. 246.
137. Edinburgh Town Council, 'Council Records', 9 February 1726 in C. Hoolihan, 'Thomas Young, M.D., 1726–83 and Obstetrical Education', *Journal of the History of Medicine,* 40 (1985): 327–45.
138. Ornella Moscucci, *The Science of Woman: Gynaecology and Gender in England, 1800–1929* (Cambridge: Cambridge University Press, 1993), p. 51.
139. Sarah Stone, *A Complete Practice of Midwifery* (London: T. Cooper, 1737), p. xix. For details on Stone's practice, see Isobel Grundy, 'Sarah Stone: Enlightenment Midwife', in Roy Porter, ed., *Medicine in the Enlightenment* (Amsterdam: Rodopi), pp. 128–44.
140. Stone, *Complete Practice,* pp. 62–4, 87, 94..
141. Smellie, *Treatise,* p. 444.
142. Elizabeth Nihell, A *treatise on the art of midwifery. Setting forth various instruments: the whole serving to put all rational inquirers in a fair way of very safely forming their own judgment upon the question; which it is best to employ, in cases of pregnancy and lying-in, a man-midwife or, a midwife* (London: 1760).
143. Ibid., pp. iv–v.
144. Ibid., pp. vi, xii, 54, 414, 417.

6. The Healing Care of Nurses

1. There is a paucity of sources dealing specifically with the role of nurses in the past. This chapter relies on a variety of sources, from ecclesiastical to medical. Many of the works written about nursing history are by nurses themselves, the most recent of which is the excellent work by Thetis M. Group and Joan I. Roberts, *Nursing, Physician Control, and the Medical Monopoly: Historical Perspectives on Gendered Inequality in Roles, Rights, and Range of Practice* (Bloomington: Indiana University Press, 2001). Older but still useful works are those by Vern Bullough and Bonnie Bullough, *The Emergence of Modern Nursing* (London: Macmillan, 1969), and Vern Bullough and Bonnie Bullough, *History, Trends and Politics of Nursing* (Norwalk, CT: Appelton-Century-Crofts, 1984)
2. Group and Roberts, *Nursing, Physician Control*, p. 9.
3. *Hippocrates*, trans. W.H.S. Jones (London: William Heinemann, 1943), II, p. 299.
4. For a summary of a number of negative stereotypes which historians of medicine had traditionally held concerning female medical practitioners in general and nurses in particular, see Margaret Connor Versluysen, 'Old Wives' Tales? Women Healers in English History', in *Rewriting Nursing History* (London: Croom Helm, 1980), pp. 175–199. She writes that 'Organised medicine, especially its most prestigious branches, has formally barred women from its ranks for most of its known past. History has reflected this sexual exclusivity and has been primarily the story of a socially privileged group of male healers' (p. 177).
5. Bullough and Bullough, *The Emergence of Modern Nursing*, pp. 226–7.
6. William L. Minkowski, 'Women Healers of the Middle Ages: Selected Aspects of their History', *American Journal of Public Health*, 82(2) (February 1992): 289.
7. *Oxford English Dictionary* online, second edition, 1989, http://dictionary.oed.com/cgi/entry/50108346.
8. Minkowski, 'Women Healers of the Middle Ages', p. 289.
9. Francisca Hernández Martín, *Historía de la enfermería en España: desde la antigüedad hasta nuestros días* (Madrid: Editorial Síntesis, 1996), p. 106.
10. Hernández Martín, *Historía*, p. 111.
11. William L. Minkowski, 'Women Healers of the Middle Ages', p. 289; Group and Roberts, *Nursing, Physician Control*, p. 24; William Morris, ed., *The American Heritage Dictionary of the English Language* (Boston: Houghton Mifflin, 1969), p. 901.
12. William Morris, ed., *The American Heritage Dictionary of the English Language*, (Boston: Houghton Mifflin, 1969), p. 901.
13. *Oxford English Dictionary*, ed. J.A. Simpson and E.S.C Weaver, vol. X, 2nd edn (Oxford: Clarendon Press, 1989), p. 603.
14. William Shakespeare, *The Comedy of Errors*, ed. T.S. Dorsch, intro. Ros King (Cambridge: Cambridge University Press, 2004), v.i.98.
15. *Oxford English Dictionary*, p. 603.
16. See Matthew 25:35–46 where he wrote: 'For I was hungry and you gave me something to eat, I was thirsty and you invited me in…' and most importantly, 'I was sick and you looked after me.' *New International Version of the Holy Bible* (Grand Rapids, MI: The Zondervan Corporation, 1984).
17. Epistle of St James 2:14–16 in *New International Version of the Holy Bible.*
18. Eliot Friedson, *Profession of Medicine: A Study of the Sociology of Applied Knowledge* (New York: Harper & Row, 1970), p. 58.
19. Paul Delaunay, *La Médecine et l'Eglise* (Paris: Editions Hippocrate, 1948), p. 50.

20. Stella Bingham, *Ministering Angels* (Oradell, NJ: Medical Economics, 1979), p. 8.
21. Delaunay, *La Médecine*, p. 51.
22. The Hôtel Dieu of Paris was founded by Saint-Landry, Bishop of Paris. It is the oldest hospital in Paris. Mary Adelaide Nutting and Lavinia L. Dock, *A History of Nursing: The Evolution of Nursing Systems from the Earliest Times to the Foundation of the First English and American Training Schools for Nurses* (New York: G.P. Putnam's Sons, 1907–1912), I, p. 292.
23. Nutting and Dock, *A History of Nursing*, I, p. 282.
24. Ibid., p. 283.
25. Ibid., pp. 284, 287.
26. Rule of St Benedict, cited in Bingham, *Ministering Angels*, p. 8.
27. Michael W. Dols, 'The Origins of the Islamic Hospital: Myth and Reality', *Bulletin of the History of Medicine*, 61 (1987): 370. Dols provides an extensive investigation into the origins of Muslim hospitals.
28. Dols, 'The Origins of the Islamic Hospital', p. 387.
29. Amin A. Khairallah, *Outline of Arabic Contributions to Medicine* (Beirut: American Press, 1946), p. 69.
30. Abdullahi Osman El-Tom, 'Healing', *Encyclopedia of Islam and the Muslim World*, ed. Richard C. Martin (New York: Macmillan Reference USA, 2004), I, p. 296.
31. Bullough and Bullough, *History, Trends and Politics of Nursing*, pp. 4–5.
32. The order was formally named and recognized on 15 February 1113 in a papal bull issued by Pope Paschal II. Raymond de Puy, who succeeded Gerard in 1120, substituted the Augustinian rule for the Benedictine and began building the power of the organization. It acquired wealth and lands and combined the task of tending the sick with defending the Crusader kingdom. After the Templars, the Hospitallers became the most formidable military order in the Holy Land.
33. Mary Ellen Snodgrass, *Historical Encyclopedia of Nursing* (Santa Barbara: ABC–CLIO, 2000), p. 129.
34. James Brodman, *Charity and Welfare: Hospitals and the Poor in Medieval Catalonia* (Philadelphia: University of Pennsylvania Press, 1998), p. 93.
35. Charles Moeller, 'Orders of the Holy Ghost', *The Catholic Encyclopedia*, vol. 7 (New York: Robert Appleton Company, 1910), http://www.newadvent.org/cathen/07415a.htm.
36. Hernández Martín, *Historía*, p. 59.
37. Third orders were fraternities or sororities of lay men and women who united under less stringent rules than the cloistered orders. Wendy Gibson, *Women in Seventeenth Century France* (New York: St Martin's Press, 1989), p. 221.
38. Patricia Ranft, *Women and the Religious Life in Premodern Europe* (New York: St Martin's Press, 1996), pp. 100–1.
39. 'Constitutions faites en 1652 pour les religieuses de l'Hôtel Dieu de Paris par le chapitre de Paris, leur Supérieur, et reçues en 1725', in *Archives de l'Hôtel Dieu de Paris (1137–1500) par Léon Brièle avec notice, appendice et table par Ernest Coyecue*, (Paris: Imprimerie nationale, 1894); Marcel Fosseyeux, *L'Hôtel Dieu de Paris au XVIIe et XVIIIe siècle* (Paris: Berger-Levrault, 1912).
40. Ernest Wickersheimer, 'Médecins et Chirurgiens dans les Hôpitaux du Moyen Âge', *Janus*, 32 (1928): 1.
41. Nutting and Dock, *A History of Nursing*, I, pp. 295–8.
42. Jean Imbert, *Histoire des hôpitaux en France* (Toulouse: Privat, 1982), p. 212.
43. Nutting and Dock, *A History of Nursing*, I, p. 302.
44. Minkowski, 'Women Healers', p. 290.

45. This took place in the mid-seventeenth century. See Delaunay, *La Médecine*, p. 85; Albin Rousselet, *Notes sur l'ancien Hôtel Dieu de Paris Relatives à la lutte des administrateurs laîques contre le pouvoir spiritual. Extraites des archives de l'Assistance publique et publiées par A. Rousselet* (Paris: E. Lecrosnier and Babé, 1888), p. 122.
46. Nutting and Dock, *A History of Nursing*, p. 303.
47. See Chapter 5 on midwifery for birthing practices. Minnie Goodnow, *Outlines of Nursing History*, 4th edn (Philadelphia: W.B. Saunders, 1929), p. 43.
48. Cited in Abbé Héylot, *Histoire des ordres monastiques religieux et militarise et des Congrégations séculières de l'un et de l'autre sexe, qui on esté establies jusqu'à present; contenant les vies de leurs fondateurs* (Paris, 1721), III, p. 185.
49. E. Coyecque, *L'Hotel Dieu de Paris au moyen age* (Paris: Champion 1889–1891), I, pp. 25–7, 31–7, 79.
50. Fol. 177 cited in Louis S. Greenbaum, 'Nurses and Doctors in Conflict: Piety and Medicine in the Paris Hotel-Dieu on the eve of the French Revolution', *Clio Medica*, 13(3–4): 254.
51. Goodnow, *Outlines*, p. 45; Gerald Joseph Griffin and H. Joanne King Griffin, *Jensen's History and Trends of Professional Nursing*, 5th edn (St Louis: C.V. Mosby), p. 72.
52. *Collection de documents pour servir à l'histoire des hôpitaux de Paris. Commencée sous les auspices de M. Michel Möring. Délibérations de l'ancien bureau de l'Hôtel Dieu*, ed. Léon Brièle (Paris, 1883), II, pp. 215–19.
53. Archives Loiret B 1477 et 1482 (procedures). Bib. Comm. Orleans, E 3911 (Recueil), Archives communales Orleans BB 5, fol. 31–34 and Joly de Fleury, 1269. Abuses denounced in 1790 to the Comité de Mendicité see Alexandre Tuetey, *L'assistance publique à Paris pendant la Révolution. Documents inédits. Recueillis et publiés par A. Tuetey* (Paris: Histoire générale de Paris. 1866), Vol. 1, no. 60.
54. Archives hospitalières du Puy, 1 E 1, folios, 17 ff., cited in René Jouanne, 'Assistance, Bienfaisance et Charité en Normandie, Orientation de Recherches et Souvenirs', *Bulletin de la Société française d'histoire des hôpitaux*, 34(1977): 39.
55. Camille Bloch, *L'Assistance et l'Etat en France à la veille de la Révolution* (Paris: Alphonse Picard, 1908), pp. 41–2.
56. *Collection de documents*, ed. Brièle, II, pp. 210–11.
57. R.P. Chalumeau, 'L'assistance aux malades pauvres au XVIIe Siècle', *Dix-Huitième Siècle*, XC–XCI (1971): 75–86.
58. These statements date from 1652 and were renewed in 1725. *Collection de documents*, ed. Brièle, II, pp. 210.
59. Greenbaum, 'Nurses and Doctors in Conflict', pp. 247–67.
60. Bingham, *Ministering Angels*, p. 10.
61. P.H. Cullum, *Cremetts and Corrodies: Care of the Poor and Sick at St. Leonard's Hospital, York in the Middle Ages* (York: University of York, 1991), pp. 13–15.
62. M. Carlin, 'Medieval English Hospitals', in Lindsay Granshaw and Roy Porter, eds, *The Hospital in History* (London: Routledge, 1989), p. 21.
63. V.C. Medvei and J.L. Thornton, *The Royal Hospital of St Bartholomew's 1123–1973* (London: St Bartholomew's and Contributors, 1974), p. 104.
64. Ibid.
65. G. Whitteridge and V. Stokes, *A Brief History of the Hospital of St Bartholomew, London* (London: The Governors of the Hospital of St. Bartholomew, 1961), p. 13.
66. Maria Lorentzon, 'Mediaeval London: Care of the Sick', *History of Nursing Journal*, 4 (1992/93): 105.

67. F.C. Parsons, *The History of St. Thomas's Hospital* (London: Methuen, 1932), pp. 14–15.
68. Delaunay, *La Médecine*, p. 51.
69. Faye Getz, *Medicine in the English Middle Ages* (Princeton, NJ: Princeton University Press, 1998), pp. 90–1.
70. Andrew Wear, *Knowledge and Practice in English Medicine, 1550–1680* (Cambridge: Cambridge University Press, 2000), p. 24.
71. For biographical information see P. Tutwiler, 'Camillus de Lellis, St', *New Catholic Encyclopedia*, 2nd edn (Detroit: Gale, 2003), II, pp. 914–16. Gale Virtual Reference Library, Gale Canadian Research Knowledge Network, 9 June 2008, http://go.galegroup.com.myaccess.library.utoronto.ca/ps/start.do?p=GVRL&u=utoronto_man.
72. Agnes E. Pavey, *The Story of the Growth of Nursing as an Art, a Vocation and a Profession* (London: Faber & Faber, 1957), pp. 222–3. David Gentilcore, '"Cradle of saints and useful institutions": Health Care and Poor Relief in the Kingdom of Naples', in Ole Peter Grell, Andrew Cunningham and Jon Arrizabalga, eds, *Health Care and Poor Relief in Counter-Reformation Europe* (New York: Routledge, 1999), pp. 139–41.
73. Nutting and Dock, *A History of Nursing*, I, pp. 278–80.
74. Bullough and Bullough, *The Emergence of Modern Nursing*, pp. 60–1.
75. Manuals for women were intended for midwives. Carmen Domínguez-Alcón, *Los cuidados y la profesión enfermera en Espana* (Madrid: Ediciones Pirámide, 1986), pp. 52–7.
76. Luis S. Granjel, *La Medicina Española Renacentista* (Salamanca: Universidad de Salamanca, 1980), p. 126.
77. Brodman, *Charity and Welfare*, p. 189.
78. The hospital's constitution dates from 1525. See Vicenta Ma. Marque de la Platay Fernández, *Mujeres Renacentistas de la Corte de Isabella la Católica* (Madrid: Editorial Castilia, 2005), pp. 127, 130, 134–5.
79. Evelyn B. Kelly, 'The Medical Role of Women: Women as Patients and Practitioners', in Neil Schlager and Josh Lauer, eds, *Science and its Times*, Vol. 3: 1450 to 1699 (Detroit: Gale, 2001), pp. 124–7, Gale Virtual Reference Library, Gale, Canadian Research Knowledge Network, 9 June 2008, http://go.galegroup.com.myaccess.library.utoronto.ca/ps/start.do?p=GVRL&u=utoronto_main.
80. Antonio García Del Moral, *El Hospital Mayor de San Sebastián de Córdoba: cinco siglos de asistencia médico-sanitaria institucional (1363–1816)* (Córdoba: Excma. Diputación Provincial, 1984), pp. 76–7.
81. Jésus Ramos Martinez, *La Salud Pública y El hospital de la Ciudad de Pamplona en el Antiguo Régmen* (Pamplona: Gobierno de Navarra, 1989), p. 302.
82. The term Béguine from the Latin *beguina* was apparently a pejorative term. They were sometimes called *mulieres vulgariter dictae beguinae*. See *Corpus Dictionary of Western Churches*, ed. T.C. O'Brien (Washington: Corpus, 1970), p. 81; Michael Cox, *Handbook of Christian Spirituality*, rev. edn (San Francisco: Harper & Row, 1985), p. 86; Fiona Bowie, introd., *Beguine Spirituality: Mystical Writings of Mechthild of Magdeburg, Beatrice of Nazareth, and Hadewijch of Brabant*, trans. Oliver Davies (New York: Crossroad, 1990), p. 12; Richard William Southern, *Western Society and the Church in the Middle Ages* (Harmondsworth: Penguin, 1970), p. 321.
83. Saskia Murk-Jansen, *Brides in the Desert: The Spirituality of the Beguines* (London: Sarton, Longman & Todd, 1998), p. 23.

84. Bowie, *Beguine Spirituality*, p. 12; Cox, *Handbook of Christian Spirituality*, p. 86.
85. Ernest Gilliat-Smith, 'Beguines & Beghards', in *The Catholic Encyclopedia*, vol. II (New York: Robert Appleton Company, 1907), online edition, Kevin Knight, 2007, http://www.newadvent.org/cathen/02389c.htm.
86. Cited in Penelope Galloway, '"Discreet and Devout Maidens": Women's Involvement in Beguine Communities in Northern France, 1200–1500', in Diane Watt, ed., *Medieval Women in their Communities* (Toronto: University of Toronto Press, 1997), p. 103.
87. Ellen L. Babinsky, 'Béguines', in William N. Kibler and Grover A. Zinn, eds, *Medieval France: An Encyclopedia* (New York and London: Garland, 1995), pp. 106–7.
88. Babinsky, 'Béguines', p. 107.
89. L.J.M. Philippen, *Béguines et béguinages: dossier accompagnant l'exposition Béguines et béguinages en Brabant et dans la province d'Anvers aux Archives générales du Royaume à Bruxelles du 27 octobre au 13 décembre 1994* (Bruxelles: Archives générales du Royaume 1994), p. 83.
90. Walter Simons, *Cities of Ladies: Beguine Communities in Medieval Low Countries 1200–1365* (Philadelphia: University of Pennsylvania Press, 2001), p. 76.
91. 'The Life of Mary Oignies, by Jacques de Vitry', in Elizabeth A. Petroff, *Medieval Women's Visionary Literature* (New York: Oxford University Press, 1986), p. 179; Ranft, *Women and Religious Life*, p. 72.
92. Snodgrass, *Historical Encyclopedia of Nursing*, pp. 150–1.
93. Simons, *Cities of Ladies*, p. 78.
94. Brodman, *Charity and Welfare*, p. 93, n. 85.
95. Hernández Martín, *Historia*, 93.
96. Ranft, *Women and Religious Life*, 107.
97. Ibid.; Mary Elizabeth Perry, 'Beatas and the Inquisition in Early Modern Spain', in Stephen Haliczer, ed., *Inquisition and Society in Early Modern Europe* (London: Croom Helm, 1986), p. 150.
98. Ranft, *Women and Religious Life*, p. 108.
99. Perry, 'Beatas and the Inquisition', pp. 150–3.
100. Ibid., p. 153, n. 36.
101. Neel, 'Origins of the Beguines', in Judith M. Bennett, ed., *Sisters and Workers in the Middle Ages* (Chicago: University of Chicago Press, 1989), p. 242.
102. Neel, 'Origins of the Beguines', p. 343.
103. Claire Guilhem, 'L'Inquisition de la Dévaluation des Discours Féminins', in Bartolomé Bennassar, ed., *L'Inquisition Espagnole XVe–XIXe Siècles* (Paris: Hachette, 1979), pp. 201, 213–16.
104. Jean Imbert, *Histoire des Hôpitaux en France* (Toulouse: Privat, 1982), p. 208.
105. Charmarie J. Blaisdell, 'Angela Merici and the Ursulines', in Richard DeMolen, ed., *Religious Orders of the Catholic Reformation* (New York: Fordham University Press, 1994), pp. 99, 107, 115, 119.
106. Blaisdell, 'Angela Merici and the Ursulines', pp. 121.
107. Jean de Viguerie, 'Une forme novelle de consacrée: enseignantes et hospitalières en France aux XVIIe et XVIIIe siècles', in Danielle Hause-Dubosc and Eliane Viennot, eds, *Femmes et Pouvoirs sous l'Ancien Régime* (Paris: Rivages, 1991), pp. 175–83.
108. Chalumeau, 'L'assistance aux malades pauvres', p. 83.
109. Martin Dinges, 'Health Care and Poor Relief in Regional Southern France in the Counter-Reformation', in Grell et al., eds, *Health Care and Poor Relief*, p. 258.

110. David Hugh Farmer, 'Chantal, Jane Frances de', *The Oxford Dictionary of Saints* (Oxford University Press 2003), Oxford Reference Online, http://www.oxfordreference.com; Susan E. Dinan, *Women and Poor Relief in Seventeenth-Century France: The Early History of the Daughters of Charity* (Aldershot, UK and Burlington, VT: Ashgate, 2006), pp. 26–7.
111. The most recent study of the Sisters of Charity is Susan E. Dinan, *Women and Poor Relief in Seventeenth-Century France*. This chapter was effectively written before Dinan's book was published. Colin Jones has studied the medical work of the Sisters of Charity in the French provinces, primarily Montpellier, in *The Charitable Imperative: Hospitals and Nursing in Ancien Régime and Revolutionary France* (New York and London: Routledge, 1989).
112. See Chapter 4 for a more detailed discussion of the Ladies of Charity, and in particular, Marie de Maupeou Fouquet.
113. Bullough and Bullough, *The Emergence of Modern Nursing*, pp. 70–1; and John E. Ryholt and Francis Ryan, Preface by Amin A. De Tarrrazi, *Vincent de Paul and Louise de Marillac: Rules, Conferences, Writings* (New York: Paulist Press, 1995), p. 41.
114. The most comprehensive biography of St Vincent de Paul remains P. Coste, *Le grand saint du Grand Siècle*, 3 vols (Paris: Desclée et cie Editeurs, 1934).
115. 'Vincent de Paul', in David Hugh Farmer, *The Oxford Dictionary of Saints* (Oxford: Oxford University Press, 2003), Oxford Reference Online, http://www.oxfordreference.com.
116. See Pierre Coste, *Saint Vincent de Paul et les Dames de la Charité* (Paris: Bloud et Gay, 1937) and Ryholt and Ryan, *Vincent de Paul and Louise de Marillac*, pp. 23–4, 40.
117. Ryholt and Ryan, *Vincent de Paul and Louise de Marillac*, p. 41.
118. Vincent de Paul, First Rule, in *Correspondance, Entretiens, Documents*, ed. Pierre Coste (Paris: Librarie Lecoffe, 1920–1926) XIV, p. 126.
119. The original manuscript copy of the regulations was discovered in 1839 in the municipal archives of Chatillon and are dated 1617. The regulations are found in Anne L. Austin, ed., *History of Nursing Source Book* (New York: G.P. Putnam's Sons, 1957), p. 136.
120. Bloch, *L'Assistance*, p. 69.
121. Vincent de Paul, 'On the Vocation of a Daughter of Charity', 5 July 1640, in *Correspondance, Entretiens, Documents*, I, p. 13.
122. Letter of Vincent de Paul to Father Deville, no date, in *Lettres et Conférences de Saint Vincent de Paul* (Suppl.), p. 167.
123. Cited in Bingham, *Ministering Angels*, p. 10.
124. *Règles ou constitutions communes de la congrégation de la Mission* (Paris: A. Le Clere, 1856), ch. VII, art 1.
125. *Conférences de S. Vincent de Paul aux filles de la Charité* (Paris: Pillet et Dumoulin,1881), II, pp. 311–12; *Règles ou constitutions communes*, ch. VII, art. 1.
126. 'On the Service of the Sick', 19 October 1659, in *The Conferences of St Vincent de Paul to the Sisters of Charity*, trans. Joseph Leonard (Westminster, MD: Newman Press, 1952), IV, p. 274.
127. 'On the Vocation', 19 July 1640, *The Conferences*, I, p. 18.
128. 'On the Service of the Sick', *The Conferences*, IV, p. 274.
129. De Marillac, *Ecrits spirituels*, Letter 521, cited in Dinan, *Women and Poor Relief*, p. 104.

130. De Marillac, 'Observations sur les regles: Soeurs employees aux Villages', in *Ecrits spirituels*, p. 727.
131. Colin Jones, 'Perspectives on Poor Relief, Healthcare and the Counter-Reformation in France', in Grell et al., eds, *Health Care and Poor Relief*, p. 232.
132. Bullough and Bullough, *History, Trends, and Politics*, pp. 277–8.
133. 'On the Service of the Sick', IV, p. 276.
134. Jones, 'Perspectives on Poor Relief', pp. 232–3.
135. *Conférences de S. Vincent de Paul aux filles*, I, p. 76.
136. Ibid.
137. *Règles ou constitutions communes*, ch. VII, arts. 1 & 3.
138. *Conférences de S. Vincent de Paul aux filles*, I, p. 76.
139. *Règles particulières aux Soeurs de Paroisses*, 24 August 1659, *Conférences de S. Vincent de Paul aux filles*, II, p. 614.
140. *Conférences de S. Vincent de Paul aux filles*, I, p. 55, No. 8, 14 June 1642; Vincent de Paul repeated these orders on several occasions. See I, p. 193, No. 19, 29 January 1645; *Règles ou constitutions communes,* ch. IV, art. 4, 346; No. 81, 2 December 1657.
141. *Règles particulières aux Soeurs de Paroisses*, ch XVIII, art. 4; *Conférences de S. Vincent de Paul aux filles*, II, p. 623.
142. Jean de Viguerie, 'Une forme novelle de consacrée', in Hause-Dubosc and Viennot, eds, *Femmes et Pouvoirs*, p. 182.
143. Domínguez-Alcón, *Los cuidados*, p. 88.
144. Ibid., p. 90.
145 Pavey, *The Story of the Growth of Nursing*, 223–4; Magaglio Riccardo, *Una patrizia genovese antesignana della moderna assistenza sociale: cenni biografici sulla serva di Dio Virginia Centurione Bracelli (1587–1651)* (Genoa: AGIS, 1972).
146. 'Catherine of Genoa', *The Oxford Dictionary of Saints*, ed. David Hugh Farmer. (Oxford: Oxford University Press 2003), Oxford Reference Online, http://www.oxfordreference.com; Jon Arrizabalaga, John Henderson and Roger French, eds, *The Great Pox: The French Disease in Renaissance Europe* (New Haven, CT: Yale University Press, 1997), pp. 145–7. Arrizabalaga et al. cite similar examples for the founding of hospitals in Naples and Venice. For a biography of Catherine of Genoa, see F. von Hugel, *The Mystical Element of Religion as studied in St. Catherine of Genoa and her Friends,* 2 vols (1908, 1961 and 1999). The 1999 edition contains a new introduction by Michael Downey.
147. Arrizabalaga et al., *The Great Pox*, pp. 158–60.
148. Ibid., p. 165.

7. The 'Irregular' Female Healer in Early Modern Europe: A Variety of Practitioners

1. See Chapter 2 for detailed information about medical licensing and its impact on female healers.
2. See the works by Margaret Pelling, Doreen Evenden Nagy and Roy and Dorothy Porter in particular.
3. Roy Porter, 'Quacks and Doctors', *The Listener*, 23 June 1983: 14–15. Porter states that nurses and midwives were excepted from being excluded from medical practice. Others were excluded from the higher education necessary to enter the medical profession until the late nineteenth century.

4. Porter, 'Quacks and Doctors', p. 15.
5. Roy Porter, 'Female Quacks in the Consumer Society', *History of Nursing Journal*, 3(1)(1990–91): 9.
6. Lucinda McCray Beier, *Sufferers and Healers: The Experience of Illness in Seventeenth Century England* (London and New York: Routledge and Kegan Paul, 1987), p. 4.
7. Beier, *Sufferers and Healers*, p. 5.
8. Margaret Pelling (with Frances White), *Medical Conflicts in Early Modern London: Patronage, Physicians and Irregular Practitioners, 1550–1640* (Oxford: Clarendon, 1993), pp. 189, 192–4.
9. Annals of the London College of Physicians, 8 July 1622, 153–4, cited in Margaret Pelling, 'Knowledge Common and Acquired: The Education of Unlicensed Medical Practitioners in Early Modern London', in Vivian Nutton and Roy Porter, eds, *The History of Medical Education in Britain* (Amsterdam: Rodopi, 1995), pp. 268–9.
10. Margaret Pelling, 'Occupational Diversity: Barber Surgeons and the Trades of Norwich', *Bulletin of the History of Medicine*, 56 (1982): 508–11.
11. Enrique Perdiguero, 'The Popularization of Medicine during the Spanish Enlightenment', in Roy Porter, ed., *The Popularization of Medicine* (London: Routledge, 1992), pp. 166–7.
12. See Roy Porter, 'Introduction', in Porter, ed., *Popularization of Medicine*, pp. 1–16 for a discussion of popular and professional medicine.
13. Charles Williams, *The Masters, Wardens and Assistants of the Gild of Barber Surgeons of Norwich, from the Year 1439 to 1723* (Norwich: 1900), p. 5.
14. Salisbury Public Documents, ccc, 75, October 1635, cited in Alice Clark, *Working Life of Women in the Seventeenth Century* (London: G. Routledge & Sons, Ltd; New York: E.P. Dutton & Co., 1919, 1968), p. 259.
15. Roy Porter and Dorothy Porter, *Patient's Progress: Doctors and Doctoring in Eighteenth Century England* (Oxford: Polity Press, 1989), p. 177. Porter's research has demonstrated that there were many females who made a living from practising some sort of medicine. Although some of these practitioners were quacks, many were not.
16. William Clowes, *Selected Writings of William Clowes*, ed. F.N.L. Poynter (London: Harvey & Blythe, 1948), pp. 22–3. But see, for example, Doreen A. Evenden, who argues that 'most studies of English medical practitioners have yielded very little information about women who practiced as licensed physicians or surgeons in the seventeenth century'. 'Gender Differences in the Licensing and Practice of Female and Male Surgeons in Early Modern England', *Medical History*, 42 (1998): 194–216.
17. Hertford County Records, Vol. 1, 435, 1698 cited in Clark, *Working Life of Women*, p. 251.
18. *Calendar of State Papers: Domestic Series, Commonwealth, 1649–1660*, M.A.E. Green (London: Longman, 1875–1886), IX, 1656, p. 23.
19. Cited in Alison Klairmont-Lingo, 'The Rise of Medical Practitioners in Sixteenth Century France: The Case of Lyon and Montpellier', unpublished PhD dissertation, University of California, Berkeley (1980), p. 218, n. 87.
20. Klairmont-Lingo, 'Women Healers', p. 89.
21. Klairmont-Lingo, 'The Rise of Medical Practitioners', pp. 90, 91, n. 219.
22. Gianna Pomata, *Contracting a Cure: Patients, Healers and the Law in Early Modern Bologna* (Baltimore and London: Johns Hopkins University Press, 1998), p. 77.
23. Edouard Nicaise, *La Grande Chirurgie de Guy de Chauliac* (Paris: F. Alcan, 1890), p. lxii.

24. Cited in Laurence Brockliss and Colin Jones, *The Medical World of Early Modern France* (Oxford: Clarendon Press, 1997), p.174.
25. Brockliss and Jones, *The Medical World*, p. 262.
26. Pierre-Jacques Brillon and Antoine-François Prost de Royer, *Dictionnaire des arrêts: ou, Jurisprudence ...*, 6 vols (Paris: Chez, Guillaume Cavelier, Pere, Michel Brunet, Nicolas Gosselin, 1727), III, p. 337.
27. Matthew Ramsey, 'From *Expert* to *Spécialiste*: The Conception of Specialization in Eighteenth- and Nineteenth-Century French Surgery', *History of Ideas in Surgery: Proceedings of the 17th International Symposium for the Comparative History of Medicine – East and West* (Tokyo, Japan: 1997), p. 77.
28. Toby Gelfand, 'Medical Professionals and Charlatans: The Comité de Salubrité enquête of 1790–91', *Social History*, 11 (1978): 62–3.
29. Roy Porter, *Health for Sale: Quackery in England, 1660–1850* (Manchester and New York: Manchester University Press, 1989), p. 3, n. 8.
30. Gelfand, 'Medical Professionals', p. 63.
31. Roy Porter, *Quacks: Fakers and Charlatans in English Medicine* (Stroud: Tempus, 2000), p. 12.
32. Collection of Advertisements (British Library, 551 a. 59), cited in Porter, 'Female Quacks in the Consumer Society', p. 6.
33. Roy Porter, 'Female Quacks in the Consumer Society', pp. 4–5.
34. *Bath Journal*, 16 January 1756, cited in Porter and Porter, *Patient's Progress*, p. 177.
35. Porter and Porter, *Patient's Progress*, p. 83. The *Gentleman's Magazine* was started in 1731 and continued into the early twentieth century. Its focus was British news but it did have a foreign affairs section, as well as reports from Parliament, biographies, poems, essays and a register of current publications. For further information about the *Gentleman's Magazine* and its coverage of health-related issues, see Roy Porter, 'Lay Medical Knowledge in the Eighteenth Century: The Evidence of the *Gentleman's Magazine*', *Medical History*, 29 (1985): 138–68. Porter correctly argues that the magazine took a middle-of-the-road, commonsense view of the issues (p. 141).
36. *Gentleman's Magazine*, August 1736.
37. Frederick F. Cartwright, *The Development of Modern Surgery from 1830* (London: Barker, 1967), p. 146.
38. *Gentleman's Magazine*, May 1738.
39. *Gentleman's Magazine*, October 1736.
40. Ibid.; Cartwright, *The Development of Modern Surgery*, p. 147.
41. *Gentleman's Magazine*, August 1736.
42. David Hartley, *Ten Cases of Persons Who Have Taken Mrs. Stephens's Medicines for the Stone* (London: S. Harding, 1738), p. 37.
43. Hartley, *Ten Cases*, pp. 38–9.
44. *Gentleman's Magazine*, October 1738.
45. Arthur J. Viseltear, 'Joanna Stephens and the Eighteenth-Century Lithontriptics: A Misplaced Chapter in the History of Therapeutics', *Bulletin of the History of Medicine*, 42 (1968): pp. 199–200.
46. This is particularly true of the older writings such as C.J.S. Thompson, *The Quacks of Old London* (New York: Bretano, 1928), pp. 295–7; Eric Jameson, *The Natural History of Quackery* (London: Michael Joseph, 1961), p. 172; E. Lee Stohl, 'Parliament Hoodwinked by Joanna Stephens', *Surgery, Gynecology and Obstetrics,* 116 (1963): 509–11. Even Roy Porter refers to Stephens in addition to Mapp as 'the

primary quacks of the age' whose motives were primarily monetary. Stephens, he argued, clinched 'the best deal ever by a quack in English history'. Porter, *Health for Sale*, pp. 34, 83. Eric J. Trimmer initially refers to Stephens as a quack, but then argues that empiric is more accurate. He writes: 'In an account of Miss Joanna Stephens I recently referred to her as a quack and there is no doubt there was a fair amount of quackery in her nature. On more mature reflection I feel she possibly was an empiric at heart and had quackery as it were, forced upon her.' Eric J. Trimmer, 'Medical Folklore and Quackery', *Folklore*, 76(3) (autumn 1965): 168. The only modern writer to give Stephens unqualified positive press is the medical historian Arthur J. Viseltear who provides the most detailed and careful analysis of the case to date. See 'Joanna Stephens and the Eighteenth-Century Lithontriptics'.

47. Morand was also a member of the Royal Society of London and the Academy of Bologna. See François Saveur Morand, *An account of the remedy for the stone: lately published in England, according to an act of Parliament, assigning a reward of 5000£ to the discoverer. Extracted from the examinations of this remedy, given into the Royal Academy of Sciences at Paris* (London: H. Woodfall, 1741).
48. Morand, *An account of the remedy for the stone*, p. 190.
49. Ibid., pp. 193–4.
50. Viseltear, 'Joanna Stephens and the Eighteenth-Century Lithontriptics', p. 199.
51. David Hartley, *Ten Cases*; see also the supplement to John Rutty's *An Account of Some Experiments and Observations on Mrs. Stephens's Medicine for Dissolving the Stone*... written by Stephen Hales and David Hartley (London: P. Manby, 1742).
52. David Hartley, *A View of the Present Evidence for and against Mrs. Stephens's Medicines, as a Solvent for the Stone, Containing a Hundred and Fifty-Five Cases with Some Experiments and Observations* (London: S. Harding et al., 1739).
53. *Le Mercure Galant*, published between 1672 and 1710, was the leading woman's review for news and culture. *Le Mercure Galant* and its supplement, *Extraordinaire du Mercure* (1678–85), featured important articles on a variety of medical subjects from the history of medicine to a discussion of diseases and their cures. Articles in the *Mercure* provide a multiplicity of perspectives from the academic to the popular. See Monique Vincent, *Le Mercure Galant* (Paris: Honoré Champion, 2005), Chapter 2.
54. *Le Mercure Galant*, September 1685 and July 1700.
55. Archives de la Bastille, dossier no. 10590, Bibliothèque de l'Arsenal, printed by Maurice Boutry, 'Les tribulations d'une guérisseuse au XVIIIe siècle', *La Chronique Médicale*, 9 (1905): 289–97.
56. Jean Verdier, *La Jurisprudence de la Médecine en France ou Trait historique et juridique*, 2 vols (Alençon: Malassis le jeune, 1762–63), I, p. 620.
57. Marilyn Bailey Ogilvie and Joy Dorothy Harvey, *The Biographical Dictionary of Women in Science: Pioneering Lives from Ancient Times to the Mid-20th Century*, 2 vols (London: Routledge, 2000), II, p. 129.
58. *Cahiers de doléances du Bailliage de Troyes*, Appendix 14, 32, cited in Wendy Gibson, *Women in Seventeenth Century France* (New York: St Martin's Press, 1989), p. 120, n. 62.
59. William Bedell, *A True Relation of the Life and Death of the Right Reverend William Bedell, Lord Bishop of Kilmore*, ed. Thomas Wharton Jones (Westminster: Camden Society, 1872), p. 2.
60. Timothy Rogers, *The character of a good woman, both in a single and marry'd state* (London, 1697), pp. 42–3.

61. Cited in John Lavicourt Anderson, *Life of Thomas Ken: Bishop of Bath and Wells*, (London: John Murray, 1854), p. 181.
62. Ralph Josselin, *The Diary of Ralph Josselin 1616–1683*, ed. Alan MacFarlane (London: Oxford University Press for the British Academy, 1976), pp. 163–4.
63. Adam Martindale, *The Life of Adam Martindale written by himself* (1632), ed. Richard Parkinson (London: Chetham Society, 1845), p. 21.
64. Hobbes is cited in Porter, 'Female Quacks in the Consumer Society', p. 6; Henry Fielding, *Journal of a Voyage to Lisbon* (Lisbon: Dent, 1864), p. 24.
65. Anthony Walker, her husband, published her diary as *The holy life of Mrs* Elizabeth Walker *giving a modest and short account of her exemplary piety and charity* (London, 1690), pp. 11, 67, 72, 89, 178.
66. Walker, *The holy life*, p. 67.
67. Ibid., p. 178.
68. Ibid., pp. 179–80.
69. Ibid., pp. 177–8.
70. Ibid., p. 35.
71. Ibid., p. 55.
72. Ibid., p. 94.
73. See Chapter 1 for details and Paul O. Kristeller, 'Learned Women of Early Modern Italy: Humanists and University Scholars', in Patricia H. Labalme, ed., *Beyond their Sex: Learned Women of the European Past* (New York: New York University Press, 1980), pp. 102–3, n. 52.
74. A. Rebière, *Les femmes dans la science* (Paris: Nony Rebière, 1894), p. 21.
75. Kate Campbell Hurd-Mead, *A History of Women in Medicine from the Earliest of Times to the Beginning of the Nineteenth Century* (Haddam: The Haddam Press: 1938), p. 431.
76. E.A. Pace, 'Elena Lucrezia Piscopia Cornaro', in *The Catholic Encyclopedia*, ed. Kevin Knight (1904; New York: Robert Appleton Company, 2003), vol. 4, http://www.newadvent.org/cathen/04373b.htm.
77. Margaret Alic, *Hypatia's Heritage* (Boston: Beacon Press, 1986), p. 135.
78. See Gianna Pomata, 'Practising between Earth and Heaven: Women Healers in Seventeenth-Century Bologna', *Dynamis*, 19 (1999): 119–43.
79. Ibid., p. 121.
80. Ibid., p. 124.
81. C.H. Fialon, 'Quelques prospectus charlatanesques du XVIIIe siècle', *Bulletin de la Société de la pharmacie*, 23 (1921); cited in Brockliss and Jones, *The Medical World*, p. 627.
82. Their numbers grew by 50 per cent between 1310 and 1335. Cited in James Brodman, *Charity and Welfare: Hospitals and the Poor in Medieval Catalonia* (Philadelphia: University of Pennyslvania Press, 1998), p. 90.
83. Pomata, 'Practising between Earth and Heaven', p. 130.
84. ASB Coll. Med. Bb. 342, 346, 224 cited in ibid., p. 131.
85. Georges Boulinier, author of a recent article on Biheron, who has conducted extensive archival research on her life and work, claims that her name is Marie Marguerite and not Cathérine. See George Boulinier, 'Une femme anatomiste au siècle des Lumières: Marie Marguerite Biheron (1719–1795)', *Histoire des sciences médicales*, 435(4)(2001): 411–23.
86. The fullest study of the life and work of Anna Morandi Manzolini in English is Rebecca Messenger, 'Waxing Poetic: Anna Morandi Manzolini's Anatomical Sculptures', *Configurations*, 9(1) (2001): 65–97. An older but still useful chapter is

'Anna Morandi Manzolini (1716–1774) Wife of Giovanni Manzolini (1712–1760)', in Josephine Rich, *Women behind Men of Medicine* (New York: Julian Messner, 1967), pp. 37–44.

87. Marilyn Bailey Ogilvie, 'Laura Maria Caterina Bassi', in Louise S. Grinstein, Rose K. Rose and Miriam Rafailovich, eds, *Women in Chemistry and Physics: A Biobibliographical Sourcebook* (Westport, CT: Greenwood, 1993), p. 308.
88. Ibid., p. 307.
89. Messenger, 'Waxing Poetic', p. 69.
90. Ogilvie, 'Laura Maria Caterina Bassi', p. 308.
91. Messenger, 'Waxing Poetic', p. 71; Maurizio Armaroli, ed., *Le cere anatomiche bolognesi del Settecento* (Bologna: Università degli Studi di Bologna, 1979), p. 33.
92. Messenger, 'Waxing Poetic', p. 75.
93. Rich, 'Anna Morandi Manzolini', p. 44.
94. Shane Agin, '"Comment se font les enfans": Sex Education and the Preservation of Innocence in Eighteenth-Century France', *Modern Language Notes*, 117 (202): 36.
95. Friedrich Melchior, Freiherr von Grimm, *Correspondance, littéraire, philosophique et critique par Grimm, Diderot, Raynal, Meister etc; revue sur les textes originaux, comprenant outre ce qui a été publié à diverses époques, les fragments supprimés en 1813 par la censure, les parties inédites conservées à la bibliothèque ducale de Gotha et à l'Arsenal à Paris. Notices, notes, table générale par Maurice Tourneux* (Paris: Garnier Frères, 1879), IX, p. 275.
96. Denis Diderot, *Correspondance* (Paris : Éditions de Minuit, 1955–1970), XII, p. 164.
97. Ibid., pp. 210–11.
98. Mélina Lipinska, *Les Femmes et le progrès des sciences médicales* (Paris: Masson et Cie), p. 67.
99. Laura Lynn Windsor, *Women in Medicine: An Encyclopedia* (Santa Barbara: ABC-CLIO, 2002), p. 27; Londa Schiebinger, *The Mind has no Sex? Women in the Origins of Modern Science* (Cambridge, MA: Harvard University Press), pp. 28–9; Lipinska, *Les Femmes et le progrès*, pp. 65–7.
100. Vittoria Ottani and Gabriella Giuliani Piccari, 'L'opera di Anna Morandi Manzolini nella ceroplastica anatomica bolognese', in *Alma mater studiorum: La presenza femminile dal XVIII al XX secolo. Ricerche sul rapport donna/cultura universitaria nell'Ateneo bolognese* (Bologna: Cooperativa Libraria Universitaria Editrice Bologna [CLUEB], 1988), p. 82.
101. Gabriella Berti Logan, 'Women and the Practice of Medicine and Teaching of Medicine in Bologna in the Eighteenth and Early Nineteenth Centuries', *Bulletin of the History of Medicine*, 77 (3) (Fall 2003): 510.
102. See Paula Findlen, 'Science as a Career in Enlightenment Italy: The Strategies of Laura Bassi', *Isis*, 84 (1993): 441–69, for a study of Bassi's career as a female scientist.
103. Schiebinger, *The Mind has no Sex?* pp. 15–16.
104. Windsor, *Women in Medicine*, p. 26; Ogilvie, 'Laura Maria Caterina Bassi', p. 24.
105. Windsor, *Women in Medicine*, pp. 26–7. The recent article by Logan, 'Women and the practice of Medicine', demonstrates the important role and contribution to medicine and teaching played by Bassi, Manzolini, Maria Dalle Donne (an educator of midwives at the University of Bologna, who lived from 1778 to 1842) and other Italian women from the mid-eighteenth to the end of the nineteenth century.

106. Ogilvie, 'Laura Maria Caterina Bassi', p. 25.
107. Cited in ibid., p. 27.
108. Laura Bassi Veratti, *Alcune lettere di Laura Bassi Veratti al Dottor Flaminio Scarselli* (Bologna: Tipi della volpe al sassi, 1836), pp. 29, 30.
109. Elizabeth Bury recorded her life and works in her diary, *An account of the life and death of Mrs. Elizabeth Bury* (Bristol: J. Penn, 1720), pp. 1, 179.
110. Bury, *An account*, p. 34.
111. Ibid., p. 179.
112. Beier, *Sufferers and Healers*, p. 5.
113. Margaret Hoby, *The Diary of Lady Margaret Hoby 1599–1605,* ed. Dorothy M. Meads (London: Routledge, 1930), pp. 49–50.
114. Kim Walker, *Women Writers of the Renaissance* (New York: Twayne, 1992), p. 39.
115. Linda Pollock, *With Faith and Physic: The Life of a Tudor Gentlewoman, Lady Grace Mildmay, 1552–1620* (New York: St Martin's Press, 1993), p. 1. Pollock has transcribed approximately 40 per cent of Mildmay's medical receipts.
116. Cited in Pollock, *With Faith and Physic*, p. 124, n. 5. Lady Grace Mildmay's recipes are discussed in Pollock's book as well as in a recent article by Jennifer Wynne Hellwarth, who uses Pollock's transcriptions as the basis of her publication. See especially Hellwarth, '"Be unto me as a precious ointment": Lady Grace Mildmay, Sixteenth-Century Female Practitioner', *Dynamis*, 19 (1999): 106–11.
117. Cited in Pollock, *With Faith and Physik*, p. 97
118. The most recent edition of the diary is edited by Joanna Moody. See Margaret Hoby, *The Private Life of an Elizabethan Lady: The Diary of Lady Margaret Hoby, 1599–1605,* ed. Joanna Moody (Stroud, Gloucestershire: Sutton Press, 1998). The original manuscript is housed in the British Library Manuscripts Department, London (BL MS Egerton, 2614). An earlier edition of the diary is Meads's 1930 publication, cited above. Both editors have left the original spelling. I have modernized it.
119. Antonia Fraser, *The Weaker Vessel: Women's Lot in Seventeenth Century England* (London: Methuen, 1985), p. 6.
120. Hoby, *Diary*, ed. Moody, p. 13.
121. Hoby, *Diary,* ed. Meads, p. 50.
122. Paul Slack, 'Hoby, Margaret Lady (1571–1633)', in C.S. Nicholls, ed., *The Dictionary of National Biography: Missing Persons* (Oxford: Oxford University Press, 1994), pp. 318–19. For biographical information about Margaret Hoby, see Beier, *Sufferers and Healers*, pp. 218–24. Beier focuses on Margaret's own illnesses and her self-medication.
123. Hoby, *Diary*, ed. Meads, pp. 168, 170, 180.
124. See entries for 4, 5, 6 January and 1, 2, 3, 4, 5, 6 February 1599 in Hoby, *Diary*, ed. Moody, pp. 58–60.
125. Monday 17, 1599, in ibid., p. 18.
126. Ibid., 58, n. 114.
127. 3 January 1599, in ibid., p. 58.
128. 26 July 1600 in Hoby, *Diary*, ed. Meads, p. 184.
129. Dacres was the daughter of Lord Thomas Dacres and Elizabeth Labourn, daughter of Sir James Labourn, a knight. She was married to Philip Howard, Earl of Arundel. *The Lives of Philip Howard, Earl of Arundel, and of Anne Dacres, his wife, edited from the original mss. By the Duke of Norfolk* (London: Hurst and Blackett, 1857), p. 168. See Chapter 8 for information on the family's recipe book compiled by Anne and other members of her family.

130. *Lives*, p. 212.
131. Ibid., pp. 213–14.
132. Lucy Apsley Hutchinson, *Memoirs of the Life of Colonel Hutchinson written by his wife Lucy*, intro. François Guizot (London: J.M. Dent, 1908), p. 146, n. 1.
133. Ibid., pp. 13–14.
134. Ibid., p. 404.
135. Ibid., pp. 145–6.
136. Ibid., p. 12.
137. *The Memoirs of Anne, Lady Halkett and Ann, Lady Fanshawe*, ed. and intro. John Loftis (Oxford: Clarendon, 1979) p. 55.
138. Ibid., p. 56.
139. George Ballard, *Memoirs of several ladies of Great Britain who have been celebrated for their writings or skill in the learned languages, arts and sciences* (Oxford: W. Jackson, 1752), p. 371.
140. Luis García-Ballester, Michael McVaugh and Augustin Rubio Vela, *Medical Licensing and Learning in Fourteenth Century Valencia* (Philadelphia: American Philosophical Society, 1989), p. 26.
141. Compared with English language studies of women in other European countries, Spain has received scant attention. See Marilyn Stone and Carmen Benito-Vessels, *Women at Work in Spain from the Middle Ages to Early Modern Times* (New York: Peter Lang, 1998), for an example of an attempt to redress this lacuna.
142. Brodman, *Charity and Welfare*, p. 91.
143. Ibid., p. 92.
144. García-Ballester et al., *Medical Licensing*, pp. 21–32.
145. Joseph Pérez, *The Spanish Inquisition: A History*, trans. Janet Lloyd (New Haven and London: Yale University Press, 2005), p. 44.
146. Pedro Aznar Cardona, *Expulsión justificada del los Moriscos espanoles y suma de las excelencias christianas de nuestro Rey D. Felipe tercero deste nombre* (Huesca: Pedro Cabarte, 1612), pp. 32, 36 and quoted in Mercedes Garcia Arenal, *Los moriscos*, (Madrid: Editoria Nacional, 1975), pp. 230, 233.
147. Mary Elizabeth Perry, 'Weaving Clio and the Moriscas of Early Modern Spain', in Susan D. Amusen and Adele Seef, eds, *Attending to Early Modern Women* (Newark: University of Delaware Press, 1998), p. 59; Pérez, *The Spanish Inquisition*, p. 49.
148. Pérez, *The Spanish Inquisition*, p. 50.
149. Perry, 'Weaving Clio and the Moriscas', p. 59.
150. AHN, libro 989, f. 21 vo and AHN libro 990, f. 372, cited in Jacqueline Fournel-Guérin, 'La femme morisque en Aragon', in *Les Morisques et Leur Temps Table Ronde International*, 4–7 July 1981, Montpellier (Paris: Editions du Centre National de la Recherche Scientifique, 1983), p. 526.
151. Historical Archives of Madrid, 'Causas de fe', cited in Ana Labarta, 'La Mujer Morisca: Sus Actitivades', in María J. Viguera, ed., *La Mujer en Al-Andalus. Reflejos historicos de su actividad y categorías sociales* (Madrid: Ediciones de la Universidad Autónoma, 1989), p. 222.
152. Appendix 2, document 1, *Cortes*, cited in García-Ballester et al., *Medical Licensing*, p. 27.
153. García-Ballester, Roger French and Jon Arrizabalaga, eds, *Practical Medicine from Salerno to the Black Death* (Cambridge: Cambridge University Press, 1994), p. 367.
154. For details, see Chapter 1.

155. James M. Anderson, *Daily Life during the Spanish Inquisition* (Westport, CT: Greenwood, 2002), pp. 90–1.

8. Motherly Medicine: Domestic Healers and Apothecaries

1. Keith Thomas, *Medicine and the Decline of Magic* (Harmondsworth: Penguin, 1971), p. 14.
2. Andrew Wear, *Knowledge and Practice in English Medicine, 1550–1680* (Cambridge: Cambridge University Press, 2000), p. 22.
3. See Wellcome MSS 160, 751, 2323, 2844, 3082, 3834. Although mother to daughter transmission is the most common, one example of male transmission is found in Wellcome MS 579. Wellcome Library Manuscripts, Wellcome Library, London. Subsequent references to these MSS are cited in the text.
4. Olivier de Serres was the author of *Le Théâtre d'agriculture et mesnage des champs* (1606; Arles: Actes Sud, 1997). This work was commissioned by the Duc de Sully, Prime Minister under Henri IV. It summarized forty years of experience as an innovative agriculturalist. De Serres brought the silkworm to France, and practised crop rotation long before the British and the Dutch. See, Maguelonne Toussaint-Samat, *History of Food* (Oxford: Blackwell, 1994), p. 612.
5. De Serres, *Le Théâtre d'agriculture*, p. 1248.
6. Vives's book was read across Europe in the sixteenth century. It was translated into French in 1542. Susan Broomhall, *Women's Medical Work in Early Modern France* (Manchester and New York: Manchester University Press, 2004), p. 138. This citation is from the French edition of that year. *Livre de l'institution de la femme chrestienne*, trans. Pierre de Changy (Paris: Jacques Kerver, 1542), p. 168.
7. For a list of manuscripts examined and the most commonly cited ailments, see the Bibliography at the end of the book.
8. In the few extant letters written by Madame de Grignan, she does not discuss her health or personal issues. Unfortunately, her letters to her mother have not been found. One biographer of Madame de Sévigné seems to think that they were intentionally destroyed. See Frances Mossiker, *Madame de Sévigné: A Life and Letters* (New York: Alfred A. Knopf, 1983), p. 77.
9. See Mary Elizabeth Perry, 'Las mujeres y su trabajo curativo en Sevilla, siglos XVI y XVII', in María Jesús Matilla and Margarita Ortega, eds, *El trabajo de las mujeres: siglos XVI–XX*, VI, *Jornadas de Investigación Interdisciplinaria sobre la Mujer* (Universidad Autónoma de Madrid, 1987), pp. 40–50.
10. Mary Elizabeth Perry, 'Weaving Clio and the Moriscas of Early Modern Spain', in Susan D. Amusen and Adele Seef, eds, *Attending to Early Modern Women* (Newark: University of Delaware Press, 1998), p. 58.
11. Mary Elizabeth Perry, *Gender and Disorder in Early Modern Seville* (Princeton, NJ: Princeton University Press, 1990), pp. 20–1.
12. Very little is known about Juan de Avignón. See Rowena Hernández Múzquiz, 'Avignón, Juan de', in *The late Medieval Age of Crisis and Renewal 1300–1500: A Biographical Dictionary*, ed. Clayton J. Drees (Westport, CT and London: Greenwood, 2001), pp. 24–5.
13. Perry, 'Weaving Clio', pp. 59–60.
14. Jennifer K. Stine, 'Opening Closets: The Discovery of Household Medicine in Early Modern England', unpublished PhD dissertation, Stanford University (1996), p. iv. Stine examined some 113 bound manuscript recipes from the seventeenth century held in various libraries including the Wellcome and British

Libraries in London, the Folger Library in Washington, DC and the Lambeth Palace archives, also in London.

15. Mary Chamberlain, *Old Wives' Tales: Their History, Remedies and Spells* (London: Virago, 1981), p. 68.
16. Lucille B. Pinto, 'The Folk Practice of Gynecology and Obstetrics in the Middle Ages', *Bulletin of the History of Medicine*, 47 (1973): 513.
17. Cited in Elaine E. Whitaker, 'Reading the Paston Letters Medically', *English Language Notes* (September 1993): 21. Whitaker cites the Paston letters from Norman Davis, ed., *Paston Letters and Papers of the Fifteenth Century* (Oxford: Published for the Early English Text Society by the Oxford University Press, 2004–05), III, p. 389, and Letter 898, in James Gairdner, ed., *The Paston Letters* (London, 1900–01), p. 1019.
18. Letter No. 70, Margaret Paston to John Paston II, 28 January 1475, in Diane Watt, *The Paston Women, Selected Letters* (Cambridge: D.S. Brewer, 2004), p. 109; Letter No. 69, Margaret Paston to Sir James Gloys, 1473, in ibid., p. 147. For more information on the Paston women and their healing practices, see Elaine E. Whitaker, 'Reading the Paston Letters Medically'.
19. Letter No. 22, Margaret Paston to John Paston I, 28 September 1443, cited in Watt, *The Paston Women*, p. 47.
20. Letter No. 490, Margaret Paston to John Paston, 8 June 1464, cited in Gairdner, *The Paton Letters*, and Letter No. 177 in Davis, *Paston Letters and Papers*.
21. Stine, 'Opening Closets', p. 17. She noted that many more recipes existed but have been lost as they were written down on scraps of paper and not bound.
22. Ibid., p. 14.
23. See Linda Pollock, *With Faith and Physic: The Life of a Tudor Gentlewoman, Lady Grace Mildmay, 1552–1620* (London: Collins & Brown, 1993); Raymond A. Anselment, '"The Want of health": An Early Eighteenth-Century Self-Portrait of Sickness', *Literature and Medicine*, 15(2) (1996): 225–43; and Leonard Guthrie, 'The Lady Sedley's Receipt Book, 1686 and other Seventeenth-Century Receipt Books', *Proceedings of the Royal Society of Medicine*, 6, 'Section of the History of Medicine' (1913): 150–70.
24. Things are changing rapidly with respect to the publication of English recipe books written in the seventeenth century. See Elizabeth Spiller, Betty S. Travitsky and Anne Lake Prescott, eds, *Seventeenth-Century English Recipe Books: Cooking, Physic and Chirugery in the Works of W.M. and Queen Henrietta Maria, and of Mary Tillinghast* (Burlington, VT: Ashgate, 2008), a vital contribution to the history of domestic medicine, cookery and receipt collection. It includes facsimiles of the recipe books written by Mary Tillinghast and Aletheia Talbot in addition to commentaries about the receipts and biographies of these women. The work is Volume 4 in the growing series of *The Early Modern Englishwoman: A Facsimile Library of Essential Works*.
25. Roy Porter and Dorothy Porter, *Patient's Progress: Doctors and Doctoring in Eighteenth-Century England* (Oxford: Polity Press, 1989), pp. 32–3.
26. Martindale was a Presbyterian minister in Roseterne, Cheshire. See Adam Martindale, *Life of Adam Martindale Written by Himself*, 1632, ed. the Reverend Richard Parkinson (Printed for the Chetham Society, 1845), p. 21.
27. Stine, 'Opening Closets', p. iv.
28. Markham (1568?–1637) wrote books on horses, husbandry, military discipline and country sports in addition to his *English Housewife*. For a modern edition of the book with an informative introduction, see Michael R. Best, *The English Housewife* (Kingston and Montreal: McGill Queens, 1986).

29. Gervase Markham, *Countrey Contentements, in Two Bookes ...The Second intituled, The English Housewife* (London, 1615), pp. 2–4.
30. Ibid., p. 4.
31. Timothy Rogers, *The Character of a Good Woman Both in a Single and Marry'd State Occasion'd by the Decease of Mrs Elizabeth Dunton Who Died May 28, 1697* (London, 1697), pp. 42–3.
32. Lucinda McCray Beier, 'In Sickness and in Health: A Seventeenth Century Family's Experience', in Roy Porter, ed., *Patients and Practitioners: Lay Perceptions of Medicine in Pre-Industrial Society* (Cambridge: Cambridge University Press, 1985), p. 29.
33. Anne Clifford, *The Diary of Anne Clifford, 1616–1619: A Critical Edition*, ed. Katherine O. Acheson (New York: Garland, 1995), p. xxii.
34. Ibid., May 1616, p. 47.
35. Kim Walker, *Women Writers of the Renaissance* (New York: Twayne, 1992), p. 33.
36. Brilliana Harley, Letter xxxvi, 'For my dear son Mr. Edward Harley in Magdeline Hall, Oxford', 26 April 1639, in *Letters of the Lady Brilliana Harley*, ed. Thomas Taylor Lewis (London: Camden Society, 1854), p. 46.
37. Harley, Letter xxxvii, 10 May 1649, ibid., p. 47.
38. The full title of Sowerby's book is *The Ladies Dispensatory, containing the Nature, Virtues, and Qualities of all Herbs and Simples usefull in Physick, reduced into a Methodical order, for their more ready use on any Sicknesse, or other accident of the Body, the like never published in English.*
39. Guthrie, 'Lady Sedley's Receipt Book', p. 163.
40. Sarah Fell, *The Household Account Book of Sarah Fell of Swarthmoor Hall*, ed. Norman Penney (Cambridge: Cambridge University Press, 1921), p. 95.
41. Charles E. Rosenberg, 'Medical Text and Social Context: Explaining William Buchan's Domestic Medicine', *Bulletin of the History of Medicine and Allied Sciences*, 57(1) (1982): 22–42. See C.J. Lawrence, 'William Buchan: Medicine Laid Open', *Medical History*, 19 (1975): 20–35 for details of Buchan's career.
42. Lawrence, 'William Buchan', pp. 21–2.
43. Ibid., p. 27.
44. These include *A new compendious dispensatory: or, a select body of the most useful, accurate, and elegant medicines, both official and extemporaneous, for the several disorders incident to the human body, to which ... is added ... a ... tables of diseases, with remedies* (London: T. Cadell, 1769); *The modern practice of physic, or, A method of judiciously treating the several disorders incident to the human body: together with a recital of their causes, symptoms, diagnostics, prognostics, and the regimen necessary to be observed in regard of them. With a variety of efficacious and elegant extemporaneous prescriptions, adapted to each particular case and circumstance*, 2 vols (London: Printed for A. Millar, and sold by T. Cadell ..., 1768); and *A treatise of fevers; wherein are set forth the causes, symptoms, diagnosticks, and prognosticks ... together with the method of cure* (London: printed by H. Cock for J. Scott, 1758).
45. John Ball, *The female physician [sic]: or, every woman her own doctor* (London: 1771), pp. 11–24.
46. Vives, cited in Perry, 'Weaving Clio and the Moriscas of Early Modern Spain', in Susan D. Amusen and Adele Seef, eds, *Attending to Early Modern Women* (Newark: University of Delaware Press, 1998), p. 61.
47. Guthrie, 'Lady Sedley's Receipt Book', p. 163.
48. Chamberlain, *Old Wives' Tales*, p. 183.

49. Lynette Hunter, 'Women and Domestic Medicine: Lady Experimenters, 1570–1620', in Lynette Hunter and Sarah Hutton, eds, *Women, Science and Medicine 1500–1700* (Phoenix Mill, Gloucestershire: Sutton, 1997), p. 89.
50. Ibid., p. 89.
51. Guthrie, 'Lady Sedley's Receipt Book', p. 163. A.S. Weber, 'Women's Early Modern Medical Almanacs in Historical Context', *English Literary Renaissance*, 33(3) (2003): 374. Quincy's *Dispensatory* was assembled by John Quincy (d. 1722), an apothecary who received an MD from the University of Edinburgh on the basis of his *Compleat English Dispensatory*. The first edition was published in 1718, and by 1742, there were twelve editions. His *Dispensatory* was the most comprehensive to date in England. See N. Howard-Jones, 'John Quincy, M.D. [d. 1722] Apothecary and Iatrophysical Writer', *Journal of the History of Medicine and Allied Sciences*, 6 (2) (1951): 149–75.
52. John Quincy, *Pharmacopoeia officinalis & extemporanea. Or, a complete English dispensary, in four parts...By John Quincy, M.D.*, 11th edn (London, 1739), pp. 495–6, Eighteenth Century Collections On-Line, Gale Group, http://galenet.galegroup.com/servelet/ECCO.
53. The full title is *Natura exenterata: or nature unbowelled by the most exquisite anatomizers of her. Wherein are contained her choicest secrets digested into receipts, fitted for the cure of all sorts of infirmities / ... Collected ... by several persons of quality ... whose names are prefixed to the book ... Whereunto are annexed many ... inventions* (London: H. Twiford [etc.], 1655).
54. Hunter, 'Women and Domestic Medicine', p. 89.
55. Ibid., pp. 93–4.
56. See Wallace Notestein, 'The English Woman, 1580–1650', in J.H. Plumb, ed., *Studies in Social History* (London: Longmans, Green and Co., 1955), p. 74 and Lester S. King, *The Medical World of the Eighteenth Century* (Chicago: University of Chicago Press, 1958), p. 31.
57. Wear, *Knowledge and Practice*, p. 23.
58. Cited in King, *The Medical World*, p. 80.
59. Walter Harris, *De Morbis Acutis Infantum*, trans. Martyn (1742), p. 61, cited in Guthrie, 'Lady Sedley's Receipt Book', p. 65.
60. James Primrose, *Popular Errours of the People in the matter of Physick. First written in Latine by the Learned Physician James Primrose, Doctor of Physick* (London: W. Willson, 1651), p. 19.
61. Sydenham cited in Guthrie, 'Lady Sedley's Receipt Book', p. 165.
62. Nicholas Culpeper, *A physicall directory, or, A translation of the London dispensatory* (London, 1649), sig. A2.
63. See F.N.L. Poynter, 'Nicholas Culpeper and his Books', *Journal of the History of Medicine*, 17 (1962): 153, 161–2.
64. Robert Burton, *The Anatomy of Melancholy* (1621), ed. Floyd Dell and P. Jourdan-Smith (New York: Tudor, 1948), p. 563.
65. Porter and Porter, *Patient's Progress*, p. 209.
66. Thomas, *Religion and the Decline of Magic*, p. 278.
67. See Faye Marie Getz, 'Charity, Translation and the Language of Medical Learning in Medieval England, *Bulletin of the History of Medicine and Allied Sciences*, 64 (1990): 3, 11; Russell Hope Robbins, 'Medical Manuscripts in Middle English', *Speculum*, XLV (July, 1970): 409; Robert S. Gottfried, *Doctors and Medicine in Medieval England, 1340–1530* (Princeton, NJ: Princeton University Press, 1986), pp. 176, 250–6.

68. H.S. Bennett, *English Books and Readers 1558–1603* (Cambridge: Cambridge University Press, 1965), p. xv.
69. Stine, 'Opening Closets', p. 76.
70. These recipes probably did not 'cure' the disease or ailment. The term 'cure' is not often used in the manuscripts. More frequent terms are 'help', 'good', 'ease', 'approved', 'sovereign'. Stine, 'Opening Closets', p. 43.
71. Michael MacDonald, *Mystical Bedlam: Madness, Anxiety, and Healing in Seventeenth-Century England* (Cambridge: Cambridge University Press, 1981), p. 29.
72. Roy Porter, *Health for Sale: Quackery in England, 1660–1850* (Manchester and New York: Manchester University Press 1989), pp. 32–3.
73. Porter and Porter, *Patient's Progress*, p. 27.
74. Guthrie, 'Lady Sedley's Receipt Book', p. 165. See Chapter 7 for details of gentlewomen as healers.
75. Ralph R. Josselin, *The Diary of Ralph Josselin, 1616–1683*, ed. Alan MacFarlane (London : Oxford University Press for the British Academy, 1976), pp. 163–4.
76. Beier, 'In Sickness and in Health', p. 121.
77. Stine, 'Opening Closets', p. 14.
78. Lady Sedley was the wife of Sir Charles Sedley, playwright and boon companion of Charles II. Guthrie, 'Lady Sedley's Receipt Book', p. 158. Her receipt book which is composed primarily of medicinal receipts with some cookery recipes, is held at the Royal College of Physicians of London archives.
79. Guthrie 'Lady Sedley's Receipt Book', p. 152.
80. John Evelyn, *Diary*, 13 June 1673, 19 January 1686, cited in Guthrie, 'Lady Sedley's Receipt Book', p. 165.
81. Two definitions of 'commonplacing' and 'commonplace books' are: 'Commonplacing is the act of selecting important phrases, lines, and/or passages from texts and writing them down; the commonplace book is the notebook in which a reader has collected quotations from works s/he has read. Commonplace books can also include comments and notes from the reader; they are frequently indexed so that the reader can classify important themes and locate quotations related to particular topics or authors.' 'Commonplacing is the practice of entering literary excerpts and personal comments into a private journal, that is, into a commonplace book or, to use a 17th century synonym, a silva rerum ('a forest of things'). Typically the excerpts were regarded as exceptionally insightful or beautiful or as applicable to a variety of situations, and as such they are often especially quotable ... The practice of commonplacing can be traced back in the European tradition to the 5th century B.C.E. and the Sophist, Protagoras.' These definitions are provided by Dr Lucia Knoles, Department of English, Assumption College, Worcester, Mass., http://www.assumption.edu/users/lknoles/commonplacebook.html.
82. See Sister Joan Marie Lechner, *Renaissance Concepts of the Commonplaces* (Westport, CT: Greenwood, 1962), pp. 2–3.
83. Ronald C. Sawyer, 'Patients, Healers, and Disease in the Southeast Midlands, 1597–1634', unpublished PhD dissertation, University of Wisconsin-Madison (1986), pp. 189–91.
84. Cited in Sawyer, 'Patients, Healers, and Disease', p. 191.
85. Cited in ibid., p. 191. Ward had studied science at Oxford and Cambridge.
86. Ibid., p. iii.
87. Cited in ibid., pp. 191–2.
88. Chamberlain, *Old Wives' Tales*, p. 69.

89. For a recent history of the regulation of apothecaries, see Penelope Hunting, *A History of the Society of Apothecaries* (London: The Society, 1998).
90. Cited in Graeme Tobyn, *Culpeper's Medicine* (Rockport, MA: Element Books, 1997), p. 9.
91. Charles Raymond Booth Barrett, *The History of the Society of Apothecaries of London* (London: E. Stock, 1905), p. xxxii.
92. Alice Clark, *Working Life of Women in the Seventeenth Century* (1919; New York: Dutton, 1968), pp. 261–2.
93. Porter, *Health for Sale*, p. 33.
94. Stine, 'Opening Closets', p.144.
95. Ibid., p. 145.
96. Linda Levy Peck, *Consuming Splendour: Society and Culture in Seventeenth-Century England* (Cambridge: Cambridge University Press, 2005), p. 127.
97. Some examples include: Elizabeth Sleigh and Felicia Whitfeld, 'Collection of medical receipts' (1647–1722; MS 751); Jane Newton and others, 'Medical and cookery receipts' (c.1675–c.1725; MS 1325); Katherine Jones, Lady Ranelagh, 'Collection of medical receipts' (c. 1675–c.1710; MS 1340); Martha Hodges and others, 'Collection of cookery receipts, including a few medical receipts' (c. 1675–1725: MS 2844); Mrs Elizabeth Hirst and others, 'Collection of medical and cookery receipts' (1684–c.1725; MS 2840); Mrs Meade and others, 'Collection of medical, veterinary and cookery receipts' (1688–1727; MS 3500); Amy Eyton and others, 'Collection of cookery receipts, with a few medical and household receipts' (1691–1738; MS 2323); Elizabeth Browne, Penelope Humphreys, Sarah Studman, Mary Dawes, 'Book of Receipts, collection of cookery and medical recipes' (c.1697–19th century; MS 785).
98. We have very little biographical information about Charlotte van Lore except that her parents were John van den Bempdé and Temperance Packer. She had two husbands: the first was Sir William Johnstone, 1st Marquess of Annandale. He was the son of James Johnstone, 1st Earl of Annandale and Hartfell and Henrietta Douglas. Van Lore married him on 20 November 1718 in London, apparently against the wishes of her father. Her second husband was Lt.-Col. John Johnstone whom she married on 1 December 1731 in St Benet's, Paul's Wharf, London. She died on 23 November 1762 in Bath. The source of this information is 'The Peerage.com: A genealogical survey of the peerage of Britain as well as the royal families of Europe', Person Page 2663, compiled by Darryl Lundy, http://thepeerage.com/p2663.htm.
99. See above and Stine, 'Opening Closets', p. 176.
100. James Primrose, *Popular Errors, or The Errours of the People in Physick*, trans. Robert Wittie (London, 1651).
101. She was born Marie de Rabutin-Chantal, the daughter of Celse Bénigne de Rabutin, Baron de Chantal and Marie de Coulanges. Her father died when she was seventeen months and her mother when she was seven. She was raised by her maternal uncle, Christophe de Coulanges, the Abbé of Livry. At the age of 19, she married Henri de Sévigné who came from an old Breton noble family. She had two children, a daughter born in 1646 and a son born in 1648. She was widowed at twenty-five when her husband was killed in a duel. Scholars are in agreement that Madame de Sévigné had an almost pathological obsession with her daughter, the future Madame de Grignan. Leonard Tancock, 'Introduction', *Madame de Sévigné: Selected Letters* (Harmondsworth: Penguin, 1982), pp. 9–10; Charles G.S. Williams, *Madame de Sévigné* (Boston: Twayne, 1981), pp. 13, 17–18.

102. The two women were acquaintances. In a letter to the Marquis de Pomponne, who was French Foreign Minister from 1671, de Sévigné relates that she had seen 'Foucquet's mother' who had sent a plaster to the queen and had healed her. Here she is referring to Nicolas Fouquet, the disgraced Surintendant of Finances, one of Madame Fouquet's sons. Letter 24 November 1664, Tancock, *Selected Letters*, p. 37.
103. Richard Aldington, *Letters of Madame de Sévigné to her daughter and her friends. Selected, with an introductory essay* (New York: Bretanos, 1927), I, p. xii.
104. Letter to Madame de Grignan, 16 September 1676, in *The Letters of Madame de Sévigné*, intro. A. Edward Newton (Philadelphia: J.P. Horn, 1927), III, p. 332. Unless indicated otherwise, all letters cited here are addressed to Madame de Grignan.
105. See letters of 26, 29 January 1676 in Tancock, *Selected Letters*, pp. 181–2.
106. Letters of 19, 29, 31 January 1676; 2, 26, February and 28 March 1676, in Newton, *Letters*, III, pp. 145–6, 151–5, 165–6, 181–2.
107. Letter, 8 June 1677, Newton, *Letters*, IV, pp. 21–2.
108. Letter, 15 December 1684, Newton, *Letters*, V, p. 278.
109. Letter to the Countess de Guitaut, 23 December 1677, in *Correspondance*, Texte établi, présenté et annoté par Robert Duchêne (Paris: Gallimard, 1972), II, p. 591.
110. Letter to the Count de Bussy, 4 January 1678, *Correspondance*, II, pp. 591–2.
111. Jeanne Ojala, *Madame de Sévigné: A Seventeenth Century Life* (Oxford: Berg, 1990), p. 9. Mossiker, *Madame de Sévigné*, p. 177.
112. Letter, 6 May 1671, *Correspondance*, I, p. 248.
113. Letters of 13, 18 May 1671, *Correspondance*, I, pp. 179, 185.
114. Letter, 27 April 1671, in *Lettres*, ed. Emile Gérard-Gailly (Paris: Gallimard, 1953–57), I, p. 275.
115. Letter to Monsieur de Grignan, 27 May 1678, *Correspondance*, II, p. 608; Augustin Cabanès, *Médecins Amateurs* (Paris: A. Michel, 1932), pp. 141–2.
116. For more details on her daughter's poor health, see Ives Marie Paul Jean Burill, *La marquise de Sévigné, docteur en medicine (honoris causa)* (Paris: A. Legrand, 1931), pp. 95–100.
117. Letter, 8 April 1671, cited in L'Aignel-Lavastine and Ives M. Burill, 'Les Cliniques de Madame de Sévigné', *Bulletin de la Société Française d'Histoire de la Médecine*, XXVI (1932): 136.
118. Letter, 27 April 1672, cited in Mossiker, *Madame de Sévigné*, p. 141.
119. Letter to Guitaut, 15 November 1677, *Correspondance*, II, pp. 586–7.
120. Letter, 29 April 1685, Newton, *Letters*, V, pp. 312–13.
121. Jacob Rosenbloom, 'Statements of Medical Interest from the Letters of Madame de Sévigné', *Medical Life*, 30 (1923): 95–6. Rosenbloom's citations are taken from *Letters of Madame de Sévigné to Her Daughter and Her Friends*, an enlarged edition translated from the Paris edition of 1806 in 9 volumes (London, 1811).
122. Letter 5 November 1672, *Correspondance*, I, p. 568.
123. Letter to Count de Guitaut, 15 November 1677, *Correspondance*, II, p. 586.
124. Rosenbloom, 'Statements of Medical Interest', p. 84.
125. Letter, 4 October 1679, *Correspondance*, II, p. 694.
126. Madame de Nesmond was Marguerite de Beauharnais de Miramon, Letter, 1 November 1679, *Correspondance*, II, p. 724.
127. 'Hungary water' is fermented rosemary (Fr. romarin). Its recipe was in a book of 'Secrets' in the possession of Queen Isabelle of Hungary. Cabanès, *Medecins Amateurs*, p. 124. Letter of 17 January 1676, in Newton, *Letters*, III, p. 143.

128. Letter of 22 July 1676, in Tancock, *Selected Letters*, p. 201.
129. Letter of 6 November 1676, ibid., p. 213.
130. Cited in Rosenbloom, 'Statements of Medical Interest', p. 244.
131. Letter of 18 September 1676, in Newton, *Letters*, III, p. 456.
132. Letter of 25 September 1676, in ibid., III, p. 460.
133. Letter of 30 September 1676, in Tancock, *Selected Letters*, pp. 206–7.
134. Letter of 7 October 1676, in Newton, *Letters*, III, p. 351.
135. Letters 10 January, 4 February 1689, in *Correspondance*, III, pp. 467, 496.
136. Amélie de Hesse-Cassel, wife of Henri-Charles de la Trémouille.
137. Letter, 2 October 1675, in Newton, *Letters*, II, p. 117.
138. The 'Capuchins of the Louvre' were apparently famous for their cures in Brittany at this time. Rosenbloom, 'Statements of Medical Interest', p. 95.
139. Letter, 16 February 1680, in Newton, *Letters*, IV, p. 327.
140. Letter, 5 November 1684, in ibid., V, p. 263.
141. Letter, 15 December 1684, in ibid., V, p. 278.
142. Letter, 5 November 1684, in ibid., V, pp. 261–2.
143. Ibid.
144. Cited in Rosenbloom, 'Statements of Medical Interest', pp. 97, 100.
145. Cited in ibid., p. 101.
146. Letter, 18 October 1679, *Correspondance*, II, p. 275.
147. Charles Delorme (1584–1678) was the first doctor of Henri IV, Marie de Médicis and Louis XII. He was a follower of contemporary medical fashions and fads such as Bourbon waters and various powders. *Correspondance*, II, p. 234. For Madame's discussion of his powders, see Letter, 21 August 1675, in Newton, *Letters*, II, p. 67.
148. Letter, 3 February 1676, *Correspondance*, II, p. 233.
149. Letter, 14 February 1685, *Correspondance*, III, p. 181.
150. Ojala, *Madame de Sévigné*, p. 9.
151. See letters about her son in Newton, *Letters*, Vol. 5, 21 August 1680, 139–42; 4 September 1680, 153–4; 2 October 1680, 178; 13 October 1680, 186. See also Mossiker, *Madame de Sévigné*, pp. 306–8.
152. George Dock, 'Robert Talbor, Madame de Sévigné, and the Introduction of Cinchona: An Episode Illustrating the Influence of Women in Medicine', *Annals of Medical History*, 4 (1922): 242.
153. Ibid., pp. 242–3.
154. Letters 29 September 1679, 17 January 1680, 17 March 1680, cited in ibid., pp. 244–6.
155. See letters of 27 September 1679 and 6 October 1679, in Newton, *Letters*, IV, pp. 200, 207.
156. Letter, 6 May 1676, in ibid., III, p. 209.
157. Letter, 30 June 1677, in ibid., IV, p. 40.
158. Cited in Rosenbloom, 'Statements of Medical Interest', p. 91.
159. Letter of 9 June 1677, in Newton, *Letters*, IV, p. 23.
160. Letter of 1 November 1679, in ibid., II, p. 29.
161. Letters of 11 and 14 March 1676, in ibid., III, pp. 172–4.
162. Letter of 16 September 1677, in ibid., IV, p. 115.
163. See letters dated 19, 21, 28 May 1676, in *Correspondance*, III, pp. 295–8, 303.
164. Letter, 28 May 1676, in Newton, *Letters*, I, 219–20.
165. L'Aignel-Lavastine and Burill, 'Les Cliniques de Madame de Sévigné', p. 131.
166. Letter of 25 September 1676, in Newton, *Letters*, I, p. 250.

167. Letter of 13 September 1677, in ibid., IV, p. 116.
168. Letter to the Count of Guitant, 9 April 1683, in *Correspondance*, III, p. 108.
169. Letter, 11 October 1679, in ibid., II, p. 700.
170. Letter, 1 November 1679, in ibid., II, p. 29.
171. Letters to Madame de Grignan, 29 April 1658, 18 May 1689, 26 June 1675, 8 July 1671, 28 July 1682, cited in L'Aignel-Lavastine and Burill, 'Les Cliniques de Madame de Sévigné', p. 132.
172. Letter to M. de Coulanges, 15 October 1695, in *Lettres*, III, pp. 892–3.
173. Letter, 8 April 1676, in Newton, *Letters*, III, p. 185.
174. Letter, 29 September 1679, in ibid., IV, p. 204.
175. Letter, 20 May 1676, in ibid., II, p. 220.
176. There are several references to taking the waters and having the pump treatment. See letters to her daughter dated 20 May 1676, 13 February 1676, 8 April 1676, 19, 20, 28 May 1676, 1, 8 June 1676 in Aldington, *Letters of Madame de Sévigné*, I, pp. 188–225.
177. Letter, 11 February 1671, Newton, *Letters*, I, p. 95.
178. Letters, 15 April, 13 May 1671, in *Lettres*, I, pp. 258–9, 290–1.
179. Letters, 15 April, 25, 28 October 1671, in *Lettres*, I, pp. 258–9, 409–10.
180. Letter, 28 October 1671, in Aldington, *Letters*, I, p. 77.
181. Letter to Bussy-Rabutin, 15 January 1687, in *Lettres*, III, pp. 140–1.
182. Marie-Louise Dufrenoy and Jean Dufrenoy, 'Coffee, the 'Exotik Drink', *The Scientific Monthly*, 70(3) (March 1950): 186.
183. Letter from Mme de Grignan, 10 January 1680, in Newton, *Letters*, IV, p. 284.
184. Letter, 16 February 1680, in ibid., IV, p. 328.
185. Letter, 8 November 1679, in ibid., IV, p. 230.
186. Letters, 8, 23 November 1688, in *Lettres*, III, pp. 239, 254.
187. Letter, 4 October 1684, in Newton, *Letters*, V, p. 258.
188. See Letter, 22 July 1685, in *Correspondance*, III, p. 217–20 and Mossiker, *Madame de Sévigné,* pp. 255–6.

9. The Wise-Woman as Healer: Popular Medicine, Witchcraft and Magic

1. Midwives come up frequently in the demonology literature but cases where women were actually prosecuted for practising midwifery are much fewer in number than those where women were accused of healing. See the provocative article by David Harley, who poignantly makes this point, arguing that 'historians have been led astray by a tradition that derives from the discredited work of Margaret Murray'. 'Historians as Demonologists: The Myth of the Mid-wife-witch', *Social History of Medicine* (1990): 99–124.
2. Primary source material for witch persecutions consists of trial records, demonology handbooks and witch-hunters' textbooks, contemporary pamphlets of eyewitness accounts, and theoretical works by believers and sceptics alike. For an excellent guide to sources, see Jean-Pierre Coumont, *Demonology and Witchcraft: An Annotated Bibliography* (Utrecht: Hes & DeGraaf, 2004).
3. This role was not unique to European society, but can also be found in the Middle East and Latin America where women's healing practices were widespread. Anne Llewellyn Barstow, *Witchcraze: A New History of European Witch Hunts* (San Francisco: Pandora, 1994), p. 207, n. 1.

4. John Henry, 'Doctors and Healers: Popular Culture and the Medical Profession', in Stephen Pumfrey, Paolo L. Rossi and Maurice Slawinski, eds, *Science, Culture and Popular Belief in Renaissance Europe* (Manchester and New York: Manchester University Press, 1991), p. 191.
5. Guido Ruggiero, *Binding Passions: Tales of Magic, Marriage, and Power at the End of the Renaissance* (Oxford: Oxford University Press, 1993), p. 17.
6. These methods are discussed in detail in Chapter 2.
7. Mary Nelson, 'Why Witches were Women', in Jo Freedman, ed., *Women: A Feminist Perspective* (Palo Alto, CA: Mayfield, 1975), p. 335.
8. Charles Goodall, ed., *The Royal College of Physicians of London Founded and Established by Law; As Appears By Letters Patents, Acts of Parliament, and Adjudged Cases, etc.* (London: M. Flesher, 1684), pp. 1–2.
9. See Richard Kieckhefer, 'The Classical Inheritance', in *Magic in the Middle Ages* (Cambridge: Cambridge University Press, 2000), ch. 2, for a discussion of magical practices in ancient Egypt, Greece and Rome.
10. See Kieckhefer, *Magic in the Middle Ages*, pp. 56–7.
11. C. Warren Hollister, *Medieval Europe: A Short History*, 7th edn (Boston: McGraw Hill, 1994), pp. 323–4. For a recent work on Catherine of Siena, see Thomas F. Luong, *The Saintly Politics of Catherine of Siena* (Ithaca: Cornell University Press, 2000).
12. Cited in Gianna Pomata, *Contracting a Cure: Patients, Healers and the Law in Early Modern Bologna* (Baltimore and London: Johns Hopkins University Press, 1998), p. 79.
13. Evelyne Berriot-Salvadore, 'The Discourse of Medicine and Science', in Natalie Zemon Davis and Arlette Farge, eds, *A History of Women, Renaissance and Enlightenment Paradoxes*, Vol. 3 (Cambridge, MA: Belknap Press of Harvard University Press, 1993), p. 354.
14. Ruggiero, *Binding Passions*, p. 17.
15. Bengt Ankarloo, Stuart Clark and William Monter, *Witchcraft and Magic in Europe: The Period of the Witch Trials*, The Athlone History of Witchcraft and Magic in Europe, Vol. 4 (London: Athlone, 2002), pp. 105, 108.
16. Mary O'Neil's work is based on the Inquisition archives in Modena, Italy. She found that the largest number of cases were those against healers. See Mary O'Neil: 'Magical Healing, Love Magic and the Inquisition in Late Sixteenth-Century Modena', in *Inquisition and Society in Early Modern Europe*, ed. and trans. Stephen Haliczer (London and Sydney: Croom Helm, 1987), pp. 80–8.
17. Francis Bacon cited in Keith Thomas, *Religion and the Decline of Magic* (Harmondsworth: Penguin, 1971), p. 14.
18. Lodowick Muggleton, *The Acts of the Witnesses of the Spirit* (London, 1699), p. 111.
19. Barstow, *Witchcraze*, pp. 109–12.
20. Danielle Piomelli and Antonino Pollio, 'A Study in Renaissance Psychotropic Plant Ointments', *History and Philosophy of Life Sciences*, 16 (1994): 248.
21. Ibid., pp. 246–7.
22. Probably *Melissa officinalis L.* (lemon balm) used today as a tranquillizer and anti-spasmodic drug (ibid., p. 249).
23. G. Cardano, *De Subtilitate, Norimbergae: I. Petreium* (1550), XVIII, p. 354, cited in ibid., p. 249.
24. Jeffrey Burton Russell, *Witchcraft in the Middle Ages* (Ithaca and London: Cornell University Press, 1972), p. 23.

25. E.E. Evans Pritchard, *Witchcraft, Oracles and Magic among the Azande* (Oxford: Oxford University Press, 1937).
26. Richard Kieckhefer, *European Witch Trials: Their Foundations in Popular and Learned Culture, 1300–1500* (Berkeley, CA: University of California Press, 1976), p. 8.
27. In addition to the demonology texts discussed in this chapter, see the numerous texts in *L'imaginaire du sabbat: édition critique des texts les plus anciens (1430c–1440c)*, collected by Martine Ostorero, Agostino Paravicini Bagliani and Kathrin Utz Tremp, in collaboration with Catherine Chène (Lausanne: Section d'histoire, Faculté des lettres, Université de Lausanne, 1999). The texts in this volume include, *Rapport sur la chasse aux sorciers et aux sorcières menée dès 1428 dans le diocèse de Sion*, Hans Fründ, *Formicarius*, Johannes Nider, *Errores gazariorum seu illorum qui scopam vel baculum equitare probantur*, Claude Tholosan, *Ut magorum et maleficiorum errors* and Martin le Franc, *Le champion des Dames*. These are the earliest known texts and are written in Latin and French. For a discussion of these texts, see Stuart Clark's chapter, 'Demonology', in *The Athlone History of Witchcraft and Magic, Vol. 4: The Period of the Witch Trials* (London: Athlone Press, 2002), pp. 122–32.
28. Christina Larner, *Witchcraft and Religion: The Politics of Popular Belief*, ed. and intro. Alan Macfarlane (Oxford: Blackwell, 1984), pp. 3–4.
29. Nelson, 'Why Witches were Women', p. 336; Anne Llewellyn Barstow, 'Witch Hunting as Woman Hunting: Persecution by Gender', in Jane Donawerth and Adele Seff, eds, *Crossing Boundaries: Attending to Early Modern Women* (Newark: University of Delaware Press, 2000), p. 129.
30. Although it is a work of fiction, Defoe (1660–1731) provides first-hand knowledge of the plague in this book first published in 1722. See *A Journal of the Plague Year: Daniel Defoe*, ed. Paula R. Backscheider (New York: W.W. Norton, 1992), p. 29.
31. Robert Burton, *The Anatomy of Melancholy*, cited in Antonia Fraser, *The Weaker Vessel: Women's Lot in Seventeenth-Century England* (London: Methuen, 1984), p. 129.
32. Brian Levack, *The Witch-Hunt in Early Modern Europe*, 2d edn (London: Longman, 1995), p. 141.
33. His *Dialogue concerning Witches and Witchcrafts* was printed in London in 1593 and again in 1603. Cited in Christina Hole, *A Mirror of Witchcraft*, (London: Chatto and Windus, 1957), p. 25.
34. Gifford, *A Dialogue concerning Witches and Witchcrafts* (London, 1603), cited in *Materials toward a History of Witchcraft*, Collected by Henry Charles Lea and arranged and edited by Arthur C. Harland, Vol. III (New York and London: Thomas Yoseloff, 1957), pp. 1308–10.
35. Diebold Schillery, *Luzerner Bilderchronik,* cited in Norman Cohn, *Europe's Inner Demons: The Demonization of Christians in Medieval Europe*, revised edn (Chicago: University of Chicago Press, 1993), p. 227.
36. This book went through thirty-four editions by 1669. Barstow, *Witch Craze*, p. 171. Kramer and Sprenger's views are discussed below.
37. Heinrich Kramer and Jacob Sprenger, *Malleus Maleficarum* (1486), in Lisa DiCaprio and Merry E. Wiesner, eds, *Lives and Voices: Sources in European Women's History* (Boston: Houghton Mifflin, 2001), pp. 224–7.
38. Jean-Michel Sallmann, 'Witches', in Natalie Zemon Davis and Arlette Farge, eds, *A History of Women: Renaissance and Enlightenment Paradoxes* (Cambridge, MA, and London: The Belknap Press of Harvard University Press, 1994), III, p. 446.

39. There is an enormous literature on the topic of the Early Modern European (including British) witch-hunts. A good starting point is the bibliography in P.G. Maxwell-Stuart's excellent and accessible introduction to the topic, *Witchcraft in Europe and the New World, 1400–1800* (Basingstoke: Palgrave, 2001), pp. 111–17.
40. Cited in Maxwell-Stuart, *Witchcraft in Europe*, p. 8.
41. Henry, 'Doctors and Healers', pp. 215–17.
42. David F. Noble, *A World without Women: The Christian Clerical Culture of Western Science* (New York and Oxford: Oxford University Press), p. 210.
43. J.A. Sharpe, *The Bewitching of Anne Gunter: A Horrible and True Story of Football, Witchcraft, Murder, and the King of England* (London: Profile, 1999), p. 46.
44. Reginald Scot, *The Discoverie of Witchcraft: being a reprint of the first edition published in 1584/by Reginald Scot,* edited with explanatory notes, glossary, and introduction by Brinsley Nicholson (East Ardsley, York: EP Publishing, 1973), Book V, p. ix; Book 4, p. 19, Chapter 3, p. 5.
45. Scot cited in Barstow, *Witchcraze*, p.176.
46. Scot, cited in Hole, *A Mirror of Witchcraft*, p. 23.
47. Scot, *Discoverie of Witchcraft*, p. 195.
48. Ibid., pp. 195–8.
49. Other critics included Henry Holland, *A Treastise against witchcraft* (1598), Robert Burton, *Anatomy of Melancholy* (1621). See Michael MacDonald, ed., *Witchcraft and Hysteria in Elizabethan London: Edward Jorden and Mary Glover Case* (London and New York: Routledge, 1991), pp. xlii, xliii.
50. Cited in Hole, *A Mirror of Witchcraft*, p. 24.
51. Levack, *The Witch-Hunt in Early Modern Europe*, p. 138.
52. Jules Michelet, *La Sorcière* (Paris: Hetzel, 1862), p. 372, n. 36.
53. Francisca Hernández Martin, *Historia de la Enfermería en Espanña* (Desde la Antiguedad hasta nuestra días) (Madrid: Síntesis, 1996), p. 63.
54. Maxwell-Stuart, *Witchcraft in Europe*, p. 8.
55. Lucinda McCray Beier, *Sufferers and Healers: The Experience of Illness in Seventeenth Century England* (London and New York: Routledge & Kegan Paul, 1987), p. 24.
56. Beier, *Sufferers and Healers*, p. 25.
57. Kieckhefer, *Magic in the Middle Ages*, pp. 75, 80.
58. Hole, *A Mirror of Witchcraft*, p. 17.
59. Ronald C. Sawyer, '"Strangely Handled in all her Lyms": Witchcraft and Healing in Jacobean England', *Journal of Social History*, 22 (Spring 1989): 471; Kieckhefer, *European Witch Trials*, p. 42.
60. Beier, *Sufferers and Healers*, p. 24.
61. Gifford, *A Discourse of the Subtle Practices of Devils by Witches and Sorcerers*, cited in Beier, *Sufferers and Healers*, pp. 46–7.
62. Johannes Oberndoerffer, *The Anatomies of the true Physician and Counterfeit Mountebank,* trans. Francis Herring (London, 1602), p. 15.
63. Cited in Levack, *The Witch-Hunt in Early Modern Europe*, p. 99.
64. Soman, 'Parlement of Paris', *Sixteenth Century Journal*, 9 (1975): 43.
65. Robert Muchembled, *La Sorcière au village* (Paris: Editions Juillard Gallimard, 1979), p. 69.
66. Barstow, *Witchcraze*, pp. 75, 89–91; William Monter and John Tedeschi, 'Toward a Statistical Profile of the Italian Inquisitions, Sixteenth to Eighteenth Centuries', in Gustav Henningsen and John Tedeschi, eds, *Inquisition in Early Modern Europe: Studies on Sources and Methods* (De Kalb: Northern Illinois University Press, 1976), pp. 133–6.

67. Edward Peters, *Inquisition* (New York: Free Press, 1988), Chapter 2.
68. Luis García-Ballester, 'The Inquisition and Minority Medical Practitioners in Counter-Reformation Spain: Judaizing and Morisco practitioners, 1560–1610', in Luis Garcia-Ballester et al., eds, *Practical Medicine from Salerno to the Black Death* (Cambridge: Cambridge University Press, 1994), pp. 158–160.
69. García-Ballester, 'The Inquisition', pp. 163–4.
70. Henry Kamen, *The Spanish Inquisition: A Historical Revision* (New Haven: Yale University Press, 1998), p. 269.
71. William Eamon, *Science and the Secrets of Nature* (Princeton, NJ: Princeton University Press, 1994), p. 204.
72. Judith Zinsser and Bonnie Anderson, *A History of their Own* (New York and Oxford: Oxford University Press, 1988), I, p. 169.
73. Ian Bostridge, *Witchcraft and its Transformation* (Oxford: Clarendon Press, 1997), p. 207.
74. Sallmann, 'Witches', p. 449. See also Robin Briggs, '"Many reasons why": Witchcraft and the Problem of Multiple Explanation', in Jonathan Barry, Marianne Hester and Gareth Roberts, eds, *Witchcraft in Early Modern Europe: Studies in Culture and Belief* (Cambridge: Cambridge University Press, 1996), pp. 49–63.
75. Noble, *A World without Women*, p. 207.
76. See J. Madule, *The Albigensian Crusade: An Historical Essay*, trans. B. Wall (New York: Fordham University Press, 1967).
77. Henry Charles Lea, *A History of the Inquisition of the Middle Ages* (New York: Russell, 1956), I, p. 151.
78. Ibid., I, p. 338.
79. Hugh Trevor-Roper, *The European Witch-Craze of the Sixteenth and Seventeenth Centuries* (New York: Harper & Row, 1970), pp. 102–3.
80. Lea, *A History of the Inquisition*, III, pp. 519–530.
81. Thomas, *Religion and the Decline of Magic*, pp. 519–21. Dominican inquisitors held that witches made a pact with the devil and ate children at their nightly gatherings. See Lea, *A History of the Inquisition*, III, pp. 401–8.
82. *Tractus de Oficio Sanctissimae Inquisitionis et modo procendi in Causis Fidei* (Lugdini, 1636, 1669), cited in Lea and Howland, *Materials toward a History of Witchcraft*, II, p. 1071.
83. Unnamed witch-hunter, cited in Barbara Ehrenreich and Deidre English, *Witches, Midwives, and Nurses: A History of Women Healers* (New York: Feminist Press, City University of New York, 1973), pp. 12–13.
84. Excerpts from the trial of 'The Enchantress', III. Sorcerers (from ASF, Atti del Esecutore, 751, fols. 25r–26r, November 5, 1375), translated in Gene Brucker, ed., *The Society of Renaissance Florence: A Documentary History* (New York: Harper & Row, 1971), p. 260.
85. Kieckhefer, *Magic in the Middle Ages*, pp. 62–3.
86. Ibid., p. 59.
87. Mattuccia's trial proceedings have been published by Domenico Mammadi in *The Record of the Trial and Condemnation of a Witch, Matteuccia di Francesco at Todi, 20 March 1428* (Rome: Res Tudertinae, 1972) and summarized by Richard Kieckhefer in *Forbidden Rites: A Necromancer's Manual of the Fifteenth Century* (Phoenix Mill: Sutton Publishing, 1997), pp. 69–70.
88. Kieckhefer, *Witch Trials*, p. 56.
89. Maria la Medica's case dates from 1480 and is cited in Jeffrey Burton Russell, *Witchcraft in the Middle Ages* (Ithaca: Cornell University Press, 1972), p. 256. For

information on Lucia Ghiai, see Carlo Ginzburg, *Night Battles, Witchcraft and Agrarian Cults in the Sixteenth and Seventeenth Centuries*, trans. John and Anne Tedeschi (Harmondsworth: Penguin, 1985), p. 81.

90. *Compendium Maleficarum, Collected in three books from many sources by Brother Francesco Maria Guazzo*, trans. E.A. Ashwin, ed. Montague Summers (London: John Rodker, 1929), Book II, Ch. XI, p. 123.
91. Mary O'Neil, 'Magical Healing', pp. 93–7.
92. This was reported by Benedetta Maranese who told the tribunal at her trial that she had been healed in this manner. SU, Sant' Uffizio, ASV Records of the Inquisition in Venice b. 68, Benedetta's first arraignment constit., 15 January 1591, cited in Ruth Martin, *Witchcraft and the Inquisition in Venice, 1550–1650* (Oxford: Blackwell, 1989), p. 13.
93. Martin, *Witchcraft*, pp. 18–19, 183.
94. Other women healers were convicted of heresy due to their methods which involved discerning bewitchment from people's clothing, not allowing patients to attend Christmas Mass, and falsely telling the inquisitors that they were healed with their blessing. See the case of Marietta Colonna in 1638, cited in Martin, *Witchcraft*, p. 187.
95. Martin, *Witchcraft*, p. 187.
96. Elena's first arraignment constit., 11 August 1571 and repeated in 1582 during her second interrogation, SU, b. 49, cited in ibid., p. 13.
97. 'Roman Inquisition Literature', in Lea and Howland, *Materials toward a History of Witchcraft*, II, pp. 970–1.
98. Kieckhefer, *European Witch Trials*, p. 18; Norman Cohn, *Europe's Inner Demons: An Enquiry Inspired by the Great Witch-Hunt* (New York: Basic Books, 1975), pp. 180–205.
99. Levack, *The Witch-Hunt in Early Modern Europe*, pp. 138–9.
100. Thomas Roger Forbes, *The Midwife and the Witch* (New Haven: Yale University Press, 1966), pp. 13–38.
101. *Malleus Maleficarum*, cited in Mary Chamberlain, *Old Wives' Tales: The History of Remedies, Charms and Spells* (Stroud: Tempus, 2006), p. 55.
102. Kramer and Sprenger, *Malleus Maleficarum*, Part II, Question, Chapter XIII: 'How Witch Midwives commit most Horrid Crimes when they either Kill Children or Offer them to Devils in most Accursed Wise'. Unabridged online republication of the 1928 edition. Introduction to the 1948 edition is also included. Translation, notes, and two introductions by Montague Summers, http://www.malleusmaleficarum.org/part_II/mm02a13a.html.
103. Gunnar Heinsohn and Otto Steiger, 'Birth Control: The Political-Economic Rationale behind Jean Bodin's *Démonomanie*', *History of Political Economy*, 31(3) (1999): 433.
104. Kramer and Sprenger, Part I, Question XI: 'That Witches who are Midwives in Various Ways Kill the Child Conceived in the Womb, and Procure an Abortion; or if they do not this Offer New-born Children to Devils', http://www.malleusmaleficarum.org/part_I/mm01_11a.html.
105. Phyllis Stock-Morton, 'Control and Limitation of Midwives in Modern France: The Example of Marseille', *Journal of Women's History*, 8(1) (Spring, 1996): 60.
106. Heinsohn and Steiger, 'Birth Control', pp. 423–48.
107. Innocent VIII (1484), p. xliv, cited in Heinsohn and Steiger, 'Birth Control', p. 432.
108. This case is cited in Ginzburg, *Night Battles*, p. 73.

109. Jarsolav Nemec, *Witchcraft and Medicine 1484–1793* (Washington, DC: Public Health Service National Institutes of Health DHEW Publication, 1974; Published in conjunction with an exhibit at the National Library of Medicine, 25 March–19 July 1973, US Department of Health, Education, and Welfare), p. 1; Lea, *A History of the Inquisition*, III, p. 497.
110. Ehrenreich and English, *Witches, Midwives, and Nurses*, p. 19.
111. Hole, *A Mirror of Witchcraft*, p.19.
112. E. William Monter, cited in Alan Charles Kors and Edward Peters, eds, *Witchcraft in Europe, 1100–1700: A Documentary History* (Philadelphia: University of Pennsylvania Press, 1972), p. 159.
113. Ehrenreich and English, *Witches, Midwives, and Nurses*, p. 13.
114. Elizabeth Brooke, *Women Healers: Portraits of Herbalists, Physicians and Midwives* (Rochester, VT: Healing Arts Press, 1995), p. 66.
115. Ibid., p. 14.
116. E. William Monter, ed., *European Witchcraft* (New York: Wiley, 1969), p. 386.
117. Julio Caro Baroja, *The World of Witches*, trans. Nigel Glendinning (London: Phoenix Press, 2001), p. 110.
118. Jean Bodin, *On the Demon-Mania of Witches*, trans. Randy A. Scott, intro. Jonathan L. Pearl, notes by Randy A. Scott and Jonathan L. Pearl (Toronto: Centre for Reformation and Renaissance Studies, 2001), p. 138.
119. Bodin, *On the Demon-Mania*, p. 101. Also cited in Heinsohn and Steiger, 'Birth Control', pp. 437–8.
120. Barstow, *Witchcraze*, pp. 25, 40–1; Alfred Soman, *Sorcellerie et Justice Criminelle: Le Parlement de Paris* (Aldershot: Ashgate, 1992), p. 36.
121. Stuart Clark, 'Protestant Demonology: Sin, Superstition, and Society (c.1520–c.1630)', in Bengt Ankarloo and Gustav Henningen, eds, *Early Modern European Witchcraft: Centres and Peripheries* (Oxford: Clarendon Press, 1990), pp. 78–9.
122. Clark, 'Demonology', pp. 116–17.
123. Forbes, *The Midwife and the Witch*, p. 12.
124. Mary O'Neil, 'Magical Healing', p. 89.
125. Case 49 I, Examination of John Devon before Hugh Darell, Esq., a Justice of the Peace for Kent', in Public Record Office, *Calendar of State Papers Domestic. Elizabeth*, Vol. 1 [1547–1580], 17 April 1561.
126. Olwen Hufton, *The Prospect Before Her: A History of Women in Western Europe, Volume One 1500–1800* (New York: Vintage, 1995), p. 337.
127. Martin Luther, *Commentary on the Epistle to the Galatians* (1535), trans. Theodore Graebner (Grand Rapids, MI: Zondervan Publishing, 1949), Chapter 3, pp. 86–106; Project Wittenberg, http://www.iclnet.org/pub/resources/text/wittenberg/luther/gal/web/gal3–01.html.
128. Hufton, *The Prospect Before Her*, pp. 347–8.
129. Thomas, *Religion and the Decline of Magic*, p. 525.
130. Chamberlain, *Old Wives' Tales*, p. 50; Thomas, *Religion and the Decline of Magic*, p. 526; Lea, ed., *Materials toward a History of Witchcraft*, III, p. 1306; Hole, *A Mirror of Witchcraft*, p. 20.
131. Lea, *Materials toward a History of Witchcraft*, III, pp. 1286–7.
132. Ibid., p. 1071.
133. Ibid., pp. 1286–7.
134. Robert Muchembled, 'The Witches of the Cambrésis', in James Obelkevich, ed., *Religion and the People 800–1700* (Chapel Hill: University of North Carolina Press, 1979), p. 255.

135. Lea, *Materials toward a History of Witchcraft,* III, 1310.
136. Noble, *A World without Women,* p. 210.
137. Johann Weyer, Book 5 Chapter 28: 'The Surest Method for Curing maleficium, i.e., evil-doing or witchcraft', in *Witches, Devils, and Doctors in the Renaissance, Johann Weyer, De praestigiis daemonum,* ed. George Mora and Benjamin Kohl, trans. John Shea (Binghampton, NY: Medieval and Renaissance Texts & Studies, 1991), pp. 446–7. Weyer (1515–1588), from Graves, Brabant, a province in the Low Countries and part of the Holy Roman Empire, studied medicine at the universities of Paris and Orléans, obtaining a medical degree in 1537. After practising for many years, he became personal physician to his ruler Duke William V of Cleve, Jülich and Berg in 1550. Mora and Kohl, 'Introduction' to Weyer, *Witches, Devils, and Doctors,* pp. xxvii–xxviii xxxii, xxxv, xlii.
138. Nemec, *Witchcraft and Medicine,* pp. 6–7.
139. Henri Boguet, *An Examen of witches: drawn from various trials of many of this sect ... edited by the Rev. Montague Summers* (London: John Rodker, 1929), pp. viii, xx.
140. Barstow, *Witchcraze,* p. 66.
141. Boguet, *An Examen of witches,* p. vi.
142. Ibid., pp. 88–9.
143. Ibid., pp. 89–90.
144. Ibid., pp. 90, 91, 94.
145. Ibid., pp. 98–101.
146. Ibid., pp. 101–2.
147. Ibid., p. 102.
148. Ibid., pp. 101–2.
149. Ibid., p. 107.
150. Ibid., p. 108.
151. Ibid., p. 110.
152. Pierre de Lancre, *Tableau de l'inconstance des mauvais anges et demons (1612),* ed. Nicole Jacques-Chaquin (Paris: Aubier, 1982), pp. 89–93.
153. Ibid., p. 84.
154. Ibid., pp. 89–91.
155. See Leigh Ann Whaley, 'The Medieval Woman in Science: Contradictions within the Church and the University', *Women's History as Scientists: a Guide to the Debates* (Santa Barbara: ABC–CLIO, 2003), Chapter 2.
156. Reverend John Gaule, *Select Cases of Conscience Touching Witches and Witchcraft* (London, 1646), cited in Hole, *A Mirror of Witchcraft,* p. 30.
157. Richard Bernard, cited in Hole, *A Mirror of Witchcraft,* p. 30.
158. See Henry Charles Lea, *A History of the Inquisition in Spain* (New York: Macmillan, 1906–07), IV, p. 209.
159. E. William Monter, *Witchcraft in France and Switzerland: The Borderlands during the Reformation* (Ithaca: Cornell University Press, 1976), p. 179.
160. Nicolas Rémy, *La Demonalatrie* (Nancy: Presses Universitaires de Nancy, 1995), Book II, ch. 2.
161. Rémy, *La Demonalatrie,* 59–60.
162. Rémy, cited in Barstow, *Witchcraze,* p. 110.

Bibliography

Primary sources

Unpublished

Archbishop of Canterbury Archives (Vicar General), Lambeth Palace Library, London, Medical Licences:

Moore (Elizabeth) VX 1A–10–259

Pemell (Jane) VX 1A–10–223

Rose (Mary) VX 1A–10–297–2

Wellcome Library Manuscripts, Wellcome Library, London: Domestic medicine and receipt books:

Sixteenth century

Anne de Croy, 'Recueil d'aulcunes confections et medicines', 1533 MS 222

Seventeenth century

Mrs Corylon, 'A Booke of divers Medecines...', 1606 MS 213

Grace Acton, Collection of cookery and medical receipts, 1621 MS 1

Jane Baber, 'A Booke of Receipts', c.1625 MS 108

Lady Frances Catchmay, 'A booke of medicens', c.1625 MS 184a

Anne Brumwich and others, 'Booke of Receipts or Medicines...', c.1625–1700 MS 160

Elizabeth Bulkeley, 'A boke of hearbes and receipts', 1627 MS 169

Joan Gibson, 'A booke of medicines', 1632–[1717] MS 311

Katherine, Countess of Chesterfield, 'A booke of severall receipts', c.1635 MSS 761–2

Jane Jackson, 'A very shorte and compendious Methode of Phisicke and Chirurgery...', 1642 MS 373

Alice Corbett, Collection of medical receipts, mid-17th century MS 212

Jane Parker, 'Mrs Jane Parker her Boock...', 1651 MS 3769

Lady Ann Fanshawe (1625–1680), Recipe book, 1651–78 MS 7113

Elizabeth Jacob and others, 'Physicall and chyrurgicall receipts', 1654–c.1685 MS 3009

Eighteenth century

Elizabeth Sleigh and Felicia Whitfeld, Collection of medical receipts, 1647–1722 MS 751

Mary Bent, Cookery book, with a few medical receipts, 1664–1729 MS 1127

Jane Newton and others, Medical and cookery receipts, c.1675–c.1725 MS 1325

Katherine Jones, Lady Ranelagh, Collection of medical receipts, c.1675–c.1710 MS 1340

Magdelaine Hanuche, Collection of medical receipts (in French), c.1750–75 MS 2777

Mrs Elizabeth Hirst and others, Collection of medical and cookery receipts, 1684–c.1725 MS 2840

Charlotte Van Lore Johnstone, 'Receipt-book', c.1725 MS 3087

Mrs Meade and others, Collection of medical, veterinary and cookery receipts, 1688–1727 MS 3500

Anne Neville, 'Collection of medical receipts', mid-18th century MS 3685

Elizabeth Okeover and others, 'Collection of medical receipts', c.1675–c.1725 MS 3712
Sarah Palmer and others, 'Collection of medical receipts', early 18th century MS 3740
Anonymous receipt book, Book of Medical Receipts in English and French dating from the later 17th century MS 4052
Frances Springatt and others, Collection of cookery and medical receipts, 1686–1823 MS 4683

Printed primary sources

By title

Archives de l'Hotel Dieu de Paris (1137–1500) par Léon Briele avec notice, appendice et table par Ernest Coyecque (Paris: Imprimerie nationale, 1894).
Collection de documents pour servir à l'histoire des hôpitaux de Paris. Commencée sous les auspices de M. Michel Möring. Délibérations de l'ancien bureau de l'Hôtel Dieu, ed. Léon Brièle, 4 vols (Paris: Imprimerie nationale, 1881–83).
L'assistance publique à Paris pendant la Révolution. Documents inédits. Recueillis et publiés par A. Tuetey, 4 vols (Paris: Histoire générale de Paris, 1895–97).
New International Version of the Holy Bible (Grand Rapids, MI: The Zondervan Corporation, 1984).
Ordonnances des rois de France de la troisième race: recueillies par ordre chronologique: avec des renvoys des unes aux autres, des sommaires, des observations sur le texte, & cinq tables, Eusèbe Jacob de Laurière, Denis François Secourses et al., 21 vols (Paris: Imprimerie nationale, 1723–1849).

By author

Agrippa von Nettehein, Heinrich Cornelius, *Sur La Noblesse, & Excellence du Sexe Féminin, de sa preeminence sur l'autre sexe, & du sacrement du marriage. Avec la traite sur l'incertitude, aussi bien que la vanite des sciences & des arts*, trans. Sr. M. de Gueudeville (Leiden: T. Haak, 1726).
Arderne, John, *Treatises of Fistula in Ano, Haemorrhoids and Clysters from an early fifteenth century manuscript translation*, ed. and trans. D'Arcy Power (London: Published for the Early English Text Society by Kegan Paul, Trench, Trübner, 1910).
Aristotle, *Generation of Animals*, in *The Complete Works of Aristotle: The Revised Oxford Translation*, ed. Jonathan Barnes, 4 vols (Princeton, NJ: Princeton University Press, 1984).
Arundel, Philip Howard, *The Lives of Philip Howard, Earl of Arundel, and of Anne Dacres, his wife*, edited from the original mss. by the Duke of Norfolk (London: Hurst and Blackett, 1857).
Augustine of Hippo, Saint, *City of God*, ed. David Knowles (Harmondsworth: Penguin, 1972).
———, *The Literal Meaning of Genesis*, trans. John Hammond Taylor SJ (New York: Newman Press, 1982).
———, *On Genesis: Two books on Genesis against the Manichees; and, On the literal interpretation of Genesis, an unfinished book*, trans. Roland J. Teske (Washington, DC: Catholic University of America Press, 1991).
Austin, Anne L., ed., *History of Nursing Source Book* (New York: G.P. Putnam's Sons, 1957).
Averroes, *Commentary on Plato's Republic*, trans. E.I.J. Rosenthal (Cambridge: Cambridge University Press, 1956).

Avicenna, *A treatise on the Canon of medicine of Avicenna, incorporating a translation of the first book*, trans. O'Cameron Gruner, 2 vols (London: Luzca, 1930).

Ball, John, *The female physician [sic]: or, every woman her own doctor. Wherein is summarily comprised, all that is necessary to be known in the cure of the several disorders to which the fair sex are liable. Together with prescriptions in English* (London, 1770; reprinted Edinburgh, 1771).

Barrington Family, *Barrington Family Letters, 1628–1632*, ed. Arthur Searle (London: Offices of the Royal Historical Society, 1933).

Bedell, William, *A True Relation of the Life and Death of the Right Reverend William Bedell, Lord Bishop of Kilmore*, ed. Thomas Wharton Jones (Westminster: Camden Society, 1872).

Bingen, Hildegard von, *Hildegard of Bingen: on natural philosophy and medicine: selections from Cause et cure*, translated from Latin, introduction, notes and interpretive essay by Margret Berger (Cambridge and Rochester, NY: D.S. Brewer, 1999).

Blackwell, Elizabeth, *A Curious Herbal, containing five hundred cuts of the most useful plants, which are now used in the practice of physick…To which is added a short description of ye plants: and their common uses in physick*, 2 vols (London: J. Nourse, 1739–1751). Eighteenth Century Collections Online (ECCO).

Bodin, Jean, *On the Demon-Mania of Witches*, trans. Randy A. Scott with an introduction by Jonathan L. Pearl, notes by Randy A. Scott and Jonathan L. Pearl (Toronto: Centre for Reformation and Renaissance Studies, 2001).

Boguet, Henri, *An Examen of witches: drawn from various trials of many of this sect … edited by the Rev. Montague Summers* (London: John Rodker, 1929).

Boix y Moliner, Miguel Marcelino, *Hippocrates aclarado, y sisterma de Galeno impugnado* (Madrid: En la Imprenta de Blds de Villabueva, 1716).

Boursier, Louise Bourgeois, *Observations diverses sur la sterilité perte de fruict foecondité accouchements et Maladies des femmes et enfants nouveaux naiz* (Paris, 1626).

———, *Apologie de Louyse Bourgeois dite Bourcier Sage femme de la Royne Mere du Roy et de feu Madame. Contre le Rapport des Médecins* (Paris, 1627).

———, *Récit véritable de la naissance de messeigneurs et dames les enfans de France; Fidelle relation de l'accouchement, maladie et ouverture du corps de feu Madame, suivie du, Rapport de l'ouverture du corps de feu Madame; Remonstrance a Madame Bourcier, touchant son apologie*, ed. and intro. Colette Winn (Genève: Droz, 2000).

Brillon Pierre-Jacques and Antoine-François Prost de Royer, *Dictionnaire des arrêts: ou, Jurisprudence universelle des parlements de France, et autres tribunaux: contenant par ordre alphabetique les matieres beneficiales, civiles, et criminelles les maximes du droit ecclésiastique, du droit romain, du droit public, des coutumes, ordonnances, édits et declarations*, 6 vols (Paris: Chez, Guillaume Cavelier, Pere, Michel Brunet, Nicolas Gosselin, 1727).

Burton, Robert. *The Anatomy of Melancholy* (1621), http://www.rc.umd.edu/cstahmer/cogsci/index.html.

Caminer Turra, Elisabetta, *Selected Writings of an Eighteenth-Century Venetian Woman of Letters*, ed. and trans. Catherine M. Sama (Chicago: University of Chicago Press, 2003).

Carbón, Damián, *Libro del Arte de las Comadres o Madrinas, del Regimento de las Preñandas y de los niños*, transcription de Francisco Susarte Molina (Alicante: Universidad de Alicante, 1995).

Cellier, Elizabeth, *Malice defeated; or a brief relation of the accusation and deliverance of Elizabeth Cellier* (London: For Elizabeth Cellier, 1680).

———, *The tryal and sentence of Eliz. Cellier* (London: T. Collins, 1680).

Chauliac, Guy de, *Chirurgia magna. English. Selections*, Ann Arbor, Mich., Early English Books Online Text Creation Partnership (2002). Originally published in London: Printed by Robert Wyer for Henry Dabbe and Rycharde Banckes (1542).

———, *La Grande Chirurgie*, ed. E. Niçaise (Paris: Felix Alcan, 1890).
———, *The Cyrugie of Guy de Chauliac*, ed. Margaret S. Ogden (London and New York: Published for the Early English Text Society by Oxford University Press, 1971).
Clifford, Anne, *The Diary of Anne Clifford, 1616–1619. A Critical Edition*, ed. Katherine O. Acheson (New York and London: Garland, 1995).
Clowes, William, *Selected Writings of William Clowes, 1544–1604* (London: Harvey & Blythe, 1948).
Comnena, Anna, *The Alexiad of the Princess Anna Comnena*, ed. and trans. Elizabeth A.S. Dawes (New York: Barnes & Noble, 1967).
Cortese, Isabella, *I Secreti* (Venice: Giacomo Fornett, 1584).
Cotta, John, *A Short Discoverie of the unobserved dangers of severall sorts of ignorant and unconsiderate practisers of physicke in England* (London: William Jones & R. Boyle, 1612).
Culpeper, Nicholas, *A physicall directory, or, A translation of the London dispensatory* (London: Peter Cole, 1649).
Defoe, Daniel, *A Journal of the plague* year, ed. Paula R. Backscheider (New York: W.W. Norton, 1992).
Denifle Heinrich and Emile Chatelain, *Chartularium Universitatis parisiensis. Sub auspiciis Consilii generalis facultatum parisiensium ex diversis bibliothecis tabulariisque collegit et cum authenticis chartis contulit Henricus Denifle auxiliante Aemilio Chatelain*, 4 vols (Paris: Delalain, 1889–97).
Depping, G.B., ed., *Réglemens sur les arts et métiers de Paris, rédigés au 13 siècle, et connus sous le nom du Livre des métiers d'Étienne Boileau. Publiés, pour la première fois en entier, d'après les manuscrits de la Bibliothèque du roi et des Archives du royaume, avec des notes et une introd., par G.B. Depping* (Paris: Imprimerie Nationale, 1837).
DiCaprio Lisa and Merry E. Wiesner, eds, *Lives and Voices, Sources in European History* (Boston: Houghton Mifflin, 2001).
Diderot, Dénis, *Correspondance*, 16 vols (Paris : Éditions de Minuit, 1955–70).
Douët-a'Arcq, L., ed., *Compte de l'Hôtel des Rois de France au XIVe et XVe siècles* (Paris: Société de l'Historie de France, 1865).
Du Châtelet, Gabrielle Émilie, Marquise, *Lettres de la Marquise du Châtelet*, ed. Theodore Besterman, 2 vols (Genève: Institut et Musée Voltaire, 1958).
Dubois, Pierre, *De Recuperatione Terre Sancte: traité de politique générale* (Paris: A. Picard, 1891).
Feijoo, Benito Jerónimo, *Defensa de la Mujer*, ed. Victoria Sau (Barcelona: Icaria, 1997).
Fielding, Henry, *Journal of a Voyage to Lisbon* (Lisbon: Dent, 1864).
Forman Cody, Lisa, 'Introduction', *Writings on Medicin: Printed Writings 1641–1700*, The Early Modern Englishwoman: A Facsimile Library of Essential Works, vol. 4 (Aldershot: Ashgate, 2000).
Géraud, Hercule, *Paris sous Philippe-le Bel, d'après des documents originaux, et notamment d'après un manuscrit contenant le role de la taille imposée sur les habitants de Paris en 1292* (Paris: Crapelet, 1837).
Goodall, Charles, ed., *The Royal College of Physicians of London Founded and Established by Law; As appears By Letters Patents, Acts of Parliament, and adjudged Cases, etc.* (London: M. Flesher, 1684).
Grant, Edward, ed., *A Sourcebook in Medieval Science* (Cambridge, MA: Harvard University Press, 1974).
Great Britain, Public Record Office, *Calendar of State Papers, Domestic. Edward VI, Mary, Elizabeth, and James I*, 10 vols (London: Longman: 1856).

———, *Calendar of State Papers Domestic Series, 1649–1660: Preserved in the State Paper Department of Her Majesty's Public Record Office*, Vol. 10, 1656–1657, ed. Mary Anne Everett Green (London: Longman, 1875–86).

Grimm, Friedrich Melchior, Freiherr von, *Correspondance littéraire, philosophique et critique par Grimm, Diderot, Raynal, Meister etc; revue sur les textes originaux, comprenant outre ce qui a été publié à diverses époques, les fragments supprimés en 1813 par la censure, les parties inédites conservées à la bibliothèque ducale de Gotha et à l'Arsenal à Paris. Notices, notes, table générale par Maurice Tourneux*, 16 vols (Paris: Garnier Frères, 1877–82)

Guazzo, Brother Francesco Maria, *Compendium Maleficarum, Collected in three books from many sources by Brother Francesco Maria Guazzo*, trans. E.A. Ashwin, ed. Montague Summers (London: John Rodker, 1929).

Guthrie, Leonard, 'The Lady Sedley's Receipt Book, 1686 and other Seventeenth-century Receipt Books', *Proceedings of the Royal Society of Medicine*, 6, 'Section of the History of Medicine' (1913): 150–70.

Halkett, Lady Anne and Lady Ann Fanshawe, *The Memoirs of Anne, Lady Halkett and Ann, Lady Fanshawe*, ed. and intro. John Loftis (Oxford: Clarendon Press, 1979).

Harley, Lady Brilliana, *Letters of the Lady Brilliana Harley* (London: The Camden Society, 1854).

Hart, James, *[Klinike], or the diet of the diseased* (London: J. Beale for R. Allot, 1633).

Hartley, David, *An account of some experiments and observations on Mrs. Stephens's medicines for dissolving the stone: ... By Stephen Hales, D.D. F.R.S. ... To which is added, a supplement to a pamphlet, intitled, A view of the present evidence for and against Mrs. Stephens's medicines* (London: Printed for T. Woodward 1740).

Hecquet, Philippe, *De l'indécence aux hommes d'accoucher les femmes et de l'obligation aux mères de nourrir leurs enfants*, ed. Hélène Rouch (Paris: Côté-femmes editions, 1990).

Henry VIII, *Herbalists' Charter of Henry the VIII: Annis Tircesimo Quarto and Tricesimo Quinto. Henry VIII Regis. Cap. VIII. An Act That Persons, Being No Common Surgeons, May Administer Outward Medicines* (1543), http://home.earthlink.net/~lifespirit23/herbcharter.htm.

Héylot, Pierre and Maximilien Bullot, *Histoire des ordres monastiques religieux et militaries et des Congrégations séculières de l'un et de l'autre sexe, qui on esté establies jusqu'à present; contenant les vies de leurs fondateurs*, 8 vols (Paris: N. Gosselin, 1714–19).

Hippocrates, *Hippocrates*, trans. W.H.S. Jones, 4 vols (Cambridge, MA: Harvard University Press, 1943–48).

Hoby, Margaret, *The Diary of Lady Margaret Hoby 1599–1605*, ed. Dorothy M. Meads (London: Routledge, 1930).

———, *The Private Life of an Elizabethan Lady. The Diary of Margaret Hoby 1599–1605*, ed. Joanna Moody (Phoenix Mill: Sutton, 1998).

Holden, Mary, *The Womans Almanac or, An Ephermerides for the Year of Our Lord 1688 being the bissextile, or leap-year: calculated for the meridian of London and may indifferently serve for any part of England* (London: Printed by J. Millet for the Company of Stationers, 1688).

———, *The womans almanack, or, An ephemeris for the year of our Lord, 1689 being the first after bissextile, or leap-year, and from the creation of the world, 5638 ... calculated for London ... and may serve for any other part of England* (London: Printed by J. Millet for the Company of Stationers, 1689).

Howard, Anne, *The Lives of Philip Howard, Earl of Arundel, and of Anne Dacres, his Wife* (London: Hurst and Blackett, 1857).

Huarte, Juan, *Examen de Ingenios or the Trial of the Wits*. trans. Mr Edward Bellamy (London: Richard Sare, 1698).

Hutchinson, Lucy Apsley, *Memoirs of the Life of Colonel Hutchinson written by his wife Lucy*, intro. François Guizot (London: J.M. Dent, 1908).

Jinner, Sarah, *The womans almanack: or, prognostication for ever: shewing the nature of the planets, with the events that shall befall women and children born under them. With several predictions very useful for the female sex* (London: Printed by J.S. for the Company of Stationers 1659).

———, *An Almanack, or prognostication for the year of our Lord 1660. Being the third after bissextile or leap year. Calculated for the meridian of London, and may without exception serve for England, Scotland, and Ireland* (London: Printed for the Company of Stationers, 1660).

Josselin, Ralph R., *The Diary of Ralph Josselin, 1616–1683*, ed. Alan MacFarlane (London: Oxford University Press for the British Academy, 1976).

Joubert, Laurent, *La Médecine et le régime de santé, ses erreurs populaires et propos vulgaires*, ed. Madeleine Tiollais, 2 vols (Paris and Montreal: L'Harmattan, 1997).

Kors, Alan Charles and Edward Peters, eds, *Witchcraft in Europe, 1100–1700: A Documentary History* (Philadelphia: University of Pennsylvania Press, 1972).

Krämer, Heinrich and James Sprenger, *Malleus Maleficarum*, an unabridged online republication of the 1928 edition, transcribed by Wicasta Lovelace and Christie Rice, intro. Wicasta Lovelace, 1998–2000, http://www.malleusmaleficarum.org/.

Lancre, Pierre de, *Tableau de l'inconstance des mauvais anges et demons (1612)*, ed. Nicole Jacques-Chaquin (Paris: Aubier, 1982).

Lea, Henry Charles and Arthur C. Harland, eds, *Materials toward a History of Witchcraft*, 3 vols (New York and London: Thomas Yoseloff, 1957).

Luis de Léon, Fray, *A Bilingual Edition of Fray Luis de Léon's La Perfecta Casada: The Role of Married Women in Sixteenth-Century Spain*, ed., trans. and intro. John A. Jones and Javier San José Lera, Spanish Studies, Vol. 2 (Lewiston, NY: Edwin Mellen, 1999).

Luther, Martin, *Commentary on the Epistle to the Galatians* (1535), trans. Theodore Graebner (Grand Rapids, MI: Zondervan, 1949), http://www.iclnet.org/pub/resources/text/wittenberg/luther/gal/web/gal3-01.html.

Maupeou Fouquet, Marie de, *Recueil de receptes, où est expliquée la manière de guerir à peu de frais toute sorte de maux tant internes, qu'externes inveterez, & qui ont passé jusqu'à present pour incurables* (Lyon: Certe, 1676).

———, *Le medecin desinteressé. Ou, l'on trouvera l'élite de plusieurs, remedes infaillibles trés-expérimentés, & à peu de frais. Le tout recueilli par les soins d'un docteur en médecine* (Limoges: Chez J. Farne, 1695).

———, *Recueil de remedes faciles et domestiques, choisis, experimentez, & trés-aprouvez pour toutes sortes de maladies internes, & externes, & difficiles à guerir* (Dijon: Jean Ressayre, 1701).

Marillac, Louise de, *Ecrits spirtuels* (Paris: Compagnie des Filles de la Charité, 1983).

Markham, Gervase, *Countrey Contentements, in Two Bookes…The Second intituled, The English Housewife* (London: J. Beale, 1623).

———, *The English Housewife*, ed. Michael R. Best (Kingston and Montreal: McGill Queen's Press, 1986).

Martindale, Adam, *Life of Adam Martindale Written by Himself, 1632*, ed. Reverend Richard Parkinson (London: Printed for the Chetham Society, 1845).

Mechthild of Magdeburg, Beatrice of Nazareth and Hadewijch of Brabant, *Beguine Spirituality: Mystical Writings of Mechthild of Magdeburg, Beatrice of Nazareth, and Hadewijch of Brabant*, intro. Fiona Bowie, trans. Oliver Davies (New York: Crossroad, 1990).

Mondeville, Henri de, *La Chirurgie de Maitre Henri de Mondeville*, ed. A. Bos, 2 vols (Paris: Firmin, Didot et cie, 1897).
Monro, Alexander, *Traité d'ostéologie, 1697–1767*, trans. Marie-Geneviève-Charlotte Thiroux d'Arconville, 2 vols (Paris: G. Cavelier, 1759).
Morand, Sauveur François, *An account of the remedy for the stone: lately published in England, according to an act of Parliament, assigning a reward of 5000£ to the discoverer. Extracted from the examinations of this remedy, given into the Royal Academy of Sciences at Paris* (London: Printed by H. Woodfall, 1741).
Muggleton, Lodowick, *The Acts of the Witnesses of the Spirit* (London, 1699).
Nantes Barrera, Oliva Sabuco de, *Nueva filosofía de la naturaleza del hombre* (Madrid: Editora Nacional, 1981).
———, *New Philosophy of Human Nature*, trans. and ed. Mary Ellen Waithe, Maria Colomer Vintro and C. Angel Zorita (Champaign, IL: University of Illinois Press, 2007).
——— and Octavio Cuartero Cifuentes, *Obras de Dona Oliva Sabuco de Nantes, escritora del siglo XVI* (Madrid: Establecimento Tipográfico de Ricardo Fé, 1888).
Nihell, Elizabeth, *A treatise on the art of midwifery. Setting forth various instruments: the whole serving to put all rational inquirers in a fair way of very safely forming their own judgment upon the question; which it is best to employ, in cases of pregnancy and lying-in, a man-midwife or, a midwife* (London: 1760).
O'Faolain Julia and Laura Martines, eds, *Not in God's Image: Women in History from the Greeks to the Victorians* (London: Temple Smith, 1973).
Oberndoerffer, Johannes, *The Anatomies of the true Physician and Counterfeit Mountebank*, trans. Francis Herring (London, 1602).
Ostorero, Martine, Agostino Paravicini Bagliani and Kathrin Utz Tremp, in collaboration with Catherine Chène, *L'imaginaire du sabbat: edition critique des texts les plus anciens (1430c–1440c)* (Lausanne: Section d'histoire, Faculté des letters, Université de Lausanne, 1999).
Paré, Ambroise, *Collected Works*, trans. Thomas Johnson (1634) (New York: Milford House, 1968).
Patin, Gui, *Lettres de Gui Patin*, ed. J.H. Reveillé-Paris, 3 vols (Paris: J.-B. Baillière, 1846).
Paul, Vincent de, *Règles ou constitutions communes de la congrégation de la Mission* (Paris: A. Le Clere, 1856).
———, *Conférences de S. Vincent de Paul aux filles de la Charité*, 2 vols (Paris: Pillet et Dumoulin, 1881).
———, *Conférences de saint Vincent de Paul aux Filles de la Charité, suivies d'avis et d'extraits de lettres de saint Vincent de Paul et de la Vénérable Louise de Marillac*, new edn (Paris: Communauté des Filles de la Charité, 1902).
———, *Correspondance, Entretiens, Documents*, ed. Pierre Coste, 14 vols (Paris : Librarie Lecoffe, 1920–26).
———, *The Conferences of St. Vincent de Paul to the Sisters of Charity*, trans. Joseph Leonard, 4 vols (Westminster, MD: Newman Press, 1952).
———, *Vincent de Paul and Louise de Marillac: Rules, Conferences, Writings*, ed. John E. Ryholt and Francis Ryan, Preface by Amin A. De Tarrazi (New York: Paulist Press, 1995).
Paston Family, *Paston Letters and Papers of the Fifteenth Century*, ed. Norman Davis, Richard Beadle and Colin Richmond, 3 vols (Oxford: Published for The Early English Text Society by the Oxford University Press, 2004–05).
———, *The Paston Letters, A.D. 1422–1509. New Complete Library*, ed. James Gairdner, 6 vols (Chatto & Windus, London: 1900–01).

———, *The Paston Women. Selected Letters*, ed. Diane Watt (Cambridge: D.S. Brewer, 2004).

Pizan, Christine de, *The Book of the City of the Ladies*, trans. Earl Jeffrey Richard, Foreword by Marina Warner (New York: Persea Books, 1972).

Poulain de la Barre, François, *De L'Education des Dames pour la conduite de l'esprit dans les sciences et dans les mœurs. Entretiens* (Paris: Jean du Puis, 1674).

———, *De L'Egalité des deux sexes* (Paris: Jean du Puis, 1673).

Primrose, James, *Popular Errours of the People in the matter of Physick. First written in Latine by the Learned Physician James Primrose, Doctor of Physick* (London: W. Willson for Nicholas Bourne, 1651).

Quincy, John, *Pharmacopoeia officinalis & extemporanea. Or, a complete English dispensary, in four parts…By John Quincy, M.D.*, 11th edn (London, 1739), Eighteenth Century Collections On-Line, Gale Group, http://galenet.galegroup.com/servelet/ECCO.

Rabelais, François, *Gargantua and Pantagruel*, ed. Donald Douglas (New York: The Modern Library, 1928), in 'Women in World History, Primary Sources, Europe', George Mason University, http://chnm.gmu.edu/wwh/p/83.html.

———, *Gargantua and Pantagruel, Complete. Five Books Of The Lives, Heroic Deeds And Sayings Of Gargantua And His Son Pantagruel*, trans. Sir Thomas Urquhart of Cromarty and Peter Antony Motteux (1653 edition), Project Guttenberg, 8 August 2004 [EBook #1200].

Raynalde, Thomas, *The birth of mankinde, otherwise named The womans booke. Set foorth in English by Thomas Raynalde phisition, and by him corrected, and augmented. Whose contents yée may reade in the table following: but most plainely in the prologue* (London: [By George Eld?] for Thomas Adams, 1604).

Rémy, Nicolas, *La Démonalâtrie* (Nancy: Presses Universitaires de Nancy, 1995).

Rogers, Timothy, *The Character of a Good Woman Both in a Single and Marry'd State Occasion'd by the Decease of Mrs Elizabeth Dunton Who Died May 28, 1697* (London, 1697).

Rosenbloom Jacob, 'Statements of Medical Interest from the Letters of Madame de Sévigné', *Medical Life*, 30 (1923): 71–108, 133–57, 291–307.

Rösselin, Eucharius, *Rosengarten*, ed. Gustav Klein (Munich: C. Kuhn, 1910).

———, *When midwifery became the male physician's province: the sixteenth century handbook: The Rose Garden for pregnant women and midwives*, trans. and intro. Wendy Arons (Jefferson, NC: McFarland & Co, 1994).

Rouvroy, Claude Henri de, comte de Saint-Simon, *Mémoires de Saint-Simon*, texte établi et annoté par Gonzague Truc, 7 vols (Paris: Gallimard, 1948–61).

Scot, Reginald, *The Discoverie of Witchcraft: being a reprint of the first edition published in 1584*, ed. with explanatory notes, glossary, and introduction by Brinsley Nicholson (East Ardsley, York: EP Publishing, 1973).

Searle, Arthur, ed., *Barrington Family Letters, 1628–1632* (London: Offices of the Royal Historical Society, 1933).

Serres, Olivier de, *Le Théâtre d'agriculture et mesnage des champs* (Arles: Actes Sud, 1997).

Sévigné, Marie de, *Letters of Madame de Sévigné to her daughter and her friends. Selected, with an introductory essay*, ed. Richard Aldington, 2 vols (New York: Bretanos, 1927; London: Routledge, 1927).

———, *The Letters of Madame de Sévigné*, intro. A. Edward Newton, 7 vols (Philadelphia: J.P. Horn, 1927).

———, *Lettres*, ed. Emile Gérard-Gailly, 3 vols (Paris: Gallimard, 1953–57).

———, *Correspondance*, texte établi, présenté et annoté par Robert Duchêne, 3 vols (Paris: Gallimard, 1972).

——, *Selected Letters*, intro. Leonard Tancock (Harmondsworth: Penguin, 1982).

Shakespeare, William, *The Comedy of Errors*, ed. T.S. Dorsch, intro. Ros King (Cambridge: Cambridge University Press, 2004).

Sharp, Jane, *The Midwives Book or the Whole Art of Midwifery Discovered*, ed. Elaine Hoby (Oxford: Oxford University Press, 1999).

Shatzmiller, Joseph, *Médecine et Justice en Provence: Médiévale Documents de Manosque* (Aix-en-Provence: Publications de l'Université de Provence, 1989).

Shaw, Peter, *Leçons de chymie, propres à perfectionner la physique, le commerce et les arts*, trans. and preface Marie-Geneviève-Charlotte Thiroux d'Arconville (Paris: J.T. Herissant, 1759).

Smellie, William, MD, *A Treatise on the theory and practice of midwifery* (London: D. Wilson, 1752).

Smith, Toulin, ed., *English gilds. The original ordinances of more than one hundred early English gilds: Together with the old usages of the cite of Wynchester; the Ordinances of Worcester; the Office of the mayor of Bristol; and the Costomary of the manor of Tettenhall–Regis. From original mss. of the fourteenth and fifteenth centuries*, with an introduction and glossary by his daughter, Lucy Toulmin Smith, and a preliminary essay 'On the history and development of gilds', by Lujo Brentano (Oxford: Early English Text Society, Oxford University Press, 1924).

Sonnet de Courval, Thomas, *Satyre contre les charlatans et les pseudo médecins empyriques* (Paris: Jean Milot, 1610).

Sowerby, Leonard, *The Ladies Dispensatory, containing the Nature, Virtues, and Qualities of all Herbs and Simples usefull in Physick, reduced into a Methodical order, for their more ready use on any Sicknesse, or other accident of the Body, the like never published in English* (London: R. Ibbitson, 1651).

Spiller, Elizabeth, Betty S. Travitsky and Anne Lake Prescott, eds, *Seventeenth-Century English Recipe Books: Cooking Physics and Chirugery in the Works of Queen Henrietta Maria and Mary Tillinghast* (Burlington, VT: Ashgate, 2008).

Stone, Sarah, *A Complete Practice of Midwifery* (London: T. Cooper, 1737).

Stubbe, Henry, *Campanella revived or, An enquiry into the history of the Royal Society, whether the virtuosi there do not pursue the projects of Campanella for the reducing England unto Popery* (London: Printed for the author, 1670). Early English Books Online.

Sydenham, Thomas, *Observationes medicae* (London: G. Kettilby, 1676).

Thiroux d'Arconville, Marie-Geneviève-Charlotte, *Essai pour servir a l'histoire de la putréfaction* (Paris: Chez P.F. Didot le jeune,1766).

Thornton, Alice, *The Autobiography of Mrs. Thornton, of East Newton, Co. York* (Durham: The Society by Andrews and co., 1875).

Trotula, *The Trotula: A Medieval Compendium of Women's Medicine*, ed. and trans. Monica H. Green (Philadelphia: University of Pennsylvania Press, 2001).

Trye, Mary, *Medicatrix, or, The woman-physician: vindicating Thomas O Dowde ... against the calumnies and abusive reflections of Henry Stubbe ... A revival of Mr. O Dowd's medicines, and other chymical remedies with an advertisement thereof* (London: Printed by T.R. & N.T. and sold by Henry Broome and John Leete, 1675).

Verdier, Jean, *La Jurisprudence de la Médecine en France ou Traité historique et juridique*, 2 vols (Alençon: Malassis le jeune, 1762–63).

Vives, Juan, *Livre de l'institution de la femme chrestienne*, trans. Pierre de Changy (Paris: Jacques Kerver, 1542).

——, *The Instruction of a Christen Woman*, ed. Virginia Walcott Beauchamp, Elizabeth H. Hageman and Margaret Mikesell, *Introduction to Juan Luis Vives* (Urbana: University of Illinois Press, 2002).

Walker, Anthony, *The vertuous wife: or, the holy life of Mrs. Elizabeth Walker* (London: John Leake, 1690). Early English Books Online, http://eebo.chadwyck.com.myaccess.library.utoronto.ca/home.

Weyer, Johann, *Witches, Devils, and Doctors in the Renaissance, Johann Weyer, De praestigiis daemonum*, ed. George Mora and Benjamin Kohl, trans. John Shea (Binghampton, NY: Medieval and Renaissance Texts & Studies, 1991).

Whitlock, Richard, *Zwotomia, Or Observations on the Present Manners of the English* (London, 1654).

———, *Observations on the Present Manners of the English Briefly Anatomizing the Living by the Dead. With an Usefull Detection of the Mountebanks of Both Sexes* (London: Thomas Roycroft, 1654).

Wickersheimer, Ernest, *Commentaires de la Faculté de médecine de l'Université de Paris (1395–1516)*, Collection de documents inédits sur l'historie de France (Paris: Imprimerie nationale, 1915).

Willughby, Percival, *Observations in Midwifery by Percival Willughby (1596–1685); Edited from the original MS. by Henry Blenkinsop, 1863*, intro. John L. Thornton (Wakefield: S.R. Publishers, 1972).

Wolley, Hannah, *The Queen-like Closet or Rich Cabinet stored with all manner of rare receipts for preserving, candying & cookery. Very pleasant and beneficial to all ingenious persons of the female sex* (London: R. Lowndes, 1670), http://www.gutenberg.org/etext/14377.

———, *The Gentlewoman's Companion to the Female Sex* (London: A. Maxwell, 1673).

Young, Sidney, *Memorials of the craft of surgery in England, from materials compiled by John Flint South*, ed. D'Arcy Power (London: Cassells, 1886).

———, *The annals of the barber-surgeons of London compiled from their records and other sources* (London: Blades, East & Blades, 1890).

Secondary sources

Unpublished

Cook, Harold John, 'The Regulation of Medical Practice in London under the Stuarts, 1607–1704', unpublished PhD dissertation, University of Michigan, 1981.

Doviak, Ronald J., 'The University of Naples and the Study and Practice of Medicine in the Thirteenth and Fourteenth Centuries', unpublished PhD dissertation, City University of New York, 1974.

Klairmont-Lingo, Alison, 'The Rise of Medical Practitioners in Sixteenth-Century France: The Case of Lyon and Montpellier', unpublished PhD dissertation, University of California at Berkeley, 1980.

Sawyer, Ronald C., 'Patients, Healers, and Disease in the Southeast Midlands, 1597–1634', unpublished PhD dissertation, University of Wisconsin-Madison, 1986.

Stine, Jennifer K., 'Opening Closets: The Discovery of Household Medicine in Early Modern England', unpublished PhD dissertation, Stanford University, 1996.

Wilson, Adrian, 'Childbirth in Seventeenth and Eighteenth Century England', unpublished PhD dissertation, University of Sussex, 1983.

Published secondary sources

Search aids, encyclopedia articles and dictionaries

Directory of Medical Licences issued by the Archbishop of Canterbury, 1535–1775, http://www.lambethpalacelibrary.org/holdings/Catalogues.

The Oxford American Dictionary of Current English, ed. Frank R. Abate (Oxford: Oxford University Press, 1999), *Oxford Reference Online*, http://www.oxfordreference.com.myaccess.library.utoronto.ca/views/GLOBAL.html.

Class, Joseph S., 'Ven. Louise de Marillac Le Gras', *New Advent Catholic Encyclopedia* (New York: Robert Appleton Company, 1907), online edition, Kevin Knight (2007), http://www.newadvent.org/cathen/09133b.htm.

Coumont, Jean-Pierre, *Demonology and Witchcraft: An Annotated Bibliography* (Utrecht: Hes & DeGraaf, 2004).

Echols, Anne and Marty Williams, *An Annotated Index of Medieval Women* (Princeton, NJ: Princeton University Press, 1993).

Farmer, David Hugh, 'Chantal, Jane Frances de', 'Vincent de Paul', 'Catherine of Genoa', in *The Oxford Dictionary of Saints* (Oxford: Oxford University Press, 2003), *Oxford Reference Online*. http://www.oxfordreference.com/.

Gilliat-Smith, Ernest, 'Beguines & Beghards', in *New Advent Catholic Encyclopedia*, Vol. II (New York: Robert Appleton Company, 1907), online edition, Kevin Knight (2007), http://www.newadvent.org/cathen/02389c.htm.

Gillispie, Charles Coulston, *Dictionary of Scientific Biography*, 18 vols (New York: Scribner, 1980–90).

Green, Monica, 'Midwives and Other Female Practitioners', in Thomas Glick, Steven J. Livesey and Faith Wallis, eds, *Medieval Science, Technology and Medicine: An Encyclopedia* (New York and London: Routledge, 2005).

Grinstein, Louise S., Rose K. Rose and Miriam Rafailovich, eds, *Women in Chemistry and Physics: A Bibliographic Sourcebook* (Westport, CT: Greenwood, 1994).

Hatch, Robert A., 'Catalog of the Scientific Community', Agrippa, Heinrich Cornelius [Agrippa von Nettesheim], in *The Scientific Revolution, Westfall Catalogue*, University of Florida (1998), http://web.clas.ufl.edu/users/rhatch/pages/03-Sci-Rev/SCI-REV-Home/resource-ref-read/major-minor-ind/westfall-dsb/SAM-A.htm.

Kibler, William N. and Grover A. Zinn, eds, *Medieval France: An Encyclopedia* (New York and London: Garland, 1995).

Lawler, Jennifer, *Encyclopedia of the Middle Ages* (London and Jefferson WI: McFarland & Co., 2001).

Lee, Sidney, ed., *Dictionary of National Biography* (London: Smith, Elder, & Co. 1909).

Martin, Richard, ed.-in-chief, *Encyclopedia of Islam and the Muslim World*, 2 vols (New York: Macmillan Reference USA, 2004).

Moeller, Charles, 'Orders of the Holy Ghost', *The Catholic Encyclopedia*, Vol. VII (New York: Robert Appleton Company, 1907), online edition, Kevin Knight (2007), http://www.newadvent.org/cathen/07415a.htm.

Morris, William, ed., *The American Heritage Dictionary of the English Language* (Boston: Houghton Mifflin, 1969).

Nicholls, Christine Stephanie and Godfrey Hugh Lancelot Le May, eds, *Dictionary of National Biography: Missing Persons* (Oxford: Oxford University Press, 1994).

O'Brien, T.C., ed., *Corpus Dictionary of Western Churches* (Washington: Corpus, 1970).

Portalié, Eugène. 'Saint Augustine', *New Advent Catholic Encyclopedia*, Vol. II (New York, Robert Appleton Company, 1907), online edition, 1999, http://www.newadvent.org/cathen/02089a.htm.

Porter, Roy, ed., *The Cambridge History of Science*, Vol. 4, *Eighteenth-Century Science* (Cambridge University Press, 2003).

Roth, Norman, ed., *Medieval Jewish Civilization: An Encyclopedia* (London and New York: Routledge, 2003).

Sartori, Eva Martin, ed., *The Feminist Encyclopedia of French Literature* (Westport, CT: Greenwood, 1999).

Schlager Neil and Josh Lauer, eds, *Science and its Times*, 8 vols (Detroit: Gale, 2000), Gale Virtual Reference Library, Gale, Canadian Research Knowledge Network, http://go.galegroup.com.myaccess.library.utoronto.ca/ps/start.do?p=GVRL&u=utoronto_main.

Shearer, Benjamin F. and Barbara S. Shearer, eds, *Notable Women in the Sciences: A Biographical Dictionary* (Westport, CT: Greenwood, 1996).

Simpson, J.A. and E.S.C Weaver, eds, *Oxford English Dictionary*, Vol. X, 2nd edn (Oxford: Clarendon Press, 1989).

Snodgrass, Mary Ellen, *Historical Encyclopedia of Nursing* (Santa Barbara: ABC–CLIO, 2000).

Touwaide, Alain, 'Galen', in Thomas Glick, Steven Livesay and Faith Willis, eds, *Medieval Science, Technology and Medicine: An Encyclopedia* (New York and London: Routledge, 2005).

Walton, John, Paul B. Beeson and Ronald Bodley Scott, eds, *The Oxford Companion to Medicine*, 2 vols (Oxford: Oxford University Press, 1986).

Windsor, Laura Lynn, *Women in Medicine: An Encyclopedia* (Santa Barbara: ABC-CLIO, 2002).

Journal articles

Abel-Halim, Rabie E., 'Ibn Zuhr (Avenzoar) and the progress of surgery', *Saudi Medical Journal*, 26(9) (2005): 1333–9.

Agin, Shane, '"Comment se font les enfants?" Sex Education and the Preservation of Innocence in Eighteenth-Century France', *MLN: Modern Language Notes*, 117 (2002): 722–36.

Allen, Phyllis, 'Medical Education in 17th Century England', *Journal of the History of Medicine & Allied Sciences* (January 1946): 115–43.

Anselment, Raymond A., '"The Want of Health": An Early Eighteenth-Century Self-Portrait of Sickness', *Literature and Medicine*, 15(2) (1996): 225–43.

Auden, G.A., 'The Gild of Barber-Surgeons of the City of York', *Proceedings of the Royal Society of Medicine*, 21(II) (May–October 1928): 1400–6.

Bancroft-Livingstone, George, 'Louise de la Vallière and the Birth of the Man-Midwife', *Journal of Obstetrics and Gynaecology of the British Empire*, LXIII (1956): 261–7.

Barkai, Ron, 'A Medieval Hebrew Treatise of Obstetrics', *Medical History*, 33(1) (January 1989): 96–119.

Bénard, Louis and Paul Delaunay, 'Le cours de sages-femmes dans la généralité d'Alençon au XVIIIe siècle. Note préliminaire', *Bulletin de la Société française d'Histoire de la Médecine*, 8 (1909): 117–20.

Benedek, Thomas, 'The Changing Relationship between Midwives and Physicians during the Renaissance', *Bulletin of the History of Medicine*, 51 (1977): 550–64.

Bennett, David, 'Medical Practice and Manuscripts in Byzantium', *Social History of Medicine*, 13(2) (2000): 279–91.

Benton, John F., 'Trotula, Women's Problems, and the Professionalization of Medicine in the Middle Ages', *Bulletin of the History of Medicine*, 59(1) (Spring 1985): 30–53.

Beya Alonso Ernesto, 'Una precursora farmacéutica del Renacimiento', *Boletin de la Sociedad Espanola de Historia de la Farmacía* (December 1984): 245–7.

Blake, John B., 'The Compleat Housewife', *Bulletin of the History of Medicine*, 49 (1975): 30–42.

Boulinier, Georges, 'Une femme anatomiste au siècle des Lumières: Marie Marguerite Biheron (1719–1795)', *Histoire des sciences médicales,* 35(4) (2001): 411–23.

Boutry, Maurice, 'Les tribulations d'une guérisseuse au XVIIIe siècle', *La Chronique Médicale,* 9 (1905): 289–97.

Bullough, Vern L., 'The Development of Medical Guilds at Paris', *Medievalia et Humanistica,* XII (1958): 33–45

———, 'Training of the Non-University-Educated Medical Practitioners in the Later Middle Ages', *Journal of the History of Medicine and Allied Sciences,* 14 (October 1959): 446–9.

———, 'The Term Doctor', *Journal of the History of Medicine,* 18 (1963): 284–7.

———, 'Medieval Medical and Scientific Views of Women', *Viator,* 4 (1973): 485–501.

Chalumeau, R.P., 'L'assistance aux malades pauvres au XVIIe siècle', *Dix-Huitième Siècle,* XC–XCI (1971): 75–86.

Chéreau, Achille, 'Procès intenté à Paris, en 1322, par la Faculté de Médecine, contre une femme exerçant illégalement la medicine', *L'Union Médicale* (7 August 1866): 241–8.

Clapper Brack, Datha, 'Displaced – the Midwife by the Male Physician', *Women and Health,* 1 (1976): 18–24.

Codellas, Pan S., 'The Pantocrator: the Imperial Byzantine Medical Center of the XIIth Century AD in Constantinople', *Bulletin of the History of Medicine,* 12 (1942): 392–410.

Cook, 'Harold J., 'The Society of Chemical Physicians, the New Philosophy, and the Restoration Court', *Bulletin of the History of Medicine,* 61 (1987): 61–87.

Cardoner, Planas A., 'Mujeres Hebreas Practicando la Medecina', *Sefarad,* 9 (2) (1949): 441–6.

Dock, George, 'Robert Talbor, Madame de Sévigné, and the Introduction of Cinchona: An Episode Illustrating the Influence of Women in Medicine', *Annals of Medical History,* 4 (1922): 241–7.

Dols, Michael W., 'The Origins of the Islamic Hospital: Myth and Reality', *Bulletin of the History of Medicine,* 61 (1987): 367–90.

Dufrenoy, Marie-Louise and Jean Dufrenoy, 'Coffee, the "Exotik Drink"', *Scientific Monthly,* 70(3) (March 1950): 185–8.

Dumas, Geneviève, 'Les Femmes et les pratiques de la santé, dans le "Registre des plaidoiries du Parlement de Paris", 1364–1427', *Canadian Bulletin of Medical History/ Bulletin canadien d'histoire de la médicine,* 13 (1996): 3–27.

Dunan, Anne, 'Mélancolie, enthousiasme et folie: pathologie et inspiration dans la littérature dissidente', *Etudes Epistémè,* 7 (spring 2005): 65–93.

Dunn, Peter M., 'Eucharius Rösslin (c.1470–1526) of Germany and the re-birth of midwifery', *Archives of Disease in Childhood,* 79 (July 1998): F77–8, http://fnbmjjournals.com/cgi/content/full/79/1/F77.

———, 'Louise Bourgeois (1563–1636): Royal Midwife of France', *Archives of Disease in Childhood and Neonatal Edition,* 89 (2004): F185, http://fn.bmjjournals.com/cgi/content/full/89/2/F185.

Eamon, William, 'From the Secrets of Nature to Public Knowledge: The Origins of the Concept of Openness in Science', *Minerva,* 23(3) (September 1985): 321–44.

———, 'Science and Popular Culture in Sixteenth Century Italy: The "Professors of Secrets" and their Books', *Sixteenth Century Journal,* 16(4) (Winter 1985): 471–85.

Evenden, Doreen A., 'Gender Differences in the Licensing and Practice of Female and Male Surgeons in Early Modern England', *Medical History*, 42(2) (April 1998): 194–216.

Findlen, Paula, 'Science as a Career in Enlightenment Italy: The Strategies of Laura Bassi', *Isis*, 84 (1993): 441–69.

Forbes, Thomas R., 'The Regulation of English Midwives in the Sixteenth and Seventeenth Centuries', *Medical History*, 8(3) (1964): 235–44.

———, 'The Regulation of English Midwives in the Eighteenth and Nineteenth Centuries', *Medical History*, 15(4) (October 1971): 352–62.

García-Ballester, Luis, 'Medical Science in Thirteenth-Century Castile: Problems and Prospects', *Bulletin of the History of Medicine*, 61 (1987): 183–202.

Gautier, Paul, 'Le typikon du Christ Sauveur Pantocrator', *Revue des Etudes Byzantines* 32 (1974): 1–147.

———, 'Le typikon de la Théotokos Kécharitôménè', *Revue des Etudes Byzantines*, 43 (1985): 5–166.

Gelfand, Toby, 'Medical Professionals and Charlatans: The Comité de Salubrité enquête of 1790–91', *Social History*, 11 (1978): 62–97.

Gélis, Jacques, 'Sages-Femmes et Accoucheurs: l'obstétrique populaire aux XVIIe et XVIIIe siècles', *Annales, Economies, Sociétés et Civilisations*, 32(5) (September–October 1977): 927–57.

Gentilcore, David, '"All that pertains to Medicine": Protomedici and Protomedicati in Early Modern Italy', *Medical History*, 38(2) (April 1994): 121–42.

Getz, Faye Marie, 'Charity, Translation and the Language of Medical Learning in Medieval England', *Bulletin of the History of Medicine*, 64 (1990): 1–17.

———, 'Medical Practitioners in Medieval England', *Social History of Medicine*, 3 (1990): 245–83.

Golinski, Jan V., 'Peter Shaw: Chemistry and Communication in Augustan England', *Ambix: The Journal of the Society for the History of Alchemy and Chemistry*, 30(1) (March 1983): 19–29

Green, Monica H., 'Women's Medical Practice and Health Care in Medieval Europe', *Signs*, 14 (1989): 434–73.

———, 'Books as a Source of Medical Education for Women in the Middle Ages', *Dynamis*, 20 (2000): 331–70.

———, 'From "Diseases of Women" to "Secrets of Women": The Transformation of Gynaecological Literature in the Later Middle Ages', *Journal of Medieval and Early Modern Studies*, 30 (1) (2000): 5–40.

Greenbaum, Louis S., 'Nurses and Doctors in Conflict: Piety and Medicine in the Paris Hôtel-Dieu on the Eve of the French Revolution', *Clio Medica*, 13(3–4): 247–67.

Guy, John R., 'The Episcopal Licensing of Physicians, Surgeons and Midwives', *Bulletin of the History of Medicine*, 56 (1982): 528–42.

Harley, David, 'Historians as Demonologists: The Myth of the Mid-wife-witch', *Social History of Medicine* (1990): 99–124.

———, '"Bred up in the Study of that Faculty": Licensed Physicians in North-West England, 1660–1760', *Medical History*, 38 (1994): 398–420.

———, 'James Hart of Northampton and the Calivinist Critique of Priest-Physicians: An Unpublished Polemic of the early 1620s', *Medical History*, 42 (1998): 362–86.

Haviland, Thomas N. and Lawrence Charles Parish, 'A Brief Account of the Use of Wax Models in the Study of Medicine', *Journal of the History of Medicine and Allied Sciences*, 25 (1970): 52–75.

Heinsohn Gunnar and Otto Steiger, 'Birth Control: The Political-Economic Rationale behind Jean Bodin's *Démonomanie*', *History of Political Economy*, 31(3) (1999): 423–48.

Hellwarth Jennifer Wynne, '"Be unto me as a precious ointment": Lady Grace Mildmay, Sixteenth-Century Female Practitioner', *Dynamis*, 19 (1999): 106–11.

Hoolihan, C., 'Thomas Young, M.D., 1726–83 and Obstetrical Education', *Journal of the History of Medicine*, 40 (1985): 327–45.

Horowitz, Maryanne Cline, 'Aristotle and Woman', *Journal of the History of Biology*, 9(2) (Fall 1976): 183–213.

Howard-Jones, N., 'John Quincy, M.D. [d. 1722] Apothecary and Iatrophysical Writer', *Journal of the History of Medicine and Allied Sciences*, 6(2) (1951): 149–75.

Huppert, M.P., 'Italian Women Doctors in the Middle Ages', *History of Medicine Quarterly*, 5(3) (Autumn 1973): 25–6.

James, R.R., 'Licences to Practise Medicine and Surgery issued by the Archbishops of Canterbury, 1580–1775', *Janus*, 41 (1937): 97–106.

Jiménez Munoz, Juan M., 'Salario de medicos, cirujanos, boticarios y enfermeras', *Asclepio: Archivo iberomaeircano de historia de la medicina y antropología médica*, 26–7 (1974–1975): 548.

Jouanne, René, 'Assistance, Bienfaisance et Charité en Normandie, Orientation de Recherches et Souvenirs', *Bulletin de la Société française d'histoire des hôpitaux*, 34 (1977): 31–45.

Kealey, Edward J., 'England's Earliest Women Doctors', *Journal of the History of Medicine and Allied Sciences*, 40 (1985): 473–7.

Klairmont-Lingo, Alison, 'Empirics and Charlatans in Early Modern France: The Genesis of the Classification of the "Other" in Medical Practice', *Journal of Social History*, 19(4) (Summer 1986): 583–604.

———, 'Women Healers and the Medical Marketplace of 16th-Century Lyons', *Dynamis*, 19 (1999): 79–94.

Kibre, Pearl, 'The Faculty of Medicine at Paris, Charlatanism, and Unlicensed Medical Practices in the Later Middle Ages', *Bulletin of the History of Medicine*, 28 (January–February 1953): 1–20.

Kristeller, Paul Oskar, 'The School of Salerno: Its Development and its Contribution to the History of Learning', *Bulletin of the History of Medicine*, 17 (1945): 138–94.

Lacquer, Thomas W., 'Sex in the Flesh', *Isis*, 94 (2003): 300–6.

L'Aignel-Lavastine and Ives M. Burill, 'Les Cliniques de Madame de Sévigné', *Bulletin de la Société Française d'Histoire de la Médecine*, XXVI (1932): 131–8.

Lander, Kathleen F., 'The Study of Anatomy by Women before the Nineteenth Century', *Proceedings of the Third International Congress of the History of Medicine* (1922): 125–34.

Langlois, Ernest, 'Le traité de Gerson contre le *Roman de la Rose*', *Romania* (1919): 29–48.

Lawence, C.J., 'William Buchan: Medicine Laid Open', *Medical History*, 19(1) (January 1975): 20–35.

Lekstrom, J.A., 'Medical Literature of Medieval Salerno: Evolution of the Modern Medical Professional', *Pharos*, 53(1) (1990): 21–7.

Logan, Gabriella Berti, 'Women and the Practice and Teaching of Medicine in the Eighteenth and Early Nineteenth Centuries', *Bulletin of the History of Medicine*, 77 (2003): 506–35.

Longo, Lawrence D., 'Classic Pages in Obstretrics and Gynecology', *American Journal of Obstetrics and Gynecology*, 173 (December 1995): 1893–4.

López de Menses, Amada, 'Cinco Catalanas Licenciadas en Medicina por Pedro el Ceremonioso (1374–1382)', *Correro Erudito*, V(37) (1957): 252–4

López-Terrada, María Luz, 'Las prácticas médicas extraacadémicas en la ciudad de Valencia', *Dynamis*, 22 (2002): 85–120.

Lorentzon, Maria, 'Mediaeval London: Care of the Sick', *History of Nursing Journal*, 4 (1992/93): 100–10.

Madge, Bruce, 'Elizabeth Blackwell – the Forgotten Herbalist?' *Health Information and Libraries Journal*, 18 (2001): 144–52.

Martensen, Robert L., 'Habit of Reason: Anatomy of Anglicanism in Restoration England', *Bulletin of the History of Medicine*, 66 (1992): 511–35.

Martin-Araguz, A., C. Bustamante-Martinez and V. Fernandez-Armayor, 'Sabuco's Suco Nerveo and the Origins of Neurochemistry in the Spanish Renaissance', *Revista de Neurologia*, 36(12) (2003): 1190–8.

Messenger, Rebecca, 'Waxing Poetic: Anna Morandi Manzolini's Anatomical Sculptures', *Configurations*, 9(1) (2001): 65–97.

Minkowski William L., 'Women Healers of the Middle Ages: Selected Aspects of their History', *American Journal of Public Health*, 82(2) (February 1992): 288–95.

———, 'Physician Motives in Banning Traditional Healers', *Women and Health*, 21(1)(1994): 83–96.

Maupeou Jacques de, 'La mere de Foucquet', *Hommes et mondes: revue mensuelle* (May 1949): 72–90.

Millar, Timothy S., 'Byzantine Hospitals', *Dumbarton Oak Papers*, 38, *Symposium on Byzantine Medicine* (1984): 53–63.

Mortimer, Ian, 'Diocesan Licensing and Medical Practitioners in South-West England, 1660–1780', *Medical History*, 48(1) (January 2004): 49–68.

Murray, Margaret, 'Historians as Demonologists: The Myth of the Mid-wife-witch', *Social History of Medicine*, 3(1) (1990): 1–26.

Olry, R., 'Medieval Neuroanatomy: The Text of Mondino dei Luzzi and the Plates of Guido da Vigevano', *Journal of the History of Neurosciences*, 6(2) (August 1997): 113–23.

Pairet, Montserrat Cabré I and Fernando Salmón Muñiz, 'Poder académico *versus* autoridad femenina: la Facultad de Medicina de París contra Jacoba Félicié (1322)', *Dynamis*, 19 (1999): 55–78.

Pelling, Margaret, 'Occupational Diversity: Barber-Surgeons and the Trades of Norwich', *Bulletin of the History of Medicine*, 56 (1982): 484–511.

———, 'Healing the Sick Poor: Social Policy and Disability in Norwich, 1550–1640', *Medical History*, 29(2) (April 1985): 115–37.

———, 'The Women of the Family? Speculations around Early Modern British Physicians', *Social History of Medicine*, 8 (1995): 383–401.

Petrelli, Richard L., 'The Regulation of French Midwifery during the Ancien Régime', *Journal of the History of Medicine and Allied Sciences*, 26 (July 1971): 276–92.

Pilcher, James E., 'Guy de Chauliac and Henri de Mondeville, A Surgical Retrospect', *Annals of Surgery*, 21(1) (January 1885): 84–102.

Pinto, Lucille B., 'The Folk Practice of Gynecology and Obstetrics in the Middle Ages', *Bulletin of the History of Medicine*, 47 (1973): 513–21.

Piomelli, Danielle and Antonino Pollio, 'A Study in Renaissance Psychotropic Plant Ointments', *History and Philosophy of Life Sciences*, 16(2) (1994): 241–73.

Pomata, Gianna, 'Practising between Earth and Heaven: Women Healers in Seventeenth Century Bologna', *Dynamis*, 19 (1999): 119–43.

Pirami, Edmea, 'La donna medico nei secoli', *Bullettino delle scienze mediche*, 138(2) (1966): 205–13.

Power, D'Arcy, 'English Medicine and Surgery in the Fourteenth Century', *Lancet*, II (1914): 176–83.

Power, Eileen Edna, 'Some Women Practitioners of Medicine in the Middle Ages', *Proceedings of the Royal Society of Medicine*, 14 (21 December 1921): 20–3.

Poynter, F.N.L., 'Nicholas Culpeper and his Books', *Journal of the History of Medicine and Allied Sciences*, 17 (1962): 152–67.

Porter, Roy, 'Female Quacks in the Consumer Society', *History of Nursing Journal*, 3(1) (1990–91): 1–25.

Raach, John H., 'English Medical Licensing in the Early Seventeenth-Century', *Yale Journal of Biology and Medicine*, 16(4) (March 1944): 267–89.

———, 'Five Early Seventeenth Century English Country Gentlemen', *Journal of the History of Medicine and Allied Sciences*, 20 (1965): 213–25.

Ramsey, Matthew, 'Traditional Medicine and Medical Enlightenment: The Regulation of Secret Remedies in the Ancien Régime', *Historical Reflections*, 9(1–2) (1982): 215–32.

———, 'From *Expert* to *Spécialiste*: The Conception of Specialization in Eighteenth- and Nineteenth-Century French Surgery', *History of Ideas in Surgery: Proceedings of the 17th International Symposium for the Comparative History of Medicine – East and West* (Tokyo, Japan: 1997): 69–117.

Richards, Penny, 'A Life in Writing: Elizabeth Cellier and Print Culture', *Women's Writing*, 7(3) (2000): 411–25.

Robb, Hunter, 'Remarks on the Writings of Louyse Bourgeois', *Johns Hopkins Hospital Bulletin*, 38 (September 1893): 1–25.

Robbins, Russell Hope, 'Medical Manuscripts in Middle English', *Speculum*, XLV (July 1970): 393–415.

Roberts, R.S., 'The Personnel and Practice of Medicine in Tudor and Stuart England: Part I. The Provinces', *Medical History* 6(4) (October 1962): 363–83.

Rosenberg, Charles E., 'Medical Text and Social Context: Explaining William Buchan's Domestic Medicine', *Bulletin of the History of Medicine and Allied Sciences*, 57(1) (1982): 22–42.

Roth, Cecil, 'Qualifications of Jewish Physicians in the Middle Ages', *Speculum*, 28 (1953): 834–43.

Rubio Vela, Agustín, 'La asistencia hospitalaria infantil en la Valencia de los siglos XIV: pobres, huérfanos y expósitos', *Dynamis*, 2 (1982): 159–91.

Sawyer, Ronald C., '"Strangely Handled in all her Lyms": Witchcraft and Healing in Jacobean England', *Journal of Social History*, 22 (Spring 1989): 461–85.

Schiebinger, Londa, 'Skeletons in the Closet: The First Illustrations of the Female Skeleton in Eighteenth Century Anatomy', *Representations*, 14 (Spring 1986): 42–82.

——, 'Skelettestreit', *Isis*, 94 (2003): 307–13.

Segré, Marcello, 'Dottoresse Ebree Nel Medioevo', *Pagina di Storia della Medicina*, 14(5) (1970): 98–106.

Seidel, Michael A., 'Poulain de la Barre's *The Woman as Good as the Man*', *Journal of the History of Ideas*, 35 (1974): 499–508.

Selig, Karl Ludwig, 'Sabuco de Nantes, Feijoo, and Robert Southey', *Modern Language Notes*, 71(6) (June 1956): 415–16.

Sigerist, H.E., 'The History of Medical Licensure', *Journal of the American Medical Association*, CIV (1935): 1057–60.

Smith, Lisa, 'Reassessing the Role of the Family: Women's Medical Care in Eighteenth Century England', *Social History of Medicine*, 16(3) (2003): 327–42.

Soman, Alfred, 'The Parlement of Paris and the Great Witch Hunt, 1565–1640', *Sixteenth Century Journal*, 9 (1978): 31–44.

Stock-Morton, Phyllis, 'Control and Limitation of Midwives in Modern France: The Example of Marseille', *Journal of Women's History*, 8(1) (1996): 60–94.

Stoffart, Henri, 'Un avortement criminal en 1660', *Histoire des sciences médicales,* 20 (1986): 67–85.

Stohl, E. Lee, 'Parliament Hoodwinked by Joanna Stephens', *Surgery, Gynecology and Obstetrics,* 116 (1963): 509–11.

Trimmer, Eric J, 'Medical Folklore and Quackery', *Folklore,* 76(3) (autumn 1965): 161–75.

Usandizaga, Manuel, 'Damían Carbón', *XV Congreso Internacional de Historia de la Medicina, Madrid* (Acala, 23–29 September 1956): 1–7.

Verma, R.L., 'Women in Arab Medicine', *Studies in History of Medicine and Science,* 1 (1977): 271–84.

Viseltear, Arthur J., 'Joanna Stephens and the Eighteenth Century Lithontripics: A Misplaced Chapter in the History of Therapeutics', *Bulletin of the History of Medicine* (1968): 199–220.

Walton, Michael T., Robert M. Fineman and Phyllis J. Walton, 'Why Can't a Woman be More Like a Man? A Renaissance Perspective on the Biological Basis for Female Inferiority', *Women and Health,* 24(4) (1996): 87–95.

Weber, A.S., 'Women's Early Modern Medical Almanacs in Historical Context', *English Literary Renaissance,* 33 (3) 2003: 358–402.

Whitaker, Elaine E., 'Reading the Paston Letters Medically', *English Language Notes* 31(3) (July–September 1993): 19–27.

Wickersheimer, Ernest, 'Médecins et Chirurgiens dans les Hôpitaux du Moyen Âge', *Janus,* 32 (1928): 1–11.

Wyman, A.L., 'The Surgeoness: The Female Practitioner of Surgery 1400–1800', *Medical History,* 28 (1984): 22–41.

Chapters in books

Bakos, Adrianna E., '"A Knowledge Speculative and Practical" The Dilemma of Midwives' Education in Early Modern Europe', in Barbara J. Whitehead (ed.), *Women's Education in Early Modern Europe: A History, 1500–1800* (New York: Garland, 1999), pp. 224–50.

Barceló, Carmen, 'Mujeres, Campesinas, Mudéjares', in María J. Viguera (ed.), *La Mujer en Al-Andalus reflejos históricos de su actividad y categorías sociales: actas de las V Jornadas de Investigación Interdisciplinaria* (Madrid: Universidad Autónoma de Madrid, 1989), pp. 213–17.

Beier, Lucinda McCray, 'In Sickness and in Health: A Seventeenth Century Family's Experience', in Roy Porter (ed.), *Patients and Practitioners: Lay Perceptions of Medicine in Pre-Industrial Society* (Cambridge: Cambridge University Press, 1985), pp. 101–28.

Benedek, Thomas G., 'The Roles of Medieval Women in the Healing Arts', in Douglas Radcliff (ed.), *The Roles and Images of Women in the Middle Ages and Renaissance,* Vol. III (Pittsburgh: University of Pittsburgh Publications on the Middle Ages and Renaissance, 1975), pp. 145–59.

Blaisdell, Charmarie J., 'Angela Merici and the Ursulines', in Richard DeMolen (ed.), *Religious Orders of the Catholic Reformation* (New York: Fordham University Press, 1994), pp. 99–136.

Carlin, M., 'Medieval English Hospitals', in Lindsay Granshaw and Roy Porter (eds), *The Hospital in History* (London: Routledge, 1989), pp. 21–39.

Dinges, Martin, 'Health Care and Poor Relief in Regional Southern France in the Counter-Reformation', in Ole Peter Grell, Andrew Cunningham and Jon Arrizabala (eds), *Health Care and Poor Relief in Counter-Reformation Europe* (London and New York: Routledge, 1999), pp. 240–79.

Elum, Pedro Lopez and Mateu Rodrigo Lizondo, 'Las mujeres medievales y su ámbitio jurídico', in *Actas de las II Jornadas de Investigación Interdisciplinaria*, introduced by Cristina Segura Graiño (Madrid: Universidad Autónoma de Madrid, 1983), pp. 125–35.

Fournel-Guérin, Jacqueline, 'La femme morisque en Aragon', in *Les Morisques et Leur Temps Table Ronde International*, 4–7 July 1981, Montpellier (Paris: Editions du Centre National de la Recherche Scientifique, 1983), pp. 525–37.

Gamelin, Adrian, 'Jacoba Félicié: Power and Privilege in Fourteenth Century Medicine', in Peter Cruse (ed.), *Proceedings of the 7th Annual History of Medicine Days* (Calgary: The University of Calgary, 1998), pp. 69–73.

Gelbart, Nina Rattner, 'Books and the Birthing Business: The Midwife Manuals of Madame du Coudray', in Elizabeth C. Goldsmith and Dena Goodman (eds), *Going Public: Women and Publishing in Early Modern France* (Ithaca: Cornell University Press, 1995), pp. 79–98.

Gentilcore, David, '"Cradle of saints and useful institutions": Health Care and Poor Relief in the Kingdom of Naples', in Ole Peter Grell, Andrew Cunningham and Jon Arrizabala (eds), *Health Care and Poor Relief in Counter-Reformation Europe* (London and New York: Routledge, 1999), pp. 132–150.

Grundy, Isobel, 'Sarah Stone: Enlightenment Midwife', in Roy Porter (ed.), *Medicine in the Enlightenment* (Amsterdam: Rodopi, 1995), pp. 128–44.

Jones, Colin, 'Perspectives on Poor Relief, Healthcare and the Counter-Reformation in France', in Ole Peter Grell, Andrew Cunningham and Jon Arrizabala (eds), *Health Care and Poor Relief in Counter-Reformation Europe* (London and New York: Routledge, 1999), pp. 215–39.

Kibre, Pearl and Nancy G. Siraisi, 'The Institutional Setting: The Universities', in David C. Lindberg (ed.), *Science in the Middle Ages* (Chicago: University of Chicago Press, 1998), pp. 120–44.

Kristeller, Paul Oskar, 'Learned Women of Early Modern Italy: Humanists and University Scholars', in Patricia Labalme (ed.), *Beyond their Sex: Learned Women of the European Past* (New York: New York University Press, 1980), pp. 91–115.

Labarta, Ana, 'La Mujer Morisca: Sus Actitivades', in María J. Viguera (ed.), *La Mujer en Al-Andalus, Reflejos históricos de su actividad y categorías sociales* (Madrid: Ediciones de la Universidad Autónoma de Madrid, 1989), pp. 219–31.

Ladero Quesada, M.A, 'Los mudéjares de Castilla en la Baja Edad Media', in *I Simposio Internacional del Mudejarismo* (Madrid: Teruel, 1981), pp. 349–90.

Lane, Joan, 'The Role of Apprenticeship in Eighteenth-Century Medical Education in England', in W.F. Bynum and Roy Porter (eds), *William Hunter and the Eighteenth Century Medical World* (Cambridge: Cambridge University Press, 1985), pp. 57–104.

Lemay, Helen, 'Women and the Literature of Obstetrics and Gynecology', in Joel T. Rosenthal (ed.), *Medieval Women and the Sources of Medieval History* (Athens and London: University of Georgia Press, 1990), pp. 189–209.

Ottani Vittoria and Gabriella Giuliani Piccari, 'L'opera di Anna Morandi Manzolini nella ceroplastica anatomica bolognese', in *Alma mater studiorum: La presenza femminile dal XVIII al XX secolo. Ricerche sul rapport donna/cultura universitaria nell'Ateneo bolognese* (Bologna: Cooperativa Libraria Universitaria Editrice Bologna [CLUEB], 1988), pp. 81–103.

Palmer, Richard, 'Physicians and the State in Post-Medieval Italy,' in Andrew W. Russell (ed.), *The Town and State Physician in Europe from the Middle Ages to the Enlightenment* (Wolfenboutel: Herzog August Bibliothek, 1981), pp. 57–63.

Pernoud, Régine, 'La Femme et la Médecine au Moyen Age', in M.J. Imbault-Huart and F. Vidal (eds), *Colloque international d'histoire de la médecine médievale* (Orléans; Société orléanaise d'histoire de la médecine, Centre Jeanne d'Arc, 1985), pp. 38–43.

Perry, Mary Elizabeth, 'Las mujeres y su trabajo curativo en Sevilla, siglos XVI y XVII', in María Jesús Matilla and Margarita Ortega (eds), *El trabajo de las mujeres: siglos XVI–XX, Jornadas de Investigación Interdisciplinaria sobre la Mujer,* VI (Madrid: Universidad Autónoma de Madrid, 1987), pp. 40–50.

Pournaropoulos, G.C., 'Hospital and Social Welfare Institutions in the Medieval Greek Empire (Byzantium)', in *XVIIe Congrès International d'histoire de la medicine,* I (Athens, The Congress, 1961, pp. 378–80.

———, 'The Real Value of Greek Medicine (Byzantium)', in *XVIIe Congrès International d'histoire de la medicine,* I (Athens, The Congress, 1961), pp. 381–2.

Rodnite Lemay, Helen, 'Anthonius Guainerius and Medieval Gynaecology', in Julius Kirsher and Suzanne F. Wemple (eds), *Women of the Medieval World: Essays in Honour of John H. Mundy* (Oxford: Blackwell, 1985), pp. 317–36.

Talbot, C.H., 'Dame Trot and her Progeny', in T.S. Dorsch (ed.), *Essays and Studies in honour of Beatrice White* (London: John Murray, 1972), pp. 1–14.

Versluysen, Margaret Connor, 'Old Wives' Tales? Women Healers in English History', in Celia Davies (ed.), *Rewriting Nursing History* (London: Croom Helm, 1980), pp. 175–99.

Viguerie, Jean de, ' Une forme novelle de consacrée: enseignantes et hospitalières en France aux XVIIe et XVIIIe siècles', in Danielle Hause-Dubosc and Eliane Viennot (eds), *Femmes et Pouvoirs sous l'Ancien Régime* (Paris: Rivages, 1991), pp. 175–83.

Books

Albistur Maité and Daniel Armogathe, *Histoire du feminisme francais,* 2 vols (Paris: Des Femmes, 1977).

Alic, Margaret, *Hypatia's Heritage: A History of Women in Science from Antiquity through the Nineteenth Century* (Boston: Beacon Press, 1986).

Allen, Sister Prudence, *The Concept of Woman* (Montreal: Eden Press, 1985).

Álvarez, Manuel Fernández, *Casadas, Monjas, Rameras y Brujas* (Madrid: Espasa, 2002).

Amusen, Susan D. and Adele Seef (eds), *Attending to Early Modern Women* (Newark: University of Delaware Press, 1998).

Amundsen, Darrel W., *Medicine, Society and Faith in the Ancient and Medieval Worlds* (Baltimore: Johns Hopkins University Press, 1996).

Anderson, Bonnie S. and Judith P. Zinsser, *A History of their Own: Women in Europe from Prehistory to the Present,* 2 vols (New York and Oxford: Oxford University Press, 2000).

Anderson, James M., *Daily Life during the Spanish Inquisition* (Westport, CT: Greenwood, 2002).

Andreski, Stanislav, *Syphilis, Puritanism and Witch Hunts* (Basingstoke: Macmillan, 1989).

Ankarloo, Bengt, Stuart Clark and William Monter, *Witchcraft and Magic in Europe: The Period of the Witch Trials,* Vol. 4, *The Athlone History of Witchcraft and Magic in Europe* (London: Athlone, 2002).

——— and Gustav Henningen (eds), *Early Modern European Witchcraft Centres and Peripheries* (Oxford: Clarendon Press, 1990).

Antonioli, Roland, *Rabelais et la Médecine. Etudes Rabelaisiennes,* Vol. 12 (Geneva: Droz, 1976).

Arrizabalaga Jon, John Henderson and Roger French, *The Great Pox: The French Disease in Renaissance Europe* (New Haven, CT: Yale University Press, 1997).

Aungier, George James, *The History and Antiquities of Syon Monastery* (London: J.B. Nichols & Son, 1840).

Aveling, J.H., MD, *English Midwives, their History and Prospects* (London: Churchill, 1872).

Azema, Xavier, *Un Prelat Janseniste: Louis Fouquet: Evêque et Comte d'Agde (1656–1702)* (Paris: J. Vrin, 1963).

Ballesteros y Beretta, *Antonio Las Cortes de 1252* (Madrid: Establecimiento Tip. de Fortanet, Impresor de la Real Academia de la Historia, 1911).

Barkai, Ron, *A History of Jewish Gynecological Texts in the Middle Ages* (Leiden: E.J. Brill, 1998).

Barrett, Charles Raymond Booth, *The History of the Society of Apothecaries of London* (London: E. Stock, 1905).

Barry, Jonathan and Colin Jones (eds), *Medicine and Charity before the Welfare State* (London: Routledge, 1994).

———, Marianne Hester and Gareth Roberts (eds), *Witchcraft in Early Modern Europe*, Studies in Culture and Belief (Cambridge: Cambridge University Press, 1996).

Barstow, Anne Llewellyn, *Witchcraze: A New History of European Witchhunts* (San Francisco: Pandora, 1994).

Baskin, Judith, R., *Jewish Women in Historical Perspective* (Detroit: Wayne State University Press, 1991).

Beck, Lois and Nikki Keddie (eds), *Women in the Muslim World* (Cambridge, MA: Harvard University Press, 1978).

Bell, Rudolph M., *How To Do It: Guides to Good Living for Renaissance Italians* (Chicago: University of Chicago Press, 1999).

Bennassar, Bartolomé (ed.), *L'Inquisition Espagnole XVe–XIXe Siècles* (Paris: Hachette, 1979).

Bennett, H.S., *English Books & Readers 1558 to 1603: Being a Study in the History of the Book Trade in the Reign of Elizabeth I* (Cambridge: Cambridge University Press, 1965).

———, *English Books & Readers 1603 to 1640* (Cambridge: Cambridge University Press, 1970).

Bennett, Judith, M. et al. (eds), *Sisters and Workers in the Middle Ages* (Chicago: University of Chicago Press, 1989).

Benson, Evelyn Rose, *As We See Ourselves: Jewish Women in Nursing* (Indianapolis: Center for Nursing Publishing, 2001).

Berger, Margaret, *Hildegard of Bingen: On Natural Philosophy and Medicine: Selections from Cause et cure*, translated from Latin with introduction, notes and interpretive essay (Cambridge and Rochester, NY: D.S. Brewer, 1999).

Berger Natalia (ed.), *Jews and Medicine: Religion Culture, Science* (Tel-Aviv: Beth Hatefutsoth 1995).

Berriot-Salvadore, Evelyne, *Les Femmes dans la Société Française de la Renaissance* (Geneva: Droz, 1990).

Best, Michael R., *The English Housewife* (Kingston and Montreal: McGill Queens, 1986).

Bingham, Stella, *Ministering Angels* (Oradell, NJ: Medical Economics, 1979).

Bloch, Camille, *L'Assistance et l'Etat en France à la veille de la Révolution* (Paris: Alphonse Picard, 1908).

Borresen, Kari Elisabeth, *Subordination and Equivalence* (Washington: University Press of America, 1981).

Bostridge, Ian, *Witchcraft and its Transformation* (Oxford: Clarendon Press, 1997).
Boucé, P.G (ed.), *Sexuality in Eighteenth Century Britain* (Manchester: Manchester University Press, 1982).
Boulding, Elise, *The Underside of History: A View of Women through Time*, 2 vols (Newbury Park, CA: Sage Publications, 1992).
Bourdillon, Hilary, *Women as Healers: A History of Women in Medicine* (Cambridge: Cambridge University Press, 1988).
Brive, Marie-France (ed.), *Les Femmes de la Révolution Française 2* (Toulouse-le-Mirail: Presses Universitaires du Mirail, 1990).
Brockliss, Laurence and Colin Jones, *The Medical World of Early Modern France* (Oxford: Clarendon Press, 1997).
Brodman, James, *Charity and Welfare: Hospitals and the Poor in Medieval Catalonia* (Philadelphia: University of Pennsylvania Press, 1998).
Brooke, Elizabeth, *Women Healers: Portraits of Herbalists, Physicians and Midwives* (Rochester, VT: Healing Arts Press, 1995).
Broomhall, Susan, *Women's Medical Work in Early Modern France* (Manchester and New York: Manchester University Press, 2004).
Brown, Judith C. and Robert C. Davis, *Gender and Society in Renaissance Italy* (Longman: London & New York, 1998).
Brucker. Gene (ed.), *The Society of Renaissance Florence: A Documentary History* (New York: Harper & Row, 1971).
Buckler, Georgina Grenfell, *Anna Comnena: A Study* (London: Oxford University Press, 1929).
Bullough Vern L. and Bonnie Bullough, *The Emergence of Modern Nursing* (London: Macmillan, 1969).
Burill, Ives M., *La marquise de Sévigné, docteur en medicine (honoris causa)* (Paris: A. Legrand, 1931).
Cabanès Augustin, *Médecins Amateurs* (Paris: A. Michel, 1932).
Cadden, Joan, *Meanings of Sex Differences in the Middle Ages* (Cambridge: Cambridge University Press, 1992).
Campaux, Antoine, *La Question des Femmes au Quinzième Siècle* (Paris: Berger-Levrault, 1865).
Capp, Bernard, *English Almanacs 1500–1800* (Ithaca: Cornell University Press, 1979).
Caro Baroja, Julio, *The World of Witches*, trans. Nigel Glendinning (London: Phoenix Press, 2001).
Carroll, Berenice A. (ed.), *Liberating Women's History: Theoretical and Critical Essays* (Urbana: University of Illinois Press, 1976).
Carson Banks, Amanda, *Birth Chairs, Midwives and Medicine* (Jackson, MS: University of Mississippi Press, 1995).
Cartwright, Frederick F., *The Development of Modern Surgery from 1830* (London: Barker, 1967).
Chaff, Sandra L. et al. (eds), *Women in Medicine: A Bibliography of the Literature on Women Physicians* (Metuchen, NJ and London: Scarecrow Press, 1977).
Chalandon, Ferdinand, *Jean II Comnène 1118–1143 et Manuel I Comnène 1143–1180*, 2 vols (New York: B. Franklin, 1960).
Chamberlain, Mary, *Old Wives' Tales: Their History, Remedies and Spells* (London: Virago, 1981).
Chambers, Mortimer, Barbara Hanawalt, Theodore K. Rabb, Isser Woloch, Raymond Grew and Lisa Tiersten, *The Western Experience*, Vol. 1: *To the Eighteenth Century*, 9th edn (Boston: McGraw-Hill, 2006).

Charles, Lindsey and Lorne Duffin (eds), *Women and Work in Pre-Industrial England* (London: Croom Helm, 1985).
Charpy, Elisabeth, *Petite vie de Louise de Marillac* (Paris: Desclée de Brouwer, 1991).
Charrier, Edmée, *L'Evolution intellectuelle féminine* (Paris: Éditions Albert Mechelinck, 1931).
Chéruel, A., *Mémoires sur la vie publique et privée de Fouquet surintendant des finances*, 2 vols (Paris: Charpentier, 1862).
Clark, Alice, *Working Life of Women in the Seventeenth Century* (New York: Dutton, 1919; reprint, 1968).
Clark, George, *A History of the Royal College of Physicians of London*, 4 vols (Oxford: Clarendon Press, 1964).
Clemente, Jose Carlos, *La Escuela Universitaria de Enfermeras de Madrid* (Madrid: Cruz Roja Española, 1999).
Cobban, Alan B., *English University Life in the Middle Ages* (London: University College of London Press, 1999).
Cohen, Esther, *The Crossroads of Justice: Law and Culture in Late Medieval France* (Leiden: E.J. Brill, 1993).
Cohn, Norman, *Europe's Inner Demons: An Enquiry Inspired by the Great Witch-Hunt* (New York: Basic Books, 1975).
Conrad, Lawrence I., Michael Neve, Vivian Nutton, Roy Porter and Andrew Wear, *The Western Medical Tradition 800 B.C. to AD 1800* (Cambridge: Cambridge University Press, 1995).
Constantelos, Demetrios J., *Byzantine Philanthropy and Social Welfare* (New Brunswick, NJ: Rutgers University Press, 1968).
———, *Byzantine Philanthropy and Social Welfare*, 2nd revised edn (New Rochelle, NY: Aristide D. Cartazas, 1991).
Coornaert, E., *Les Corporations en France avant 1789*, 2nd edn (Paris: Les Editions ouvrières, 1968).
Cosman, Madeleine Pelner, *Women at Work in Medieval Europe* (New York: Facts on File, 2000).
Coste, Pierre, *Le Grand Saint du Grand Siècle*, 3 vols (Paris: Desclée et cie Editeurs, 1934).
———, *Saint Vincent de Paul et les Dames de la Charité* (Paris: Bloud et Gay, 1937).
———, *The Life and Works of Saint Vincent de Paul (Monsieur Vincent: Le grand saint du grand siècle)*, trans. Joseph Leonard, 2 vols (Westminster, MD: The Newman Press, 1952).
Coyecque, E., *L'Hôtel Dieu de Paris au Moyen Âge moyen âge*, 2 vols (Paris: H. Champion, 1889–91).
Cox, Michael, *Handbook of Christian Spirituality* (San Francisco: Harper & Row, 1985).
Cuartero, Octavio, *Obras de Dona Oliva Sabuco de Nantes* (Madrid: Ricardo Fé, 1888).
Cullum, P.H., *Cremetts and Corrodies: Care of the Poor and Sick at St Leonards Hospital, York in the Middle Ages*, Borthwick Papers No. 79 (York: University of York, 1991).
Dakin, Theodora P., *A History of Women's Contribution to World Health* (Lewiston, NY: Edwin Mellen Press, 1991).
Dall'ava-Santucci, Josette, *Des Sorcières aux Mandarines: Histoire des femmes médicins* (Paris: Calmann-Lévy, 1989).
Dalven, Rae, *Anna Comnena* (New York: Twayne Publishers, 1972).
Dangler, Jean, *Mediating Fictions: Literature, Women Healers and the Go-between in Medieval and Early Modern Iberia* (Lewisburg: Bucknell University Press, 2001).

Debus, Allen G., (ed.), *Medicine in Seventeenth Century England: A Symposium Held at UCLA in Honor of C.D. O'Malley* (Berkeley: University of California Press, 1974).

———, *The Chemical Philosophy: Paracelsian Science and Medicine in the Sixteenth and Seventeenth Centuries*, 2 vols (New York: New York Science History Publications, 1977).

Delaunay Paul, *La Maternité de Paris* (Paris: Jules Rousset, 1909).

———, *La Médecine et l'Eglise* (Paris: Editions Hippocrate, 1948).

De Renzi, Salvatore, *Storia documentata della Scuolo Medica di Salerno* (Naples, 1857; reprinted Naples: M. D'Auria, 2002).

Drees, Clayton J. (ed.), *The Late Medieval Age of Crisis and Renewal 1300–1500: A Biographical Dictionary* (Westport, CT, and London: Greenwood, 2001).

Dinan, Susan E., *Women and Poor Relief in Seventeenth-Century France: The Early History of the Daughters of Charity* (Aldershot, Hampshire and Burlington, VT: Ashgate, 2006).

Dobson, Jessie and R. Milnes Walker, *Barbers and Barbers-Surgeons in London: A History of the Barbers' and Barber-Surgeons' Companies* (London: Blackwell Scientific Publications for the Worshipful Co. of Barbers, 1979).

Domínguez-Alcón, Carmen, *Los cuidados y la profesión enfermera en España* (Madrid: Ediciones Pirámide, 1986).

Donawerth, Jane and Adele Seff (eds), *Crossing Boundaries: Attending to Early Modern Women* (Newark: University of Delaware Press, 2000).

Donegan, Jane N., *Women and Men Midwives: Medicine, Morality, and Misogyny in Early America* (Westport, CT: Greenwood, 1978).

Donnison, Jean, *Midwives and Medical Men: A History of Inter-Professional Rivalries and Women's Rights* (New York: Schoken Books, 1977).

Eamon, William, *Science and the Secrets of Nature* (Princeton, NJ: Princeton University Press, 1994).

Ehrenreich, Barbara and Deirdre English, *Witches, Midwives, and Nurses: A History of Women Healers* (New York: Feminist Press, 1973).

Evans Pritchard, E.E., *Witchcraft, Oracles and Magic among the Azande* (Oxford: Oxford University Press, 1937).

Evenden, Doreen, *The Midwives of Seventeenth-Century London* (Cambridge and New York: Cambridge University Press, 2000).

Feldman, David M., *Health and Medicine in the Jewish Traditions* (New York: Crossroad, 1976).

Fenster, Thelma S. and Claire A. Lees (eds), *Gender and Debate from the Early Middle Ages to the Renaissance* (New York: Palgrave, 2002).

Forbes, Thomas Roger, *The Midwife and the Witch* (New Haven, CT: Yale University Press, 1966).

Forster, Robert and Orest Ranum (eds), *Medicine and Society in France*, Vol. 6 of *Selections from Annales, Economies, Sociétés, Civilisations*, trans. Elborg Forster and Patricia M. Ranum (Baltimore and London: Johns Hopkins University Press, 1980).

Fosseyeux Marcel, *L'hôtel Dieu de Paris au XVIIe et XVIIIe siècle* (Paris: Berger-Levrault, 1912).

Fraser, Antonia. *The Weaker Vessel: Women's Lot in Seventeenth-Century England* (London: Methuen, 1984).

Freedman, Jo (ed.), *Women: A Feminist Perspective* (Palo Alto, CA: Mayfield Publishing Co., 1975).

French, Marilyn, *Beyond Power: On Women, Men and Morals* (New York: Summit Books, 1986).

French, Roger and Andrew Wear (eds), *The Medical Revolution of the Seventeenth Century* (Cambridge: Cambridge University Press, 1989).
French, Roger, Jon Arrizabalaga, Andrew Cunningham and Luis García-Ballester (eds), *Medicine from the Black Death to the French Disease* (Aldershot: Ashgate, 1998).
Friedenwald, Harry, *The Jews and Medicine: Essays*, 2 vols (Baltimore: Johns Hopkins University Press, 1944).
Friedson, Eliot, *Profession of Medicine: A Study of the Sociology of Applied Knowledge* (New York: Harper & Row, 1970).
Furst, Lilian R. (ed.), *Women Healers and Physicians: Climbing a Long Hill* (Lexington: The University Press of Kentucky, 1997).
Gage, Matilda Joslyn, *Women, Church and State* (Salem, NH: Ayer Co. 1985).
García-Ballester, Luis, *Medicine in a Multi-Cultural Society: Christian, Jewish and Muslim Practitioners in the Spanish Kingdoms, 1222–1610* (Aldershot: Ashgate, 2001).
———, Roger French and Jon Arrizabalaga (eds), *Practical Medicine from Salerno to the Black Death* (Cambridge: Cambridge University Press, 1994).
———, Michael McVaugh and Augustin Rubio Vela, *Medical Licensing and Learning in Fourteenth Century Valencia* (Philadelphia: American Philosophical Society, 1989).
Gelbart, Nina Rattner, *The King's Midwife: A History and Mystery of Madame du Coudray* (Berkeley: University of California Press, 1998).
Gelfand, Toby, *Professionalizing Modern Medicine: Paris Surgeons and Medical Science and Institutions in the 18th Century* (Westport, CT: Greenwood, 1980).
Gélis, Jacques, *La sage-femme ou le médecin: une nouvelle conception de la vie* (Paris: Fayard: 1988).
Gentilcore, David, *Healers and Healing in Early Modern Italy* (Manchester: Manchester University Press, 1998).
Getz, Faye Marie, *Medicine in the English Middle Ages* (Princeton, NJ: Princeton University Press, 1998).
Gibson, Wendy, *Women in Seventeenth Century France* (New York: St Martin's Press, 1989).
Giles, Mary, E. (ed.), *Women in the Inquisition: Spain and the New World* (Baltimore and London: Johns Hopkins University Press, 1999).
Ginzburg, Carlo, *The Night Battles: Witchcraft and Agrarian Cults in the Sixteenth and Seventeenth Centuries*, trans. John and Anne Tedeschi (Harmondsworth: Penguin, 1985).
Goodnow, Minnie, *Outlines of Nursing History*, 4th edn (Philadelphia: W.B. Saunders, 1929).
Gottfried, Robert S., *Doctors and Medicine in Medieval England, 1340–1530* (Princeton, NJ: Princeton University Press, 1986).
Granjel, Luis, *La Medicina Española del siglo XVII* (Salamanca: Ediciones Universidad de Salamanca, 1978).
Granshaw, Lindsay and Roy Porter, *The Hospital in History* (London: Routledge, 1989).
Grell, Ole Peter, Andrew Cunningham and Jon Arrizabala (eds), *Health Care and Poor Relief in Counter-Reformation Europe* (London and New York: Routledge, 1999).
Green, Monica H., *Women's Healthcare in the Medieval West: Text and Contexts* (Aldershot: Ashgate, 2000).
Griffin, Gerald Joseph and H. Joanne King Griffin, *Jensen's History and Trends of Professional Nursing*, 5th edn (St Louis: C.V. Mosby, 1965).
Group, Thetis M. and Joan I. Roberts, *Nursing, Physician Control, and the Medical Monopoly: Historical Perspectives on Gendered Inequality in Roles, Rights, and Range of Practice* (Bloomington: Indiana University Press, 2001).

Guthrie, Shirley, *Arab Women in the Middle Ages* (London: Saqi Books, 2001).
Hacquain François, *Histoire de l'art d'accouchement en Lorraine de temps anciens aux Xxe siècle* (Saint-Nicolas-de-Port: Star, 1979).
Hahn, André, *Commentaires sur dix grands livres de la Médecine Française* (Paris: Au Cercle du Livre Précieux, 1968).
Haliczer, Stephen (ed.), *Inquisition and Society in Early Modern Europe* (London and Sydney: Croom Helm, 1987).
Hawley, Richard and Barbara Levick (eds), *Women in Antiquity: New Assessments* (London and New York: Routledge, 1995).
Hellman, Alfred Myer, M.D., *A Collection of Early Obstetrical Works* (New Haven, CT: Yale University Press, 1952).
Henningsen, Gustav and John Tedeschi (eds), *Inquisition in Early Modern Europe: Studies on Sources and Methods* (De Kalb: Northern IllinoisUniversity Press, 1976).
Hernández Alcántara, Antonio, *Estudio historico de la obra toco-ginecológica y pediátrica de Damián Carbón* (Salamanca: Seminario de Historia de la Medicina, Universidad de Salamanca, 1957).
Hernández Martín, Francisca, *Historía de la enfermería en España: desde la antigüedad hasta nuestros días* (Madrid: Editorial Síntesis, 1996).
Hobby, Elaine, *Virtue of Necessity: English Women's Writing: 1649–88* (Ann Arbor: University of Michigan Press, 1989).
Hole, Christina, *A Mirror of Witchcraft* (London: Chatto and Windus, 1957).
Hollister, C. Warren, *Medieval Europe: A Short History*, 7th edn (Boston: McGraw Hill, 1994).
Hufton, Olwen, *The Prospect Before Her: A History of Women in Western Europe, Volume One 1500–1800* (New York: Vintage, 1995).
Hughes, Muriel Joy, *Women Healers in Medieval Life and Literature* (Freeport, NY: Books for Libraries Press, 1968).
Hunter, Lynette and Sarah Hutton (eds), *Women, Science and Medicine 1500–1700* (Gloucester: Sutton Publishing, 1997).
Hunting, Penelope, *A History of the Society of Apothecaries* (London: The Society, 1998).
Hutson, Lorna (ed.), *Feminism and Renaissance Studies* (Oxford: Oxford University Press, 1999).
Imbert Jean, *Histoire des hôpitaux en France* (Toulouse: Privat, 1982).
Jacob, James R., *Henry Stubbe, Radical Protestantism and the Early Enlightenment* (Cambridge: Cambridge University Press, 1983).
Jacquart, Danielle, *Le milieu médical en France du XIIe au XVe siècle* (Geneva: Droz, 1981).
———, *La Médecine médiévale dans le cadre parisien: XIVe-XVe siècle* (Paris: Fayard, 1998).
Jameson, Eric, *The Natural History of Quackery* (London: Michael Joseph, 1961).
Jones, Colin, *Montpellier in the Charitable Imperative: Hospitals and Nursing in Ancien Régime and Revolutionary France* (New York and London: Routledge, 1989).
Jordan, Brigitte, *Birth in Four Cultures* (Montreal: Eden Press, 1978).
Kamen, Henry, *The Spanish Inquisition: A Historical Revision* (New Haven: Yale University Press, 1998).
Kavey, Allison, *Books of Secrets: Natural Philosophy in England 1550–1600* (Chicago and Urbana: University of Illinois Press, 2007).
Kersey, Ethel M., *Women Philosophers: A Bio-Critical Source Book* (Westport, CT: Greenwood, 1989).

Khairallah, Amin A., *Outline of Arabic Contributions to Medicine* (Beirut: American Press, 1946).
Kibre, Pearl, *Scholarly Privileges in the Middle Ages* (Cambridge, MA: Mediaeval Academy of America, 1962).
———, *Studies in Medieval Science, Alchemy, Astrology, Mathematics and Medicine* (London: Hambeldon Press, 1984).
Kieckhefer, Richard, *European Witch Trials: Their Foundations in Popular and Learned Culture, 1300–1500* (Berkeley: University of California Press, 1976).
———, *Magic in the Middle Ages* (Cambridge: Cambridge University Press, 2000).
King, Helen, *Hippocrates' Women: Reading the Female Body in Ancient Greece* (London and New York: Routledge, 1998).
King, Lester S., *The Medical World of the Eighteenth Century* (Chicago: University of Chicago Press, 1958).
King, Margaret L., *Women of the Renaissance* (Chicago: University of Chicago Press, 1991).
Kitts, Sally-Ann, *The Debate on the Nature, Role and Influence of Woman in Eighteenth-Century Spain* (Lewiston: Edwin Mellen Press, 1995).
Knibiehler, Yvonne and Catherine Fouquet, *La Femme et les Médecins Analyse Historique* (Paris: Hachette, 1983).
Knoles, Lucia, 'Commonplace Books', http://www.assumption.edu/users/lknoles/commonplacebook.html.
Labarge, Margaret Wade, *Women in Medieval Life* (London: Hambledon Press, 1986).
Laget, Mireille, *Naissances: L'accouchement avant l'âge de la clinique* (Paris: Seuil, 1982).
Laissus, Yves and Jean Torlais, *Le Jardin du Roi et le Collège royal dans l'enseignement des sciences au XVIIIe siècle* (Paris: Hermann, 1986).
Lane Furdell, Elizabeth, *The Royal Doctors 1485–1714: Medical Personnel at the Tudor and Stuart Courts* (Rochester: University of Rochester Press, 2001).
———, *Publishing and Medicine in Early Modern England* (Rochester: University of Rochester Press, 2002).
Lanning, John Tate, *The Royal Protomedicato* (Durham, NC: Duke University Press, 1985).
Larner, Christina, *Witchcraft and Religion: The Politics of Popular Belief*, ed. Alan Macfarlane (Oxford: Blackwell, 1984).
Le Maguet, Paul Émile, *Le monde médical parisien sous Le Grande Roi [Louis XIV] suivi du portefeuille de Vallant* (Paris: A. Maloine, 1899).
Le Naour, Jean Yves and Catherine Valenti, *Histoire de l'avortement XIXe–XXe siècles* (Paris: Seuil, 2003).
Lea, Henry Charles, *A History of the Inquisition in Spain*, 4 vols (New York: Macmillan, 1906–07).
———, *A History of the Inquisition of the Middle Ages*, 3 vols (New York: Russell, 1956).
Lebrun, François, *Se Soigner d'autrefois: Médecins, saints et sorciers aux 17e et 18e siècles* (Paris: Temps Actuels, 1983).
Lechner, Sister Joan Marie, *Renaissance Concepts of the Commonplaces* (Westport, CT: Greenwood, 1962).
Leclair, Edmond, *Un chapitre de l'histoire de la chirurgie à Lille: les accouchements* (Lille: H. Morel, 1910).
Lespinasse, René de, *Les métiers et corporations de la ville de Paris, 14e–18e siècle* (Paris: Impr. Nationale, 1886–97).
Levack, Brian, *The Witch-Hunt in Early Modern Europe*, 2nd edn (London: Longman, 1995).

Levin, Beatrice, *Women and Medicine*, 3rd edn (Lanham, MD: Scarecrow Press, 2002).
Lévy-Valensi, J., *La Médecine et les Médecins Français au XVIIIe Siècle* (Paris: J.B. Baillière et Fils, 1933).
Lewin, Linda, *Surprise Heirs: Illegitimacy, Patrimonial Rights and Legal Nationalism in Luso-Brazilian Inheritance 1750–1821*, 2 vols (Stanford: Stanford University Press, 2003).
Lindemann, Kate, Women-philosophers.com, http://www.women-philosophers.com/Oliva-Sabuco.html.
Lindemann, Mary, *Medicine and Society in Early Modern Europe* (Cambridge and New York: Cambridge University Press, 1999).
Lipinska, Melina, *Histoire des Femmes Médecins depuis l'antiquité jusqu'à nos jours* (Paris : Librairie Jacques et Cie, 1900).
———, *Les Femmes et le progrès des sciences médicales* (Paris: C. Jacques, 1930).
Lough, John, *An Introduction to Seventeenth Century France* (London: Longmans, Green & Co., 1995).
Luchaire, Achille, *Social France at the Time of Philip Augustus*, intro. John W. Baldwin, trans. Edward Benjamin Krehbiel (New York: Harper & Row, 1967).
Luong Thomas F., *The Saintly Politics of Catherine of Siena* (Ithaca: Cornell University Press, 2000).
MacDonald, Michael, *Mystical Bedlam: Madness, Anxiety, and Healing in Seventeenth-Century England* (Cambridge: Cambridge University Press, 1981).
MacDonald, Michael (ed.), *Witchcraft and Hysteria in Elizabethan London: Edward Jorden and Mary Glover Case* (London and New York: Routledge, 1991).
Maclean, Gerald (ed.), *Culture and Society in the Stuart Restoration: Literature, Drama, History* (Cambridge: Cambridge University Press, 1995).
Maclean, Ian, *The Renaissance Notion of Woman* (Cambridge: Cambridge University Press, 1990).
Madule, J., *The Albigensian Crusade: An Historical Essay*, trans. B. Wall (New York: Fordham University Press, 1967).
Marland, Hilary, *The Art of Midwifery: Early Modern Midwives in Europe* (London and New York: Routledge, 1993).
——— and Margaret Pelling (eds), *Task of Healing: Medicine, Religion, and Gender in England and the Netherlands, 1450–1800* (Rotterdam: Erasmus, 1996).
——— and Ann Marie Rafferty (eds), *Midwives, Society, and Childbirth: Debates and Controversies in the Modern Period* (London and New York: Routledge, 1997).
Marshall, Sherrin (ed.), *Women in Reformation and Counter Reformation Europe: Private and Public Worlds* (Bloomington and Indianapolis: Indiana University Press, 1989).
Martin, Ruth, *Witchcraft and the Inquisition in Venice, 1550–1650* (Oxford: Blackwell, 1989).
Martinez, Cándida and Reyna Pastor (eds), *Mujeres en la Historia de España* (Barcelona: Planeta, 2000).
Marty, Martin E. and Kenneth L. Vau, *Health/Medicine and the Faith Traditions: An Inquiry into Religion and Medicine* (Philadelphia: Fortress Press, 1982).
Maxwell-Stuart, P.G., *Witchcraft in Europe and the New World, 1400–1800* (Basingstoke: Palgrave, 2001).
McClelland, Ivy Lilian, *Benito Jerónimo Feijóo* (New York: Twayne, 1969).
McLeod, Enid, *The Order of the Rose: The Life and Ideas of Christine de Pizan* (Totowa, NJ: Rowan and Littlefield, 1976).
McTavish, Lianne, *Childbirth and the Display of Authority in Early Modern France* (Aldershot, Hampshire, and Burlington, VT: Ashgate, 2005).

McVaugh, Michael R., *Medicine before the Plague: Practitioners and their Patients in the Crown of Aragon, 1285–1345* (Cambridge: Cambridge University Press, 1993).
Mead, Kate Campbell (Hurd), *A History of Women in Medicine* (Haddam, CT: The Haddam Press, 1938).
Medici, Michele, *Compendio storico della Scuola Anatomica di Bologna dal rinascimento dell scienze e delle lettere a tutto secolo XVII: con un paragone fra la sua antichità a quella delle scuole di Salerno e di Padova* (Bologna: Tipografia governativa Della Volpe e del Sassi, 1857).
Medvei, V.C. and J.L. Thornton, *The Royal Hospital of St Bartholomew's 1123–1973* (London: St Bartholomew's and Contributors, 1974).
Michelet, Jules, *La Sorcière* (Paris: Hetzel, 1863).
Miller, Timothy, S., *The Birth of the Hospital in the Byzantine Empire* (Baltimore: Johns Hopkins University Press, 1997).
Monter, E. William (ed.), *European Witchcraft* (New York: Wiley, 1969).
———, *Witchcraft in France and Switzerland: The Borderlands during the Reformation* (Ithaca: Cornell University Press, 1976).
Morin, Bruce T., *Distilling Knowledge: Alchemy, Chemistry, and the Scientific Revolution* (Cambridge, MA: Harvard University Press, 2005).
Moscucci, Ornella, *The Science of Woman: Gynaecology and Gender in England, 1800–1929* (Cambridge: Cambridge University Press, 1993).
Mossiker, Frances, *Madame de Sévigné: A Life and Letters* (New York: Alfred A. Knopf, 1983).
Mozans, H.J., *Women in Science* (Notre Dame, IN: University of Indiana Press, 1991).
Murk-Jansen, Saskia, *Brides in the Desert: The Spirituality of the Beguines* (London: Sarton, Longman & Todd, 1998).
Muchembled, Robert, *La Sorcière au village* (Paris: Editions Juillard Gallimard, 1979).
Murphy, Lamar Riley, *Enter the Physician: The Transformation of Domestic Medicine 1760–1830* (Tuscaloosa, AL: University of Alabama Press, 1991).
Nagy, Doreen Evenden, *Popular Medicine in Seventeenth-Century England* (Bowling Green, OH: Bowling Green State University Popular Press, 1988).
Needham, Joseph, *A History of Embryology*, 2nd edn (New York: Abelard-Schuman, 1959).
Nemec, Jarsolav, *Witchcraft and Medicine 1484–1793*, Published in conjunction with an exhibit at the National Library of Medicine, 25 March–19 July 1973, US Department of Health, Education, and Welfare (Washington, DC: Public Health Service National Institutes of Health DHEW Publication, 1974).
Nevins, Michael, *The Jewish Doctor* (London: Jason Aronson, 1996).
Nicaise, Edouard, *La Grande Chirurgie de Guy de Chauliac* (Paris: Alcan, 1890).
Noble, David F., *A World without Women: The Christian Clerical Culture of Western Science* (Oxford and New York: Oxford University Press, 1992).
Nutting, Mary Adelaide and Lavinia L. Dock, *A History of Nursing: The Evolution of Nursing Systems from the Earliest Times to the Foundation of the First English and American Training Schools for Nurses*, 4 vols (New York: G.P. Putnam's Sons, 1907–12).
Nutton, Vivian and Roy Porter (eds), *The History of Medical Education in Britain* (Amsterdam: Rodopi, 1995).
O'Brien, T.C. (ed.), *Corpus Dictionary of Western Churches* (Washington: Corpus, 1970).
O'Day, Rosemary, *The Professions in Early Modern England, 1450–1800: Servants of the Commonweal* (Harlow, Essex: Pearson Education, 2000).

Obelkevich, James (ed.), *Religion and the People 800–1700* (Chapel Hill: University of North Carolina Press, 1979).

Ogilvie, Marilyn Bailey, *Women in Science: Antiquity through Nineteenth Century, a Biographical Dictionary with Annotated Bibliography* (Cambridge, MA: MIT Press, 1986).

——— and Joy Dorothy Harvey, *The Biographical Dictionary of Women in Science: Pioneering Lives from Ancient Times to the Mid-20th Century*, 2 vols (London: Routledge, 2000).

Ojala, Jeanne, *Madame de Sévigné: A Seventeenth Century Life* (Oxford: Berg, 1990).

Olivier-Martin, François, *L'Organisation corporative de la France d'Ancien régime* (Paris: Recueil Sirey, 1938).

Ouin-Lacroix, Charles, *Histoire des anciennes corporations d'arts et métiers et des confréries religieuses de la capitale de la Normandie* (Rouen: Lecointe, 1850).

Owst, G.R., *Literature and the Pulpit in Medieval England* (Oxford: Oxford University Press, 1933).

Packard, Francis R., *Guy Patin and the Medical Profession in Paris in the XVIth Century* (New York: Paul B. Hoeber, 1925).

Park, Katharine, *Doctors and Medicine in Early Renaissance Florence* (Princeton, NJ: Princeton University Press, 1985).

Parsons, F.C., *The History of St Thomas's Hospital* (London: Methuen, 1932).

Pavey, Agnes E., *The Story of the Growth of Nursing as an Art, a Vocation and a Profession* (London: Faber & Faber, 1957).

Peck, Linda Levy, *Consuming Splendour: Society and Culture in Seventeenth-Century England* (Cambridge: Cambridge University Press, 2005).

Pelling, Margaret, *The Common Lot: Sickness, Medical Occupations, and the Urban Poor in Early Modern England* (London; New York : Longman, 1998).

——— (with Frances White), *Medical Conflicts in Early Modern London: Patronage, Physicians and Irregular Practitioners, 1550–1640* (Oxford: Clarendon, 2003).

Pérez, Joseph, *The Spanish Inquisition, A History*, trans. Janet Lloyd (New Haven and London: Yale University Press, 2005).

Perkins, Wendy, *Midwifery and Medicine in Early Modern France: Louise Bourgeois* (Exeter: University of Exeter Press, 1996).

Perry, Mary Elizabeth, *Gender and Disorder in Early Modern Seville* (Princeton, NJ: Princeton University Press, 1990).

Peters, Edward, *Inquisition* (New York: Free Press, 1988).

Petitfils, Jean-Christian, *Fouquet* (Paris: Perrin, 1998).

Petroff, Elizabeth A., *Medieval Women's Visionary Literature* (New York: Oxford University Press, 1986).

Philippen, L.J.M., *Béguines et béguinages: dossier accompagnant l'exposition Béguines et béguinages en Brabant et dans la province d'Anvers aux Archives générales du Royaume à Bruxelles du 27 octobre au 13 décembre 1994* (Bruxelles: Archives générales du Royaume, 1994).

Piaget, Arthur, *Martin Le Franc: Prévôt de Lausanne* (Lausanne: Payot, 1858).

Plumb, J.H. (ed.), *Studies in Social History* (London: Longmans, Green and Co., 1955).

Pollock, Linda, *With Faith and Physic: The Life of a Tudor Gentlewoman, Lady Grace Mildmay, 1552–1620* (London: Collins & Brown, 1993).

Pomata, Gianna, *Contracting a Cure: Patients, Healers and the Law in Early Modern Bologna* (Baltimore and London: Johns Hopkins University Press, 1998).

Popkin, Richard H. (ed.), *The Columbia History of Western Philosophy* (New York: Columbia University Press 1999).

Porter, Roy, (ed.), *Patients and Practitioners: Lay Perceptions of Medicine in Pre-Industrial Society* (Cambridge and New York: Cambridge University Press, 1985).
———, *Patient's Progress : Doctors and Doctoring in Eighteenth-Century England* (Oxford: Polity, 1989).
———, *Health for Sale: Quackery in England, 1660–1850* (Manchester and New York: Manchester University Press, 1989).
——— (ed.), *The Popularization of Medicine, 1650–1850* (London and New York: Routledge, 1992).
———, *Medicine and the Enlightenment* (Amsterdam: Rodopi, 1995).
——— (ed.), *The Cambridge Illustrated History of Medicine* (Cambridge and New York: Cambridge University Press, 1996).
——— *Quacks: Fakers and Charlatans in English Medicine* (Stroud : Tempus, 2000).
——— and W.F. Bynum (eds), *Medical Fringe and Medical Orthodoxy 1750–1850* (London: Croom Helm, 1987).
——— and Lindsay Granshaw (eds), *The Hospital in History* (London and New York: Routledge, 1989).
Pouchelle, Marie-Christine, *The Body and Surgery in the Middle Ages*, trans. Rosemary Morris (Cambridge: Polity, 1990).
Powell James M. (ed.), *Muslims under Latin Rule 400–1300* (Princeton, NJ: Princeton University Press, 1990).
Power, Eileen Edna, *Medieval Women*, ed. M.M. Postan (New York: Cambridge University Press, 1975).
Power, Kim, *Veiled Desire: Augustine's Writing on Women* (New York: Continuum, 1996).
Prost M. Aug, *Corneille Agrippa sa vie et ses oeuvres*, 2 vols (Paris: Champion, 1881).
Pumfrey, Stephen, Paolo L. Rossi and Maurice Slawinski (eds), *Science, Culture and Popular Belief in Renaissance Europe* (Manchester and New York: Manchester University Press, 1991).
Queirel, Auguste, *Histoire de la Maternité de Marseille* (Marseille: Ballatier et Berthelet, 1899).
Ramsey, Matthew, *Professional and Popular Medicine in France, 1770–1830* (Cambridge: Cambridge University Press, 1988).
Ranft, Patricia, *Women and the Religious Life in Premodern Europe* (New York: St Martin's Press, 1996).
Rashdall, Hastings, *The Universities of Europe in the Middle Ages: A New Edition in Three Volumes*, ed. F.M. Powicke and A.B. Emden (Oxford: Oxford University Press, 1967).
Rawcliffe Carole, *Sources for the History of Medicine in Late Medieval England* (Kalamazoo: Western Michigan University, 1995).
———, *Medicine and Society in Later Medieval England* (Phoenix Mill: Sutton, 1997).
Read, Malcolm R., *Juan Huarte de San Juan* (Boston: Twayne, 1981).
Rebière, A., *Les femmes dans la science* (Paris: Nony Rebière, 1894).
Riccardo, Magaglio, *Una patrizia genovese antesignana della moderna assistenza sociale: cenni biografici sulla serva di Dio Virginia Centurione Bracelli (1587–1651)* (Genova: AGIS, 1972).
Richardson, Lula McDowell, *The Forerunners of Feminism in French Literature of the Renaissance from Christine of Pisa to Marie de Gournay* (Baltimore: Johns Hopkins University Press, 1929).
Rich, Josephine, *Women behind Men of Medicine* (New York: Julian Messner, 1967).
Rigaud, Rose, *Les Idées Féministes de Christine de Pisan* (Geneva: Slatine Reprints, 1973).

Rosenthal, Joel, *Medieval Women and the Sources of Medieval History* (Athens: University of Georgia Press, 1990).

Rousselet, Albin, *Notes sur l'ancien Hôtel Dieu de Paris Relatives à la lutte des adminstrateurs laïques contre le pouvoir spiritual. Extraites des archives de l'Assistance publique et publiées par A. Rousselet* (Paris: E. Lecrosnier & Babé 1888).

Rousselot, Paul, *La Pédagogie Féminine* (Paris, Delgrave, 1881).

Ruderman, David B., *Science, Medicine and Jewish Culture in Early Modern Europe* (Tel-Aviv: Tel-Aviv University, 1987).

Ruggiero, Guido, *Binding Passions: Tales of Magic, Marriage, and Power at the End of the Renaissance* (Oxford: Oxford University Press, 1993).

Ruíz Moreno, Aníbal, *La medicina en la legislaction medioeval española* (Buenos Aires: El Ateneo, 1946).

Russell, Jeffrey Burton, *Witchcraft in the Middle Ages* (Ithaca and London: Cornell University Press, 1972).

Sánchez Sánchez, Teresa, *La mujer sin identidad: un ciclo vital de sumisíon femenina durante del Renacimento* (Salamanca: Aramu Ediciones, 1996).

Saint-Saëns, Alain (ed.), *Religion, Body and Gender in Early Modern Spain* (San Francisco: Mellen Research University Press, 1991).

Schiebinger, Londa, *The Mind has no Sex? Women in the Origins of Modern Science* (Cambridge, MA: Harvard University Press, 1991).

Sharpe, J.A., *The Bewitching of Anne Gunter: A Horrible and True Story of Football, Witchcraft, Murder, and the King of England* (London: Profile,1999).

Shatzmiller, Joseph, *Jews, Medicine and Medieval Society* (Berkeley: University of California Press, 1994).

Shorter, Edward, *Women's Bodies: A Social History of Women's Encounters with Health, Ill-Health and Medicine* (New Brunswick, NJ: Transaction Publishers, 1981).

Simons, Walter, *Cities of Ladies: Beguine Communities in Medieval Low Countries 1200–1365* (Philadelphia: University of Pennsylvania Press, 2001).

Singer, Charles, *From Magic to Science: Essays on the Scientific Twilight* (New York: Boni & Liveright, 1928).

Siraisi, Nancy G., *Medieval and Early Renaissance Medicine: An Introduction to Knowledge* (Chicago and London: University of Chicago Press, 1990).

———, *Medicine and the Italian Universities, 1250–1600* (Leiden and Boston: Köln Brill 2001).

Smith, Hilda, *Reason's Disciples: Seventeenth-Century English Feminists* (Urbana: University of Illinois Press, 1982).

Smith, Theresa Ann, *The Emerging Female Citizen: Gender and Enlightenment in Spain* (Berkeley: University of California Press, 2006).

Solomon, Michael, *The Literature of Misogyny in Medieval Spain: The Arcipreste de Talavera and the Spill* (Cambridge: Cambridge University Press, 1997).

Soman, Alfred, *Sorcellerie et Justice Criminelle: Le Parlement de Paris* (Aldershot: Ashgate, 1992).

Southern, Richard William, *Western Society and the Church in the Middle Ages* (London: Penguin, 1970).

Stone, Marilyn and Carmen Benito-Vessels (eds), *Women at Work in Spain: From the Middle Ages to Early Modern Times* (New York: Peter Lang, 1998).

Surtry, Muhammed Ibrahim, *Muslims' Contribution to the Development of Hospitals* (Birmingham: Qu'ranic Arabic Foundation, 1996).

Talbot, C.H. and E.A. Hammond, *The Medical Practitioners in Medieval England: A Biographical Register* (London: Wellcome Historical Medical Library, 1965).

Thillaud, Paul, *Les Malades et la Médecine en Pays Basque nord à la fin de l'ancien régime* (Geneva: Droz, 1993).
Thomas, Keith, *Medicine and the Decline of Magic* (Harmondsworth: Penguin, 1971).
Thomson, C.J.S., *The Quacks of Old London* (London: Brentano's, 1928).
Thorndike, Lynn, *A History of Magic and Experimental Science*, 2 vols (New York: Columbia University Press, 1923; reprint 1964).
———, *University Records and Life in the Middle Ages* (New York: Octagon Books, 1971).
Tobyn, Graeme, *Culpeper's Medicine* (Rockport, MA: Element Books, 1997).
Tomasi, Lucia T., *An Oak Spring Flora: Flower Illustration from the Fifteenth Century to the Present Time* (Upperville, VA: Oak Spring Garden Library, 1997).
Toussaint-Samat, Maguelone, *History of Food* (Oxford: Blackwell, 1994).
Trevor-Roper, H., *The European Witch-Craze of the Sixteenth and Seventeenth Centuries* (New York: Harper & Row, 1970).
Underwood, E.A. (ed.), *Science, Medicine and History: Essays on the Evolution of Scientific Thought and Medical Practice Written in Honour of Charles Singer*, 2 vols (London: Oxford University Press, 1953).
Wade Labarge, Margaret, *Women in Medieval Life* (London: Hamish Hamilton, 1986).
Waddington, Raymond B and Arthur H. Williamson (eds), *The Expulsion of the Jews: 1492 and After* (New York: Garland, 1994).
Waithe, Mary Ellen (ed.), *A History of Women Philosophers*, Vol. 2, *Medieval, Renaissance and Enlightenment Women Philosophers A.D. 500–1600* (Dordrecht: Kluwer Academic Publishers, 1989).
Walker, Kim, *Women Writers of the Renaissance* (New York: Twayne, 1992).
Walsh, James J., *Medieval Medicine* (London: A & C Black, 1920).
Wear, Andrew (ed.), *Health and Healing in Early Modern Europe* (Aldershot: Ashgate, 1998).
———, *Knowledge and Practice in English Medicine, 1550–1680* (Cambridge: Cambridge University Press, 2000).
Webster, Charles (ed.), *Health, Medicine and Mortality in the Sixteenth Century* (Cambridge: Cambridge University Press, 1979).
Wiesner, Merry E., *Women and Gender in Early Modern Europe* (Cambridge: Cambridge University Press, 1993).
Whaley, Leigh Ann, *Women's History as Scientists: A Guide to the Debates* (Santa Barbara: ABC-CLIO, 2003).
Whitelock, Dorothy, *The Beginnings of English Society* (Harmondsworth: Penguin, 1979).
Whitteridge, G. and V. Stokes, *A Brief History of the Hospital of St Bartholomew, London* (London: The Governors of the Hospital of St Bartholomew, 1961).
Wickersheimer, Ernest, *La médecine et les médecins en France à l'Epoque de la Renaissance* (Paris: A. Malaine, 1906).
———, *Dictionnaire biographique des Médecins en France au Môyen Age*, 2 vols (Paris: E. Droz, 1936).
Wilson, Adrian, *The Making of Man-Midwifery: Childbirth in England, 1660–1770* (Cambridge, MA: Harvard University Press, 1994).
Williams, Charles G.S., *Madame de Sévigné* (Boston: Twayne Publishers, 1981).
Witkowsky, Gustave-Joseph, *Histoire des accouchements chez tous les peuples* (Paris: G. Steinheil, 1887).
Zemon Davis, Natalie and Arlette Farge (eds), *A History of Women*, Vol. 3, *Renaissance and Enlightenment Paradoxes* (Cambridge, MA: The Belknap Press of Harvard University Press, 1993).

Index

GPSR Compliance
The European Union's (EU) General Product Safety Regulation (GPSR) is a set of rules that requires consumer products to be safe and our obligations to ensure this.

If you have any concerns about our products, you can contact us on

ProductSafety@springernature.com

In case Publisher is established outside the EU, the EU authorized representative is:

Springer Nature Customer Service Center GmbH
Europaplatz 3
69115 Heidelberg, Germany

www.ingramcontent.com/pod-product-compliance
Ingram Content Group UK Ltd.
Pitfield, Milton Keynes, MK11 3LW, UK
UKHW020154290926
15471UKWH00005B/875

* 9 7 8 1 3 4 9 3 2 8 7 0 3 *